Little, Brown's Paperback Book Series

Basic Medical Sciences

Albers, Agranoff, Katzman, & Siegel	Basic Neurochemistry
Colton	Statistics in Medicine
Hine & Pfeiffer	Behavioral Science
Levine	Pharmacology
Peery & Miller	Pathology, 2nd Ed.
Selkurt	Physiology, 3rd Ed.
Sidman & Sidman	Neuroanatomy
Snell	Clinical Anatomy for Medical Students
Snell	Clinical Embryology for Medical Students, 2nd Ed.
Valtin	Renal Function
Watson	Basic Human Neuroanatomy

Clinical Medical Sciences

Clark & MacMahon	Preventive Medicine
Eckert	Emergency-Room Care, 2nd Ed.
Grabb & Smith	Plastic Surgery, 2nd Ed.
Green	Gynecology, 2nd Ed.
Judge & Zuidema	Methods of Clinical Examination, 3rd Ed.
Keefer & Wilkins	Medicine
MacAusland & Mayo	Orthopedics
Nardi & Zuidema	Surgery, 3rd Ed.
Thompson	Primer of Clinical Radiology
Ziai	Pediatrics, 2nd Ed.

Nursing Sciences

DeAngelis	Basic Pediatrics for the Primary Health Care Provider
Sana & Judge	Physical Appraisal Methods in Nursing Practice
Selkurt	Basic Physiology for the Health Sciences

Manuals and Handbooks

Arndt	Manual of Dermatologic Therapeutics
Children's Hospital Medical Center, Boston	Manual of Pediatric Therapeutics
Condon & Nyhus	Manual of Surgical Therapeutics, 3rd Ed.
Friedman & Papper	Problem-Oriented Medical Diagnosis
Massachusetts General Hospital	Manual of Nursing Procedures
Neelon & Ellis	A Syllabus of Problem-Oriented Patient Care
Spivak & Barnes	Manual of Clinical Problems in Internal Medicine: Annotated with Key References
Wallach	Interpretation of Diagnostic Tests, 2nd Ed.
Washington University Department of Medicine	Manual of Medical Therapeutics, 21st Ed.
Zimmerman	Techniques of Patient Care

Little, Brown and Company
34 Beacon Street
Boston, Massachusetts 02106

MANUAL OF
SURGICAL
THERAPEUTICS

MANUAL OF SURGICAL THERAPEUTICS

THIRD EDITION

**Departments of Surgery
The Medical College of Wisconsin
and University of Illinois**

EDITED BY

Robert E. Condon, M.D.
Professor of Surgery, The Medical College of Wisconsin, Milwaukee, and Chief, Surgical Services, Veterans Administration Center, Wood, Wisconsin

Lloyd M. Nyhus, M.D.
Professor of Surgery and Head of the Department, The Abraham Lincoln School of Medicine of the University of Illinois at the Medical Center, Chicago

Little, Brown and Company
Boston

PREFACE TO THE
THIRD EDITION

The *Manual of Surgical Therapeutics* has been widely accepted by those for whom it was intended—surgical students and surgical house officers—and also has gained a large and cosmopolitan readership among more senior surgeons and physicians. Our colleagues who have reviewed the *Manual* for professional journals have found it to be very worthwhile. We are, of course, pleased and grateful.

Much new and revised material in this third edition of the *Manual* is the result of valued suggestions from those who use it every day. New chapters and sections discuss acute respiratory insufficiency and its treatment, parenteral alimentation and tube feedings, eye injuries, epistaxis, and gynecological emergencies. An important new chapter, constituting a small atlas of minor surgical techniques, also has been added at the request of many readers.

The chapters and sections on resuscitation from shock and trauma, upper gastro-intestinal hemorrhage, preoperative evaluation of renal, cardiac, and pulmonary function, anesthesia and anesthetic premedication, acute renal insufficiency, infections and antibiotics, coagulation disorders, burns, pediatric surgery, and cancer chemotherapy have been rewritten in their entirety. The entire *Manual* has been extensively revised, updated, and rechecked by contributors, old and new.

Another new feature in this edition is the inclusion of a short list of "Suggested Reading" after many sections. The purpose of these references is to provide for the student desiring more detailed information entry to review articles and key references in the literature. A standard surgical text also should be consulted by all readers for discussion in depth which cannot be provided in the outline format of the *Manual*.

To our colleagues, whose expertise is recorded in the pages of the *Manual,* our thanks and appreciation of their efforts and diligence. We continue to beg the for-bearance of our contributors for our sometimes extensive exercise of editorial pre-rogatives. Most of the drawings in the third edition of the *Manual* are the work of Ms. Carole Russell; we thank her and Mr. George Spuda, Chief of the Medical Illustration Service at the Wood Veterans Administration Hospital, for their valued addition to the utility of the *Manual*.

Mrs. Ann Haddick Napoletan undertook the heavy responsibilities of typing and retyping the manuscript and checking the proofs with her usual good humor and grace; we are most grateful and appreciative of her capable help and devotion, without which it would not have been possible to complete this third edition. To Mr. Fred Belliveau of Little, Brown and Company, his skilled editorial staff, and, in particular, Mrs. Anne N. Merian, our thanks and continued admiration.

Robert E. Condon
Lloyd M. Nyhus

PREFACE TO THE FIRST EDITION

In the *Manual of Surgical Therapeutics* the student or house officer will find the essentials of day-to-day care of the surgical patient. It is a manual for the *man on the firing line,* and as such it is a readily available source of information on the pathophysiologic, pharmacologic, and nonoperative aspects of the care of the surgical patient. Discussion will be found on drug usage and administration, dosages and side effects, as well as on diagnostic maneuvers and the management of complications should they arise. No attempt has been made to be all-inclusive, however, since inclusiveness itself is a presumptuous goal. It is expected that when the frenetic pace of the Surgical Service slackens, the user of this *Manual* will undertake to find in standard surgical textbooks the in-depth coverage he seeks.

For a number of years, the value of another manual, the *Manual of Medical Therapeutics,* has been apparent wherever medical students and house staff are in evidence. Its edges often frayed, the medical manual is seen in the pockets of many white coats throughout the nation as well as in many dictating and nursing stations where harried medical students or house officers have temporarily misplaced it. But much of the information which the student or house officer on the Surgical Service needs is not to be found in the medical manual.

Thus the need for a surgical manual made itself apparent. This *Manual* has been prepared by the members of the Department of Surgery of the University of Illinois College of Medicine and reflects our methods and judgment in the management of selected surgical problems. We thank all the contributors for their assistance and for their understanding acceptance of the considerable exercise of editorial prerogative which the published version of their contributions represents.

Deep appreciation is due Mr. Fred Belliveau of Little, Brown and Company, his editorial staff, and, in particular, Mrs. Anne N. Merian. Special thanks are due Mrs. Ann Napoletan and Mrs. Barbara Getz, editorial assistants of the Department of Surgery, University of Illinois College of Medicine, without whose capable help and devotion it would not have been possible for us to complete this *Manual.*

Robert E. Condon
Lloyd M. Nyhus

CONTENTS

MANUAL OF
SURGICAL
THERAPEUTICS

NOTICE

1. RESUSCITATION FROM SHOCK AND TRAUMA

I. GENERAL PRINCIPLES

A. **Priorities of management** In acute trauma, diagnostic and therapeutic measures are carried out concurrently rather than sequentially. The first objective in the care of an injured person is the preservation of life. Treatment of airway obstruction, shock, or cardiorespiratory failure often must be started without exact knowledge of the cause of these disorders. Once the patient is stable, etiological evaluation can be undertaken as a secondary objective.

1. **Establish and maintain an airway** Look for signs of obstruction: stridor, retraction, wheezing, or cyanosis. Sweep a finger deep into the oropharynx to remove clotted blood, mucus, vomitus and any loose teeth or dentures. Insert an **oropharyngeal airway** if the patient is obtunded or if unstable facial fractures cause obstruction. After these measures have been taken, ventilatory assistance with a mask is possible. When a patient makes violent efforts to sit up, he should be allowed to do so since this action usually is a reflex response to maintain an open airway.

   In comatose patients, an **endotracheal tube** may reduce aspiration and facilitate respiratory support. In a patient alert enough to make endotracheal intubation impractical, close observation and frequent suctioning are essential.

   Examine for evidence of sucking chest wounds, flail chest, tension pneumothorax, or lung injury. Treat airway obstruction (suction and intubation) and respiratory insufficiency (oxygen and positive-pressure ventilation). Direct injury to the larynx or trachea may make endotracheal intubation impossible. In such rare instances, be ready to perform an emergency tracheostomy.

   Position is important. The possibility of cervical or spinal cord injury necessitates immobilization and negates other positional considerations. Otherwise, keep the patient in a semiprone position. The patient must not lie or be restrained flat on his back.

2. **Assess and support cardiopulmonary function** Hypoxia and acidosis can cause cardiac arrest. If arrest has occurred, mouth-to-mouth ventilation and closed chest massage is started immediately. Time should not be wasted attempting a difficult endotracheal intubation during the early stages of resuscitation from cardiac arrest. Ventilation with an oral airway and a mask is sufficient in most patients (see Chap. 4). If the chest wall is unstable (flail chest) or rigid (advanced emphysema) and closed

1

chest massage is not effective, thoracotomy and direct manual cardiac compression may be necessary.

Metabolic **acidosis** should be anticipated in every patient with hypoperfusion and corrected with IV sodium bicarbonate. Early arterial blood gas analyses are helpful. Electrocardiographic (ECG) monitoring is essential for the diagnosis of specific arrhythmias (see Chap. 3).

3. **Control hemorrhage**   External hemorrhage is best controlled by **direct pressure over the site of bleeding.** Pressure is maintained until proximal control can be obtained in association with definitive treatment in the operating room. The use of tourniquets or of blind clamping in the depths of a wound is not advisable, as further injury may ensue.

Internal hemorrhage may be identified by thoracentesis or paracentesis. Peritoneal lavage, interpreted by an experienced observer, increases diagnostic accuracy. Blood loss due to fractures, even without major vessel injury, can be appreciable.

4. **Treat shock**   Hypovolemic shock is treated by blood replacement. Loss of less than 1,500 ml may be replaced by blood substitutes, but a more major blood loss should be replaced by blood. Patients with a loss of over 45% of blood volume become severely hypotensive and hypoxic and will progress to cardiopulmonary arrest if not resuscitated vigorously. Clinical guides to assessment of blood loss are given in Table 9-4.

The **essential steps in the management of hemorrhagic shock** are:

a. **Insert intravenous catheters**   Several catheters should be inserted using sterile techniques. At least one must be in the central venous pool. Vessels potentially involved by trauma are avoided. The clinical situation dictates which veins to use—almost always above the nipple line.

b. **Draw blood samples for typing and crossmatching** before giving plasma expanders. Determinations of arterial blood gases and hematocrit at this time provide baseline values and insight into the volume of bicarbonate buffering needed and the efficacy of respiratory support.

c. **Administer IV fluids**   Colloid and isotonic crystalloid solutions are administered very rapidly at first, with the rate of infusion slowed as the blood pressure and central venous pressure (CVP) begin to rise.

d. **Transfuse** as soon as compatible cross-matched blood is available. Maintain the hematocrit at 30–35%. In extreme cases in which colloid and crystalloid blood substitutes are not adequate for resuscitation, or when the hematocrit is below 15%, small amounts of type-specific or universal donor (O-neg) packed red blood cells may be given to maintain minimal oxygen-carrying capacity until cross-matched blood is available (see Chap. 15).

5. **Monitor CVP**   Fluctuation of the saline column in the manometer with respiration is a good indication that the tip of the central venous catheter

rests in the central venous pool. The catheter tip should be within the thorax but outside the pericardium. Pulsation coincidental with the pulse indicates placement in the right ventricle, and the catheter should be withdrawn to an appropriate position. All catheters should be checked for position by chest x-ray when this becomes clinically feasible. Initial placement of a catheter (Swan-Ganz) in the pulmonary artery is not necessary, although such a catheter may be helpful later in treating those patients who develop cardiac failure or myocardial infarction.

Monitoring the CVP requires **serial observation of changes** with fluid replacement. The absolute value of the CVP measured in a hypovolemic patient is less meaningful than the change in CVP with therapy. A rise in CVP paralleling that of systolic blood pressure is seen with adequate volume replacement. A low CVP persisting after volume replacement may indicate continued occult bleeding. A significant elevation of CVP in the face of continued hypotension suggests cardiac tamponade, myocardial infarction, or congestive heart failure.

6. **Catheterize the bladder** with a Foley catheter   Measure urine output hourly. Decreased urine output with elevated specific gravity (above 1.030) or osmolality (above 700 mOsm/kg) reflects hypovolemia. Later, low urine output with low specific gravity and osmolality in the face of normal vital signs may reflect renal tubular damage (see Chap. 11).

7. **Immobilize fractures**   "Splint 'em where they lie" remains the best rule. Protection of associated soft tissues—especially neurovascular structures—is of prime importance (see Sect. VII).

8. **Dress soft tissue wounds**   Elevation, compression for hemostasis, and sterile dressings protect against further injury and contamination. Tetanus prophylaxis and antibiotics, if appropriate, should be given. Definitive therapy can be carried out when anesthesia is available for adequate debridement and repair.

9. **Establish the etiology of shock**   Inability to restore blood pressure and circulating volume by adequate blood volume replacement indicates that a source of uncontrolled hemorrhage is present. Hematuria, hemoptysis, bloody nasogastric suction, or rectal bleeding suggests internal sources of blood loss. Thoracentesis, paracentesis, peritoneal lavage, pyelography, or endoscopy may define the hidden bleeding site. Pelvic fractures frequently account for occult loss of as much as 10 units of blood. Continuing major hemorrhage usually requires operative exploration. *Prolonged preoperative attempts to stabilize the circulation in such cases may result in failure of resuscitation.*

10. **Make repeated examinations of the patient,** with special attention to pulse rate, pulse pressure, skin temperature and color, and state of consciousness. A rapid pulse, narrow pulse pressure, blanched cool skin, and combativeness are signs of recurrent hypovolemia and hypoxia.

    After successful resuscitation, the patient enters a critical phase requiring continuous observation and general evaluation to note changes in the level of consciousness, spontaneous motion of the extremities, chest excursions, and abdominal habitus. A nasogastric tube is inserted, the aspirate inspected, and the stomach emptied and kept on intermittent suction.

All patients must be completely disrobed. A rapid assessment of the extent of injuries is performed by gentle but firm palpation of all body parts, especially those areas where injuries are suspected. Obvious deformities, asymmetry, lacerations, and contusions require special attention. Palpation of the scalp, facial bones, trachea, and vertebral column, as well as gentle compression of the thorax, pelvis, and extremities, usually will elicit signs of hidden fractures or dislocations. A careful abdominal examination is mandatory; particular attention is paid to the presence of tenderness and the character of bowel sounds. Rectal examination is performed in all patients, with particular attention to the presence or absence of blood. Peripheral pulses and the neuromuscular status of the extremities are assessed. Chest auscultation and percussion may demonstrate signs of pleural collapse, rub, or effusion as well as cardiac changes consistent with injury.

11. **Obtain** as thorough **a history** as possible   Previous medical problems, allergies, and medications used, as well as conditions concerning the accident, are important. Sources other than the patient may be necessary for an adequate history. During this period, serial determinations of blood gases and hematocrit, as well as indicated laboratory and x-ray evaluations, are carried out.

B. Pathophysiology of shock

1. **Definition**   Shock is a state of hypoperfusion secondary to decreased effective circulating blood volume. Sympathetic neural responses, diverting blood so that perfusion to vital tissues is maintained, produce physiological and metabolic changes in poorly perfused tissues which eventually have profound general effects.

2. **Classification**   Shock associated with trauma is primarily hypovolemic; associated problems may induce other forms of shock concurrently or subsequently.

   a. **Hypovolemic shock** is due to loss of blood volume either from hemorrhage of whole blood or from "third space" losses of plasma seen in peritonitis, pancreatitis, intestinal obstruction, and burns.

   b. **Endotoxin shock** is the result of peripheral pooling of blood in capacitance (primarily venous) vessels, impairing circulating blood volume without actual volume loss.

   c. **Cardiogenic shock** represents pump failure with inadequate output, and, therefore, inadequate tissue perfusion, in spite of normal blood volume.

   d. **Neurogenic shock** results from loss of sympathetic control of resistence vessels with resultant dilation of arterioles and venules; the decrease in effective circulating volume produces shock. Hypotension due to spinal anesthesia is an example of this phenomenon.

3. **Endocrine response**   Release of adrenocorticotropic hormone (ACTH), antidiuretic hormone (ADH), and aldosterone during hypotension results in renal retention of sodium, chloride, and water, enforcing renal potassium loss and a decreased urinary volume output. Release of epinephrine and norepinephrine from the adrenal medulla produces peripheral vasoconstriction, maintaining blood pressure by decreasing the volume of the vascular space as well as by mobilizing intravascular fluid from peripheral tissues to the central pool. With prolonged peripheral vasoconstriction, anaerobic metabolism results in accumulation of acidic metabolites (Fig. 1-1).

Hyperglycemia develops during shock and generally has been attributed to the glycogenolytic properties of corticosteroids and epinephrine. Recent studies demonstrating depression of insulin secretion in shock imply more intricate relationships.

4. **Metabolic effects**   A normally perfused cell utilizes glucose in the glycolytic and citric acid pathways to form energy through adenosine triphosphate (ATP). Without oxygen, pyruvate is transformed anaerobically to lactic acid (see Fig. 1-1), which then accumulates and results in acidosis. Amino acids and fatty acids which normally would enter oxidative pathways for energy production also accumulate in shock, compounding the metabolic acidosis. Oxygen deficit and acidosis eventually interfere with cell membrane function. Potassium is lost; sodium and water move into the cell, producing cellular edema.

5. **Cardiorespiratory response**   The intense sympathetic response during shock increases cardiac output by augmenting the rate and force of cardiac contraction in addition to increasing peripheral resistance. Since myocardial perfusion occurs primarily during diastole, tachycardia depresses myocardial perfusion, resulting in myocardial acidosis with prolonged shock. Although metabolic acidosis is compensated initially by increasing ventilation to augment carbon dioxide elimination, profound acidosis combined with hypoxia (both primary and secondary to de-

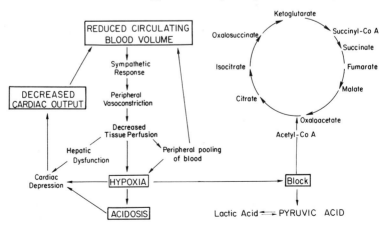

Figure 1-1. Shock leads to tissue hypoxia, with blockage of normal aerobic metabolism. Lactic acid accumulates, resulting in tissue acidosis.

creased myocardial perfusion) results in myocardial depression, irritability, and susceptibility to arrythmias.

C. Choice of replacement fluids in hypovolemia

1. **Crystalloid solutions** Initial volume replacement with normal saline or Ringer's lactate provides effective intravascular expansion. There are theoretical advantages to a buffered salt solution such as Ringer's lactate; concern about accumulation of lactate has not proved to be clinically important. Diffusion of noncolloid salt solutions out of the intravascular space is relatively rapid, so that a volume of up to four times the amount of blood lost must be infused as crystalloid solution to restore circulating blood volume.

   It is desirable to maintain the hematocrit above 30% and serum total protein above 6 gm/100 ml. At these values, the oxygen-carrying capacity and oncotic pressure of blood can protect against further hypoxia and tissue edema. Thus, dilution of hemoglobin and plasma protein are the factors that limit the volume of crystalloid solutions to be administered. **There is no place for salt-free crystalloid solutions (dextrose in water) in primary resuscitation.** When these solutions are given in acute post-traumatic states, water is retained because of the action of ADH and severe hypo-osmolality may result.

2. **Albumin** Human serum albumin in various concentrations is readily available and free of the risk of hepatitis. It is an effective plasma expander and has other advantages, one of which is that this protein is easily metabolized and spares body muscle proteins from catabolism.

3. **Plasma and plasma protein fraction** (Plasmanate) may be given without cross matching and are excellent blood volume expanders. Their use also should be considered when plasma losses are anticipated, as in burns, peritonitis, and pancreatitis. The use of fresh-frozen plasma provides coagulation factors for patients with clotting abnormalities. There is a risk of hepatitis transmission by plasma. This risk is reduced by use of single donor units, but cannot be entirely eliminated. Plasma protein fraction carries no risk of hepatitis and is preferred for most clinical situations.

4. **Dextrans** Both clinical dextran and low molecular weight dextran are effective plasma expanders; they also decrease blood viscosity and improve microcirculatory flow. Dextrans may interfere with platelet function, alter coagulation mechanisms, and interfere with cross-match reactions. The use of dextrans prior to exploration of soft tissue injuries is ill-advised. Although often effective in preventing renal failure, low molecular weight dextran also can be responsible for renal failure due to "tubular burn" resulting from the very hyperosmolar urine formed if dextran is excreted in an inadequate volume of urine. No more than 1 liter of dextran solution should be given each day.

5. **Blood transfusion** Major losses of whole blood may be replaced with whole blood or, preferably, with packed red cells and a plasma substitute (albumin, Plasmanate). It is generally possible to provide adequate vol-

ume expansion initially with crystalloid solutions and plasma substitutes until crossmatching can be accomplished. The use of matched blood minimizes reactions due to blood group incompatibilities and isosensitization.

Banked blood becomes progressively acidic and hyperkalemic, and there is a rapid loss of many coagulation factors (see Chap. 15). Massive transfusion (over 20 units), in addition to having a high incidence of transfusion reactions, carries a potential of development of wet lung due to pulmonary entrapment of fibrin and other aggregates in the blood; the use of a microaggregate filter is advisable.

6. **Buffer therapy**   The development of metabolic acidosis during shock can be countered by administration of buffer agents such as sodium bicarbonate. Generally, sodium bicarbonate is a sufficient adjunct to volume replacement in the treatment of shock. Tromethamine (THAM) is an effective intracellular and extracellular buffer and may be used if acidosis is severe (arterial pH below 7.2). The side effect of central respiratory arrest has limited the clinical use of THAM. Rapid changes in pH may be induced and cause cardiac arrhythmias, so that patients receiving rapid infusions of buffers should have continuous ECG monitoring.

D. Adjunctive therapy in shock

1. **Oxygen therapy and ventilatory support**   All patients who display dyspnea or tachypnea should be given oxygen. Remember that the important mechanism of oxygen transport (over 95%) is the hemoglobin in erythrocytes. A normal hemoglobin of 15 mg/100 ml provides transport for 20 vol% of oxygen; a hemoglobin of 7 gm/100 ml (hematocrit 21%) carries only 10 vol%, which is the critical reserve level of oxygen consumption for most tissues, especially the myocardium and brain.

Oxygen given by a properly applied mask or by nasal catheter at 8 liters/min will increase inspired oxygen concentrations by 10%, and improve hemoglobin saturation and oxygen delivery to the tissues. Oxygen administered via a T-adapter and an endotracheal or tracheostomy tube will increase the inspired oxygen concentration to 40%. Oxygen delivery in concentrations above 50% is unnecessary in the management of most patients. Pulmonary oxygen toxicity may result if 100% oxygen is administered continuously for 24 hr. It should be remembered that cyanosis, a generally reliable clinical sign of inadequate oxygenation, may be absent if blood loss has reduced the circulating hemoglobin concentration below 5 gm/100 ml.

Ventilatory support is indicated whenever voluntary respiratory volumes are inadequate and for specific conditions such as cardiopulmonary arrest, mechanical chest wall dysfunction, atelectasis, or pulmonary edema (see Chap. 12). Repeated examinations for hemothorax or pneumothorax prior to and during ventilatory support are especially important. Previously undetected injury may be responsible for the development of a tension pneumothorax when positive-pressure ventilation is employed.

High inspiratory pressure, continuous positive pressure, and the use of expiratory retarding devices all may contribute to increased resistance to pulmonary blood flow. The positive pressure is transmitted to the alveolar space, pulmonary capillaries are compressed, and blood flow through the pulmonary circulation is diminished. Decreased return to the left side of the heart causes a fall in cardiac output and may prolong or increase shock, especially in a hypovolemic patient.

2. **Thermal support** Hyperpyrexia can contribute to the deleterious cellular metabolic effects of shock and appears frequently in endotoxin shock. The patient should be kept at normal temperature by means of a hypothermia blanket and administration of acetaminophen, aspirin, or sodium salicylate.

3. **Antibiotics** Massive trauma and shock are associated with depression of reticuloendothelial function. During the early post-traumatic period, the ability of the body to clear bacteria from the circulation is depressed. Prophylactic antibiotic therapy frequently is indicated in such circumstances. The choice of antibiotic therapy depends on the type of injury involved. A cephalosporin is recommended for initial therapy, with the addition of gentamicin in selected cases. Antibiotic therapy is discussed more thoroughly in Chapter 14.

4. **Diuretics** Maintenance of adequate urinary output (30–50 ml/hr) is a prime aim in the management of shock and major trauma and is accomplished by providing adequate volumes of intravenous fluids and blood. Generally speaking, an inadequate urine output reflects inadequate volume replacement. Until there is reliable clinical evidence that volume expansion has been adequate, diuretics should be avoided. With persistent depression of urinary output in the face of a rising CVP and normal pulse and blood pressure, osmotic diuresis may be indicated. Mannitol, a monosaccharide which is filtered but not resorbed by the kidney, induces an obligate excretion of filtered water which helps maintain renal tubular flow and patency. Inasmuch as mannitol also acts as a plasma expander, monitoring of CVP during therapy is essential. If no response is obtained to mannitol, ethacrynic acid or furosemide may be used intravenously; however, the fact that these agents will enforce urine output even in the face of hypovolemia, aggravating the shock state, makes it essential that these diuretics be avoided until stable normovolemia is obtained.

5. **Vasoactive drugs** Profound vasoconstriction secondary to the sympathetic response in shock worsens the primary problem of hypoperfusion. Vasoconstrictor drugs aggravate this response and generally have no role in the therapy of septic or hypovolemic shock.

Theoretically, agents that block sympathetic vasoconstriction should provide increased perfusion, decreasing tissue hypoxia and acidosis. However, because of the systemic effects of such agents, it is *essential that the blood volume be restored prior to their use and that fluid administration be continued* during their administration. Without these precautions, a precipitous drop in blood pressure can be anticipated due to the opening of peripheral capillary beds. Once adequate volume has been administered, chlorpromazine (Thorazine), 3 mg every 2–3 hr, may produce an appreciable improvement in tissue perfusion. Phenoxybenzamine hydrochloride (Dibenzyline) is a potent alpha-adrenergic blocker; however, it has not yet been approved for parenteral administration.

6. Cardiac drugs   In most cases of traumatic shock, one is dealing with an otherwise normal myocardium which has become hypoxic. Digitalis is generally unnecessary, since cardiac function will improve with successful treatment of the blood volume deficit. However, older patients who may have underlying primary myocardial disease, patients who develop a very rapid tachycardia which persists after volume replacement, and, certainly, patients who develop cardiac failure or exhibit a rising CVP in the face of persistent hypotension are candidates for digitalization. Hypokalemia should be corrected before digitalis is administered. Rapidly acting preparations, such as lanatoside C (Cedilanid) and digoxin, are preferable. Contraindications to digitalization include the presence of conduction abnormalities (partial or complete heart block) and irritability of the myocardium (ventricular ectopic beats or ventricular tachycardia).

Isoproterenol (Isuprel) increases myocardial contractility and heart rate. Isoproterenol also stimulates beta-receptors in peripheral muscle beds, causing vasodilation and improved flow to these tissues. The total effect is decreased blood pressure and peripheral resistance and increased cardiac output. A serious drawback to the use of isoproterenol is that many patients develop a very rapid tachycardia and administration of the drug must be decreased or discontinued.

The combination of hypoxia and acidosis frequently leads to cardiac arrhythmias which require therapy (see Chap. 3). Digitalis is the drug of choice for the treatment of atrial arrhythmias. Ventricular arrhythmias may be treated with 50-100 mg of lidocaine IV.

7. Steroids   Pharmacological doses of corticosteroids frequently are helpful in low-flow states refractory to ordinary resuscitative measures such as volume replacement and pH buffering. Dexamethasone (1-3 mg/kg) or methylprednisolone (1-2 gm) is given in a single IV injection. Proposed but unproved mechanisms of action of steroids include increased tissue perfusion by capillary vasodilation, improved oxygen and micronutrient uptake by cells, augmented conversion of lactic acid to glycogen through unknown metabolic pathways, protection of lysosomal membranes against pH changes, and decreased aminoaciduria and hyperphosphatemia accomplished through induced transamination, converting amino acid carbon skeletons to energy-producing trioses or citric acid intermediates, replenishing the citric acid cycle, yielding ATP, and increasing utilization of free phosphates.

SUGGESTED READING

Carey, L. C., Lowery, B. D., and Cloutier, C. T.   Hemorrhagic shock. *Curr. Probl. Surg.* 3:48, 1971.

Moore, F. D., and Ball, M. R.   *The Metabolic Response to Surgery.* Springfield, Ill.: Thomas, 1952.

Moss, G. S., and Saletta, J. D.   Traumatic shock in man. *N. Engl. J. Med.* 290:724, 1974.

Skillman, J. J., Lauler, D. P., Hickler, R. B., Lyons, J. H., Olson, J. E., Ball, M. R., and Moore, F. D.   Hemorrhage in normal man: Effect on renin, cortisol, aldosterone, and urine composition. *Ann. Surg.* 166:865, 1967.

II. FACIAL INJURIES   Patients with facial trauma may have associated mortal injuries, but facial injuries in themselves need rarely cause death. The most common serious injuries associated with facial injuries involve the brain, cervical spine, and eye. Despite frequently published statements to the contrary, *serious facial injury alone is not an indication for emergency tracheostomy.* Patients with facial injury who require tracheostomy have associated injury of the head, neck, or chest.

The common causes of facial trauma are automobile accidents and accidents occurring in and about the home. The most serious injuries are sustained from automobile accidents and accidents at work. Learning the direction and type of injuring force as well as the nature of the injuring object is valuable in anticipating injuries not obvious at first examination.

A. Classification of facial injury   To avoid overlooking subtle forms of injury, a scheme of organization of common facial injuries should be kept in mind. The simplest scheme divides both soft tissue areas and facial bones into zones and forms of injury, as follows:

1. Soft tissue facial injuries

a. Type of injury

(1) Contusions and abrasions, with or without hematoma.

(2) Accidental tattoo (numerous small foreign particles embedded in dermis) or retained larger foreign bodies.

(3) Puncture wounds.

(4) Lacerations—simple, beveled, tearing, or bursting (stellate).

(5) Avulsion injury, either with complete loss of tissue or as a flap (undermined laceration).

b. Location of injury—forehead, eyelids, ears, nose, cheek, chin, lips, intraoral.

2. Facial bone fractures

a. Type of fracture—closed (simple), open (compound), greenstick, comminuted, undisplaced, displaced.

b. Location of fracture

(1) Upper third of face: frontal bone, frontal sinuses, glabella, and supraorbital ridge.

(2) Middle third of face: nasal bones and septum, maxillary sinuses (antrum), orbital bones, zygoma and zygomatic arch, transverse maxilla (Le Fort I), pyramidal maxilla (Le Fort II), craniofacial disjunction (Le Fort III), alveolar processes, and maxillary dentition.

       (3) Lower third of face: mandibular dentition, alveolar process, symphysis, body, angle, ascending ramus, condyle, and coronoid process.

B. Priorities of treatment   Though facial injuries may be extensive, the patient first must be evaluated completely, using those priorities which always apply in trauma and which are outlined in Section I of this chapter. Extensive facial injuries seldom cause great pain. When pain seems to be severe, associated injuries should be suspected.

Most facial hemorrhage can be controlled by direct pressure or ligation of the bleeding vessel. One real danger of facial hemorrhage is obstruction of the upper airway. The volume of hemorrhage from facial injuries alone is seldom sufficient to cause shock or to require emergency blood transfusion. Associated cerebral, cervical, or ocular injuries are more apt to be the cause of shock.

C. Diagnosis of facial injury is established by observation, palpation, and x-ray examination.

    1. Observation   In addition to obvious soft tissue injuries, asymmetry of the face caused by underlying fractures often can be detected early, before the masking effects of soft tissue swelling occur. The eyelids always should be opened to look for ocular injury, and the mouth opened to observe dental occlusion.

    2. Palpation   Observation of facial symmetry is reinforced by palpation of bony prominences. These landmarks may be masked by overlying hematoma or edema. Comparing the height of the malar eminences (zygoma) is especially informative in diagnosing depressed fractures of that bone. Tenderness usually can be elicited at the site of a fracture, but seldom is the discomfort extreme. Systematic bilateral palpation, even in the presence of obvious injury, helps to detect subtle deformities and should be performed in the following order: supraorbital and lateral orbital rims, infraorbital rims, malar eminences, zygomatic arches, nasal bones, maxilla, and mandible.

    3. X-ray examination   Gross facial bone fractures can be diagnosed without x-ray confirmation. Indeed, some grossly displaced facial bone fractures do not visualize well on x-rays. The most informative x-ray views should be obtained initially: posteroanterior (PA), lateral, and occipitomental (Waters') projections. After review of these films and as indicated by the nature of the injury, special views of the nasal bones, mandible, and zygoma may be needed. In addition to routine x-ray studies, laminography (tomography) is useful in diagnosing fractures about the orbit. Sialography may be helpful if laceration of the parotid duct is a possibility and cannot be confirmed by direct observation.

    4. Documentation of injury should include a record of the type of injury and measurement of any wounds. A photograph of extensive facial injuries should be taken before treatment begins. Such a photograph can be invaluable in understanding and explaining secondary problems and the nature of final healing.

D. Triage and treatment of facial injury   Once life-threatening problems have been resolved, soft tissue injuries amenable to repair under local anesthesia are treated first. Complex facial injuries with tissue loss and extensive fractures seldom can be treated immediately, since these patients usually are poor candidates for a general anesthetic. When definitive care must be postponed, the simplest accurate tissue approximation will promote a better end result. If necessary, soft tissue injuries can wait without repair up to 24 hr without compromising the final result, provided that bleeding has been controlled and the wounds properly cleansed and dressed. Systemic antibiotics are advisable when delay in soft tissue repair is anticipated.

Reduction and fixation of facial bone fractures almost never need to be carried out as an emergency operation, but facial fractures can be difficult to reduce more than 2 wk after injury and should be treated definitively before this time. As facial bones are membranous in origin, healing begins with fibrous union which can be overcome by manipulation and sharp dissection, even if delayed reduction is necessary. Healing in children is accelerated and reduction of their fractures should be attempted within 7-10 days of injury whenever possible.

E. Operative care   Repair of facial injuries should be oriented toward anatomical repositioning of soft and bony tissues. If this is accomplished, normal features, symmetry, dental occlusion, and functions of the face will be restored.

1. Anesthesia   Patients with acute extensive facial injuries are poor candidates for general anesthesia, often arriving in the emergency room with their stomachs filled with food, alcohol, or blood. Given a reasonably cooperative patient, local anesthesia is unquestionably superior for the management of most facial injuries. Local anesthesia allows the surgeon far greater ease, as endotracheal intubation for general anesthesia almost invariably results in restricted access to the patient's face and distortion of his features. Sedation appropriate to the age and condition of the patient will make local anesthesia more successful.

Repair of the deep structures of the face and open reduction of most major facial bone fractures are best performed under general anesthesia. A weak solution of epinephrine can be infiltrated into the face to facilitate hemostasis and shorten operating time.

2. Operating room   A scrub nurse and a circulating nurse are minimum assistance when repairing facial injuries. Attempting soft tissue repair unassisted in an emergency room invites frustration and second-rate results.

3. Tissue loss   Extensive tissue losses can wait definitive repair for 24 hr or more. Repair with adjacent tissue, if it can be moved without distortion of features, is preferred. If skin grafts are needed, full-thickness postauricular grafts serve best to match the color and texture of facial skin. Rotation and transposition flaps often can be used to cover defects immediately following injury, but tubed pedicle flaps, direct pedicle flaps, and island flaps are techniques ordinarily reserved for later, reconstructive procedures.

SUGGESTED READING
Kazanjian, V., and Converse, J. M.   *The Surgical Treatment of Facial Injuries* (3rd ed.). Baltimore: Williams & Wilkins, 1974.
Schultz, R. C.   *Facial Injuries.* Chicago: Year Book, 1970.

III. **HEAD AND CERVICAL INJURIES**   The most important observation of head injury is change in the state of consciousness since injury. Record the present level of consciousness, preferably in terms of what the patient does spontaneously or to what he responds. Prompt and lucid conversation implies alert consciousness. Memory loss for the accident commonly occurs with concussion. Memory loss for such items as address, occupation, or year means intellectual impairment and represents an early change in consciousness. In progressive stupor leading to coma, lack of verbal response to questioning occurs sooner than does lack of accurate avoidance of painful stimuli. In coma there is absence of purposeful movements, either spontaneous or evoked.

A. General care

1. **Vital signs** (blood pressure, pulse, and respiratory rate) are important indicators of change in the patient's status. Record them frequently and post them in a prominent place; a blackboard on the wall is a help.

2. A good **airway,** oxygenation, and humidification are of the utmost importance, since hypoxia will increase cerebral edema. If secretions pool or breathing becomes labored, an endotracheal tube should be inserted or a tracheostomy done. A lateral position with no elevation of the head is superior to the supine position.

3. **Nothing by mouth** should be given until it is clear that no operation is to be performed.

4. **Intravenous infusion** should be started and a **Foley catheter** introduced if the patient is not alert or if an operation is considered likely. Watch for development of water excess (dilutional hyponatremia), a common sequela of head injury.

5. **Restraint** of the patient in spread-eagle fashion is dangerous. If restraints are unavoidable, the patient should be positioned on either side, alternating the sides every 3 hr, with both legs and arms strapped to the same side of the bed. Very large bandages wrapped in boxing-glove fashion around the hands and up the forearm will prevent pulling at tubings or dressings.

6. **Sedation** interferes with evaluation of consciousness and **should be avoided.**

7. **Anticonvulsants** are given to all patients who have had a cerebral contusion or an intracranial hematoma. Diphenylhydantoin (Dilantin), 100 mg tid, is given IV after a loading dose of 500 mg. IM administration is avoided because of poor absorption.

8. **Changes in pupil size or reaction to light** may be caused by pressure on the third nerve or to pontine damage. Dilated or unequal pupils indicate transtentorial shift resulting from increased intracranial pressure (coning). Constricted pupils that do not react to light are signs of brain stem damage, either primary (e.g., contusion) or secondary to increased pressure.

9. If immediate **reduction in intracranial pressure** is needed while the operating room is being prepared, give mannitol (100 ml of 20% solution) or urea (125 ml of 30% solution) IV. Hyperosmolar solutions are otherwise avoided, lest brain shrinkage permit increased bleeding.

10. **Cerebral angiography** is the most versatile diagnostic study in the evaluation of craniocerebral injury, but may not always be available or without hazard. Lateralizing signs may indicate the presence of an expanding clot, but just as often they point to cerebral contusion and edema. Angiograms may help define the nature of the injury.

11. **Echoencephalography** is an easily applied noninvasive test that entails no risk to the patient. It may permit determination of the probable presence of a clot or mass with sufficient accuracy to lead to exploratory bur holes. Rapid deterioration of consciousness may indicate the need for exploratory operation without either angiography or echoencephalography.

B. **Definitions and suggestions**

1. **Cerebral concussion** means temporary disruption in cerebral activity resulting from injury, reflected in transiently altered consciousness or other *temporary* loss of neural function (e.g., blindness).

2. **Cerebral contusion** means damage to a portion of the brain and is characterized by dulled mentation, pink cerebrospinal fluid (CSF), and a sensory or motor deficit. Contused frontal or temporal lobes may need to be resected if sufficient swelling occurs.

3. **Linear fractures** of the cranial vault usually are clearly visible in films of the skull. If a linear fracture is present, suspect (a) an *arterial epidural hematoma* in an adult if the fracture crosses any branch of the middle meningeal artery, (b) a *venous epidural hematoma* if it crosses the superior longitudinal or a lateral sinus, and (c) a *diploic epidural hematoma* if there is a large separation of fractured bone fragments in an infant or toddler.

4. **Depressed skull fracture** is an impaction of fragmented calvaria which may result in penetration of the underlying dura and brain. These fragments should be elevated depending on location, depth of depression, and overlying scalp laceration.

5. **Basilar fractures** may be diagnosed roentgenographically; by the leakage of CSF from the nose or ear; more often by bleeding from the ear in the absence of obvious cutaneous cause; or by severe ecchymosis of the

eyelids or over the mastoid process (Battle's sign). Broad-spectrum antibiotics are indicated with CSF leak, but not with nasal or aural bleeding alone. The ear canal should not be packed with anything, as it might hinder egress of fluid or blood.

6. **Intracerebral hematoma** may result from severe acute injury or progressive damage secondary to contusion. These hematomas should be removed if they threaten life or well-being.

7. **Epidural hematoma** may be of arterial, venous, or diploic origin. When change of neural function indicates continued bleeding, craniotomy is performed to evacuate the clot and stop the source of bleeding.

8. **False intracranial aneurysm,** or "pseudoaneurysm," is a cavity with walls composed of clots which are becoming organized with fibroconnective tissue. Such clots must be evacuated and the source of bleeding arrested.

9. In **acute subdural hematoma** there is a variable amount of freshly clotted blood in the subdural space, accompanied by severe contusion of the underlying brain. Usually it is the severely contused brain which is responsible for the patient's compromised clinical state, not the clot in the subdural space. This type of hematoma is fatal in 95% of patients.

10. **Subacute subdural hematoma** implies large amounts of recently clotted blood in the subdural space, with either no contusion of the underlying brain or, at most, punctate cortical hemorrhages and small patches of subarachnoid blood. The clot is responsible for the neurological deficit, and its timely removal almost invariably results in good recovery.

11. **Chronic subdural hematoma** is mentioned in connection with acute head injuries because, although present and asymptomatic for months, it can present very acutely. Fluid similar in appearance to crankcase oil is located within a capsule which, in turn, is within the subdural space. Bur holes, followed by drainage of the fluid and irrigation of the cavity, almost always result in a cure.

12. **Acute subdural hygroma**   The origin of the blood-tinged fluid present in these collections and the reason why such small amounts cause severe neurological deficits are not known. The fluid is indistinguishable from CSF. Drainage of the fluid results in impressive improvement.

C. **Clinical evaluation**

1. **Signs of progressive increase in intracranial pressure are:**

a. Steady slowing of the pulse.

b. Change in size and symmetry of the pupils and their reaction to light.

c. Progressive diminution in level of consciousness.

d. Irregularities of respiration.

The presence of one or more of these signs is adequate justification for bilateral carotid angiography. Cranial exploration is indicated if signs of a clot or lobar contusion are found.

2. **Adult: previous loss of consciousness; now alert**   If there is a definite history of head injury and loss of consciousness, the patient should be admitted to the hospital for observation. If the patient is alert at the time of examination, order skull films: anteroposterior (AP), right and left lateral, and Towne's views.

   a. If **no fracture** is seen, 24 hr of observation is probably adequate.

   b. If there is a **linear fracture over the convexity** of the skull, and especially if it crosses a venous sinus, observation should be prolonged. If the level of consciousness declines, echoencephalography or cerebral angiography should be done to diagnose hematoma, as a prelude to its evacuation.

   c. If the **linear fracture crosses the pterion,** longer observation is necessary. Angiography and operation are indicated if the patient becomes obtunded or if a rapid pulse slows to less than 60/min. Displacement of meningeal or cerebral vessels seen in the angiogram should lead to exploratory craniotomy.

   d. If skull films show a **fracture depressed 5 mm or more,** it should be elevated as an elective procedure. If it overlies a venous sinus, the possibility of air embolism from opening the sinus may require use of the Trendelenburg position or positive-pressure ventilation during operation.

   e. If there is **scalp laceration and a depressed fracture,** the patient should be taken directly to the operating room. If there is to be any delay, lacerations should be sutured temporarily in the emergency room. The wound should be irrigated, the edges debrided, the depressed fragments removed and discarded, and the scalp sutured. If the defect is sizable or over a vital area, an elective cranioplasty should be performed later. Some neurosurgeons wash the bone fragments and replace them, using antibiotic coverage.

   f. If there is **scalp laceration and linear fracture,** irrigate and debride the scalp wound and repair the laceration.

3. **Adult: previous loss of consciousness; now irritable or confused**   If there is definite history of head injury and loss of consciousness in a patient who is irritable or confused, with or without a neurological deficit, order skull films and observe the patient for several days or a week. Loss of consciousness means there has been concussion and perhaps contusion. If the patient becomes more obtunded or develops more neurological findings, consider angiography to determine if there is a clot or contusion with edema. Lobar resection may be needed if the patient's condition worsens.

Lumbar puncture may be advised by some neurosurgeons; it is probably safe if no fluid is allowed to escape when pressure is over 200 mm in the lateral decubitus position, and may be useful if the patient is not too restless to prevent proper estimation of pressure.

a. Pink CSF implies cerebral contusion, but also may be present with subdural hematoma or lobar swelling.

b. Clear CSF may be present with epidural hematoma.

c. Increased pressure may be present with contusion or hematoma, with or without blood in the CSF.

d. Normal pressure may be present with concussion or contusion, and sometimes with hematoma.

The presence or absence of fracture does not correlate with CSF pressure, or with presence or absence of blood in the CSF.

4. Adult: responsive only to painful stimuli   Skull films should be taken only if they can be done conveniently and quickly. Echoencephalography is more rapid than angiography and may be repeated frequently.

a. If **echoencephalography** shows a **shift of midline structures** and the patient's condition is stable, cerebral angiography may reveal a hematoma or indicate contusion of the brain. If the state of consciousness is rapidly deteriorating, if the pupils become unequal, or if the pulse rate falls below 60/min, **exploratory bur holes** may supplant angiography as an urgent procedure.

(1) If there is a **contusion of the temporal lobe,** cerebral angiography will show an elevation of the middle cerebral artery in the AP and lateral projections and, sometimes, also a shift of the anterior cerebral artery. Treatment is resection of the tip of the temporal lobe.

(2) Subacute subdural hematoma is impossible to distinguish from epidural hematoma. If there is no visible medial displacement of the middle meningeal artery to indicate the latter diagnosis, bur holes or craniotomy with removal of the fresh clot is indicated.

(3) If an **acute subdural hematoma** is present, angiography will show an irregularly outlined filling defect over the surface of the brain with evidence of intraparenchymal swelling in either the underlying or the contralateral hemisphere. Removal of the subdural hematoma through bur holes is the only treatment. Unfortunately this lesion usually is fatal.

b. If **echoencephalography** shows **no shift,** serial observations of clinical signs and repeated echoencephalography are indicated.

c. If echoencephalography and angiography are unavailable, any sign of clinical worsening indicates the need for cranial exploration.

d. Lumbar puncture is more meaningful in the comatose patient responsive only to painful stimuli.

(1) If the **pressure is elevated over 200 mm** H_2O in the lateral decubitus position, edema, contusion, or hematoma is probable, and angiography or operation may be urgently needed.

(2) If the **pressure is normal,** hematoma is less likely, and observation for change in clinical condition is indicated.

(3) If the **pressure is below 50 mm** H_2O, there probably is herniation of brain at the tentorial notch or foramen magnum. If the pupils are not dilated and fixed, immediate exploration is indicated, but with a poor prognosis. If the pupils are dilated and fixed, operation is fruitless.

e. Steroids may combat edema, especially when no operable lesion is found. A loading dose of 12 mg dexamethasone is followed by 4 mg every 4–6 hr.

5. **Infants under 2 yr of age**   Unconsciousness at the time of examination is extremely rare in infants. Neurological deficits or changes in pupil size often do not occur even with major trauma. A rapid pulse secondary to severe blood loss may occur in a child with only a subgaleal hematoma as well as in one with a diploic epidural hematoma. Lost blood should be replaced immediately. Corticoids and mannitol should be used to reduce cerebral edema if there is intracranial injury. If a child has only a subgaleal hematoma, it should not immediately be tapped, since it almost always will resorb within a 2-wk period. Skull films should be obtained (AP, lateral, and Towne's projections).

a. If the skull films reveal a **linear fracture,** the child is to be admitted to a hospital and observed for 48 hr. He should then be followed as an outpatient for 3 mo to exclude a chronic subdural hematoma. Subsequent roentgenograms are needed to ensure absence of enlarging fracture.

b. If the **skull fracture is depressed** more than 5 mm, the child should be admitted to a hospital and the fracture elevated as an elective procedure.

c. If the **skull fracture is stellate** and there is wide diastasis of the fracture edges, the child is to be observed in a hospital for accumulation of an epidural hematoma.

d. If there is no clear history of trauma, but there is evidence of a bulging fontanelle, split sutures, vomiting, and failure to thrive, or if convulsions are present in any irritable child, one must consider the possibility of a chronic subdural hematoma or a postmeningitic subdural effusion. Bilateral subdural taps should be performed. Do not aspirate fluid but allow it to flow spontaneously. Do not drain more than 10 ml from each side the first time, since rapid decompression may tear arachnoid venous channels and cause fatal bleeding.

6. **Children 2-10 yr of age**   The principle to be remembered in this age group is that the level of consciousness, vital signs, and degree of neurological deficit are most compromised immediately after injury, but spontaneous recovery may be rapid and dramatic. General supportive measures (airway, bladder catheter, and IV fluids) are to be emphasized in the immediate post-traumatic period, and consideration of angiography or operation is made during 2-12 hr of observation.

D. **Cervical injury**   Fracture dislocation of cervical vertebrae may result from direct trauma or from deceleration injury. Vertebral column and spinal cord damage often is overlooked in the presence of more obvious injuries to the head, thorax, or abdomen. The comatose or confused patient is not a good subject to examine for neck stiffness, quadriplegia, or sensory deficit. Diaphragmatic breathing, paralytic ileus, or acute urinary retention may be the only signs of cervical cord damage in the unconscious patient.

1. The patient who has a **stiff neck but no motor or sensory deficit** should have the neck immobilized in a plastic collar and cervical spine films taken. If the x-rays show displacement of one cervical vertebra on another, cranial tongs and traction should be applied. If they show either a teardrop or a compression fracture, the patient should be left in the plastic collar.

2. Patients who have a **sensory or motor deficit** at the level of the clavicle or involving the upper extremities should be placed immediately in cranial tongs and connected to 15-25 lb of traction. The amount depends on the degree of malalignment of vertebrae. Portable x-rays can be taken with the patient still on the examining table or stretcher, or in bed, without turning the head and neck. Lateral turning of the patient from supine to prone position may cause sudden death. The supine position is safest, since it allows free diaphragmatic breathing. If possible, a turning frame should be used to turn the patient every 2 hr. Decubitus ulcers are better prevented than treated. If paralytic ileus develops, nasogastric tube suction should be instituted. An indwelling Foley catheter should be inserted to keep the bladder decompressed. The patient should not be allowed to eat.

    If the cervical cord injury is at the C5 level, there will be complete quadriplegia, a sensory level at the clavicle, and the patient will breathe only with his diaphragm. Hypoxia may then cause the patient to be confused or delirious. If the injury is at the C6 level, there will be paraplegia and paralysis in extension of both arms. If the injury is at the C7 level, the patient will be able to flex his arms well but extend them only poorly. If extension is preserved, the injury is at or below the T1 level.

3. The patient who demonstrates a **rising sensory or motor level** after cervicovertebral trauma should have a decompressive laminectomy, since he may have either an extramedullary hematoma or an extension of intra-

medullary contusion. Lumbar puncture and manometric studies are not reliable and are not advisable in this situation. Dexamethasone (3-4 mg every 4 hr after a loading dose of 12 mg) may be used to combat edema of the spinal cord. Diskectomy and anterior spine fusion may be employed if disk protrusion is responsible for paraplegia with retention of some posterior column sensation.

4. **The newborn child with respiratory difficulty** who does not writhe when pinched or become startled when stimulated may have cervical cord injuries secondary to craniocervical hyperextension during birth. Test for sensory level by slowly passing a pinwheel up the body and watching the face. The child will wince when he feels pain, indicating the level of cord damage. X-rays of the spine are not helpful. Scalp traction, using 2-in. tape connected to 5 lb of weight, provides excellent immobilization. The tape should be applied to both sides of the scalp with the center of the tape in the same coronal plane as the external auditory canal. Tracheostomy is often necessary to establish a free airway, and a gastrostomy may be required temporarily to provide nutrition.

5. **The infant who develops ileus** after a fall or deceleration injury should be tested and treated as outlined in paragraph **4**, above.

SUGGESTED READING

Committee on Trauma, American College of Surgeons   A guide to evaluation of serious head injuries. *Bull. Am. Coll. Surg.* 59:21, 1974.

Hooper, R.   *Patterns of Acute Head Injury.* Baltimore: Williams & Wilkins, 1969.

Jamieson, K. G., and Yelland, J. D. N.   Surgically treated traumatic subdural hematomas. *J. Neurosurg.* 37:137, 1972.

IV. **CHEST INJURY**   Chest injury is common, sometimes misunderstood, and occasionally misdiagnosed. If impaired ventilation and circulation are not restored expeditiously, the patient may die. Infection is not an immediate threat but its prevention is an essential part of adequate therapy. There are **three major steps in managing a patient with chest trauma: resuscitation, decision about early thoracotomy, and establishing a complete diagnosis.** Nonoperative management of thoracic trauma will suffice for most patients, but thoracotomy is indicated for some and may be urgent (Table 1-1).

A. **Initial evaluation and therapy**

1. **Clear the airway, assist ventilation, treat shock**—these three imperative initial steps in trauma therapy are discussed in Section I, above.

2. **Look for tension pneumothorax**   Air hunger and a hyperresonant hemithorax should immediately raise a suspicion of tension pneumothorax. **Needle thoracentesis** (see Chap. 25), using a medium- or large-bore needle thrust into the affected hemithorax, may be a life-saving maneuver. Air escapes until the excess pressure is relieved. After conversion of tension to a simple pneumothorax, place a chest tube to manage any continuing air leak from the lung.

TABLE 1-1. Indications for Thoracotomy

Type of Injury	Diagnostic Aids
Open wound into pleural space	Visual inspection
Failure of initial resuscitation	
Continued bleeding	Record volume of blood loss
Continued air leak	Unexpanded lung on x-ray; bronchoscopy
Ruptured diaphragm	GI tract (gas) in chest on x-ray; confirm with contrast roentgenography examination
Foreign body	Visual inspection; PA and lateral x-ray views
Traumatic aortic aneurysm	Wide mediastinum on x-ray; depressed left main bronchus; angiography imperative
Ruptured esophagus	Barium swallow

3. **Look for cardiac tamponade**   Beck's triad—falling arterial pressure, rising venous pressure, and a small, quiet heart—indicates the possible presence of cardiac tamponade due to hemopericardium. A **paradoxical pulse** occasionally is seen in a patient with grunting respirations due to chest wall pain, but a paradoxical pulse should alert one to look for evidence of cardiac tamponade. Hemopericardium rarely is evident on chest x-ray.

    Needle pericardiocentesis (see Chap. 25) is the urgent initial temporary treatment of acute cardiac tamponade due to hemopericardium. The catheter is left in place while the patient is taken to the operating room. If the removal of 25-50 ml of blood does not restore arterial pressure, the diagnosis of acute cardiac tamponade is in doubt. Remember that blood in the pericardium may clot and cannot be removed through a needle and also that heart wounds may occur without cardiac tamponade.

4. **Physical diagnosis**   Look for clinical signs of respiratory insufficiency (stridor, cyanosis) and for asymmetrical or paradoxical movement of the chest with respiratory effort. Subcutaneous emphysema usually indicates a bronchial or pleural tear with a pneumothorax, but also occurs with a fractured larynx or tracheal or esophageal rupture and may require early operative care.

    Physical diagnosis has severe limitations in defining chest injuries and must be supplemented by **x-ray examination.** A physician should always accompany the injured patient during x-ray examinations. Upright PA and lateral films are ideal. A portable AP film taken with the head of the bed elevated is better than no film at all. A lateral film with the patient supine is a compromise but may be essential in planning treatment. Angiography and barium contrast studies may be necessary for definitive diagnosis.

5. **Tracheostomy** is not necessary for the initial treatment of chest trauma. The only indication for an urgent tracheostomy is upper airway obstruction which cannot be removed or managed by intubation.

6. **Endotracheal intubation** with a cuffed tube is the preferred method of establishing and maintaining an airway that is severely compromised. The oral or nasal route may be used, but the latter is preferable for the trained operator. Topical anesthesia reduces patient discomfort.

7. **Mechanical ventilation and oxygen therapy** are required in most serious chest injuries but are not substitutes for enforced coughing and tracheal suctioning in preventing atelectasis. A manual bag ventilator is useful when the patient must be moved about the hospital. Pressure-controlled ventilators are satisfactory for initial resuscitation. Assistance may be intermittent or continuous, depending on the degree of impairment. A volume-controlled ventilator is necessary for definitive treatment of a flail chest or severely contused lung. Positive end expiratory pressure must be added for the drowned lung syndrome. *Patients on ventilators must be carefully observed for increased airway resistance and diminished tidal volume, which are signs of tension pneumothorax.*

8. **Arterial blood gas determinations** should not delay initiation of obvious resuscitative measures, but should be obtained at the first opportunity. Maintain arterial oxygen tension (Pa_{O_2}) between 70 and 100 mm Hg, keeping the inspired oxygen concentration (FI_{O_2}) as low as possible. Weaning should be begun as soon as Pa_{O_2} can be maintained without support. Management of progressive or continued respiratory insufficiency is discussed in Chapter 12.

9. A baseline **ECG** is important. Ischemia and arrhythmias from blunt trauma respond to standard therapy (see Chap. 3). Cardiac wounds require thoracotomy for correction.

10. **Bronchoscopy** may be needed if intubation and tracheal suctioning do not remove obstructing secretions or aspirated blood. The flexible bronchoscope is sometimes useful for this task.

11. Strapping of chest wall injuries with adhesive tape or elastic bandages is not done since it interferes with ventilation. Intercostal nerve blocks also are not part of the emergency armamentarium, though rarely they may be useful in later management.

12. Small doses of morphine sulfate, administered intravenously once resuscitation is completed and the patient's condition is stable, relieve pain and allow more adequate voluntary ventilation and coughing.

B. **Trauma to the lung and associated structures**   A classification of injuries useful in establishing a framework for therapy is listed in Table 1-2. Judging which patient needs a thoracotomy may be aided by the discussion below and by the clues listed in Table 1-1. The management of respirator-supported ventilation is outlined in Chapter 12.

1. **Tension pneumothorax** may occur with sucking chest wounds or with a lung laceration. Lung laceration is the more common cause of tension pneumothorax; large volumes of air may enter the pleural space during

TABLE 1-2. Classification of Chest Trauma

Type of Injury	Typical Source	Effects	Comment
Chest wall defect	Shearing trauma (shotgun blast, explosion, flying objects, automobile hood ornament)	Circulation deficit; ventilation deficit; pleural infection; pulmonary infection	Occlusive dressing; chest tube(s); thoracotomy (urgent)
Major blunt trauma	Automobile accident; fall from a height	Ventilation deficit; possible circulation deficit; esophageal or diaphragmatic injury; pulmonary infection (later)	Usually multiple injuries; major resuscitative effort needed; need for thoracotomy indicated by failure of resuscitation
Perforating wound	Bullet	Circulation deficit (life-threatening); possible ventilation deficit	Frequent associated abdominal injuries requiring celiotomy; need for thoracotomy indicated by failure of resuscitation
Penetrating wound	Knife	Circulation deficit (usually life-threatening)	Resuscitative measures usually suffice; extent of damage frequently not evident until after 8–12 hr of observation
Minor blunt trauma	Simple fall	Decreased ventilation and impaired removal of tracheobronchial secretions because of pain; pulmonary infection (later)	Morbidity if not vigorously treated, especially in aged and alcoholic patients

inspiration. The air is prevented from escaping during expiration by collapse of soft lung tissue, occluding the laceration. Sucking chest wounds that produce tension pneumothorax are very unusual; air enters the hemithorax during inspiration owing to negative intrapleural pressure but it cannot escape during expiration owing to a one-way flap-valve effect of the injured chest wall tissue.

    a. High pressure in the pleural cavity produces collapse of the ipsilateral lung, compression of the contralateral lung, and obstruction of blood flow in the great veins and pulmonary vessels. Myocardial dysfunction due to anoxia produces a further fall in cardiac output.

    b. Relief of tension must be accomplished at once by inserting a large-bore needle or catheter anteriorly through the second intercostal space in the midclavicular line. Follow by inserting a chest tube (see Chap. 25).

2. Flail chest develops after fracture of several ribs or of the sternum in more than one place.

    a. The unstable chest wall segment develops **paradoxical movement,** pushed in during inspiration (negative intrapleural pressure) and pushed out during expiration (positive intrapleural pressure). The flail chest may become apparent only after continued examination. It can cause serious ventilatory impairment if anterior or lateral, but may cause little difficulty if posterior. Traction, compression, and operative fixation are no longer recommended therapy.

    b. The flail segment causes **hypoventilation.** Atmospheric pressure pushes the unstable area inward during inspiration, diminishing the effect of the decreased intrapleural pressure required to move air into the lungs, i.e., the pressure gradient from bronchus to pleural space across the lung surface is lost. During exhalation the unstable area is pushed outward, diminishing the effect of the increased intrapleural pressure required to move air out of the lung. Essentially, the same mechanism accounts for the ventilatory deficit in open pneumothorax and tension pneumothorax. As with any injured lung, atelectasis leads to arterial oxygen desaturation because of the functional right-to-left shunt created by hypoventilation of perfused lung.

    c. It formerly was thought that failure of the lungs to fill and empty synchronously caused the mediastinum to swing back and forth, and that decreased cardiac output caused by the compromise of venous return resulted from the instability of the mediastinum. The laws of fluid physics confirmed by multiple clinical observations make this concept obsolete. Similarly, in the absence of a rigid mediastinum due to prior disease, the pendelluft theory that air enters the compressed lung from the functioning lung defies the laws of fluid physics and should be abandoned.

    d. Effective **coughing is impaired** owing to pain and the abnormal chest wall movement, resulting in retention of secretions.

   e. **Ventilatory support with a volume respirator** is definitive treatment for most flail defects. It may be needed for 1-4 wk, until the patient is able to maintain Pa$_{O_2}$ without respirator support. The ventilator must be able to deliver sufficient volume at whatever pressures may be necessary to ventilate the lungs. Contusion of the lung frequently accompanies a flail chest; although usually apparent on admission, its effects may not appear for 12-24 hr. The ventilatory defect secondary to direct lung injury may be severe. Therapy must be evaluated frequently by measuring ventilation volumes and blood gases.

3. **Pneumothorax** occurs when air enters the pleural cavity from an injured lung or through a penetrating thoracic injury, reducing the normal negative intrapleural pressure and permitting partial collapse of the lung. Since air is readily compressible, the normal pressure changes essential to ventilation of the lung are damped in pneumothorax. A functional shunt results from the ventilation-perfusion imbalance and adds to the hypoxemia of impaired ventilation. All forms of traumatic pneumothorax are treated definitively by insertion of a chest tube (see Chap. 25) connected to underwater seal drainage or to suction.

   In the absence of continued air leak, the chest tube frequently will be blocked early by clot. Since the tube is so easily blocked, surveillance cannot be relaxed even when the tube is used prophylactically in an injured patient at risk of pneumothorax because of anesthesia or assisted ventilation.

4. **Hemothorax** is an accumulation of blood within the pleural cavity. Because blood is not compressible, there is less interference with ventilation in hemothorax than with a pneumothorax of equivalent size.

   A large hemothorax can compress the lung and impair ventilation. Needle thoracentesis through an intercostal space is useful in the treatment of a small- or medium-sized hemothorax. Insert the needle through the fifth intercostal space in the anterior axillary line, the sixth intercostal space in the midaxillary line, or the eighth interspace infrascapularly. Avoid the liver and the spleen. A major hemothorax is drained with a chest tube and suction. The chest tube should be placed in a dependent position, the best location being through the sixth or seventh intercostal space in the midaxillary line, about 1 in. below the level of the nipple in the midaxillary line, directing the tube posterior to the lung (see Chap. 25).

   Hemothorax requires emergency thoracotomy and operative control of the bleeding source if adequate blood replacement does not correct shock or if measured blood loss from the chest tube continues at a rate greater than 250 ml/hr after the first 2 hr or is greater than 1,000 ml/24 hr. A large hemothorax that remains visible on the chest x-ray after a chest tube is placed and is functioning is probably clotted and may be an indication for early thoracotomy.

5. **Laceration of the lung** may result from spicules of fractured ribs puncturing the lung or from other shearing forces. Pneumothorax and hemothorax of varying degrees always are present and are treated as outlined above. The best method of controlling blood and air leaks from lacerated lung is to remove all the air and clot from the pleural space and

expand the lung completely via chest tube suction. Continued bleeding or continued air leaks may indicate a need for suturing or resection by open thoracotomy.

6. **Contusion of the lung** and other thoracic viscera is a common sequela of blunt chest trauma. Contusion of the lung with hemorrhage reveals itself as an area of increased density in the chest x-ray and usually is apparent on admission, but sometimes becomes apparent 12-72 hr after injury. Areas of cavitation may appear later.

7. Chest trauma patients seem particularly vulnerable to development of the **adult respiratory distress syndrome.** A falling Pa_{O_2} in spite of increasing FI_{O_2}, a white lung on x-ray examination, and an increase in pressure required to move a given volume of air (stiff lungs) characterize the syndrome.

   The etiology remains speculative but *excessive IV fluid administration* is the most frequently documented event. The excess fluids usually are administered in the emergency room although the syndrome becomes evident only 48-72 hr later. Prevention is a primary goal. Once the respiratory distress syndrome is present, restriction of fluids, administration of salt-poor serum albumin and diuretics, and use of positive end expiratory pressure with a volume ventilator are sometimes effective (see Chap. 12).

8. **Tracheal or bronchial rupture or laceration** produces pneumomediastinum or pneumothorax. Tension pneumothorax may occur. The presence of subcutaneous emphysema, especially in the mediastinum or neck, indicates the possibility of major airway injury. Bronchoscopy is helpful to establish the diagnosis. Chest tubes should be inserted if a pneumothorax is present. Unless the volume of air leak is small, operative repair of the tracheal or bronchial laceration should be done as soon as the patient's general condition permits in order to maintain function of the affected lung and to prevent sequestration and recurrent infection.

9. **Splinting,** due to the pain of rib fractures, results in decreased tidal volume and may lead to atelectasis and pneumonia. A diagnosis of rib fracture may be made if point tenderness and splinting are present; x-ray evidence of rib fractures may not develop for up to 10-14 days. Injection of the involved intercostal nerves occasionally may be used to relieve pain and to permit a player to finish a game, but patients are more effectively managed with analgesics, ambulation, and enforced coughing.

10. **Esophageal rupture** may occur with either blunt or penetrating chest trauma. Pain may be substernal, epigastric, or cervical, but more commonly is in the back. Pneumomediastinum and pneumohydrothorax may be seen on the chest x-ray. The diagnosis is confirmed by x-ray studies performed with thin contrast media. Repair and drainage must be done promptly if the patient is to survive.

11. **Chylothorax** is a rare complication of chest trauma and is caused by injury to the thoracic duct. Accumulating chylous fluid should be

drained by needle thoracentesis or via a chest tube to prevent pulmonary compression. Most chylous fistulas close spontaneously and only removal of the fluid from the chest is needed; recurrent chylothorax persisting longer than 3 wk may require direct control of the leak at thoracotomy.

12. **Rupture of the diaphragm** is seen after blunt trauma to either the chest or the abdomen. The diagnosis is frequently missed even after laparotomy. The chest x-ray most often shows an air-fluid level in the lower chest.
The torn diaphragm no longer provides a barrier between the thorax and the abdomen. The derangements caused by diaphragmatic rupture or paralysis are the same as those seen in flail chest except for the absence of pain and splinting. During inspiration (increased negative intrathoracic pressure), abdominal viscera are pushed into the chest, preventing normal inflation of the lung, which then becomes atelectatic. In addition to impairing ventilation, the ruptured diaphragm poses a threat of compromised circulation to the herniated viscera. A ruptured diaphragm should be promptly repaired operatively.

C. Trauma to the heart, aorta, and vena cava

1. **Contusion of the heart** is manifest by ECG changes of epicardial injury or myocardial ischemia and typically is the result of severe anterior chest injury caused by a steering wheel. Heart contusion is treated as a myocardial infarction, details of treatment being dependent on the magnitude of ECG and serum enzyme changes.

2. **Cardiac perforation** may involve the walls of the cardiac chambers, the septa, or the valves and can produce cardiac tamponade. While it is true that some small perforations of the heart seal spontaneously and may be treated effectively by observation, all heart wounds should be explored if a cardiac surgical team is available. If the more radical treatment of observation is elected, recurrent cardiac tamponade is an absolute indication for thoracotomy. Pressure and oxygen saturation should be measured in the cardiac chambers during operation to help delineate intracardiac injury.

3. **Cardiac tamponade** should be differentiated from simple hemopericardium. Cardiac tamponade is present when the hemopericardium is of sufficient size to produce Beck's triad of falling arterial pressure, rising venous pressure, and a small, quiet heart. Hemopericardium usually is not evident on a chest x-ray. The basic hemodynamic derangement in cardiac tamponade is impaired filling of the low-pressure chambers on the right side of the heart. Therefore, additional IV fluid therapy in spite of an elevated CVP is rational. Always consider the possibility of cardiac tamponade in chest trauma when the patient fails to respond to appropriate therapy and when a high CVP is associated with shock, decreased pulse pressure, or low cardiac output. Needle pericardiocentesis (aspiration) is the initial treatment of cardiac tamponade. The patient should be transferred immediately to the care of an experienced thoracic surgeon, in case definitive therapy becomes necessary.

4. Injury to the aorta   Blunt chest trauma, especially of the deceleration type, may lead to aortic rupture, usually just distal to the origin of the left subclavian artery. A widened mediastinum and depression of the left main bronchus seen on an upright PA chest x-ray must be considered suggestive of aortic injury and should lead to aortography to rule out this potentially fatal injury. Fractures of the scapula, the first and second ribs, and the medial third of the clavicle all suggest severe trauma and should lead to a consideration of aortography. Aortic injuries require emergency thoracotomy with cardiopulmonary bypass or a shunt.

5. Traumatic asphyxia is a condition produced by prolonged compressive thoracic trauma. Characteristically the patient is cyanotic only about the face. Cerebral dysfunction almost invariably is present but clears within 24 hr. The significance of this injury is that one should not be misled by the facial cyanosis into giving unneeded ventilatory assistance while overlooking other possible intrathoracic injuries.

SUGGESTED READING

Beall, A. C., Patrick, T. A., Okies, J. E., Bricker, D. B., and DeBakey, M. E. Penetrating wounds of the heart: Changing patterns of surgical management. *J. Trauma* 12:468, 1972.

Tector, A. J., Reuben, C. F., Hofmann, J. F., Gelfand, E. T., Keelan, M., and Worman, L.   Coronary artery wounds treated with saphenous vein bypass grafts. *J.A.M.A.* 225:282, 1973.

V. ABDOMINAL INJURY

A. General comments

1. Any patient involved in an automobile, industrial, or sports accident should be considered to have an abdominal injury until proven otherwise. Serious intra-abdominal injury can occur from very minor trauma.

2. **Patients with blunt abdominal trauma are more difficult to evaluate,** the signs of their injury can be delayed, and the consequences of injury, particularly to solid organs, can be difficult to manage.

3. Signs and symptoms of intra-abdominal injury can be masked by injuries elsewhere. The presence of fractured ribs with secondary splinting makes examination of the abdominal wall difficult. A serious central nervous system (CNS) injury also can mask abdominal wall findings.

4. Decisions must be made based on **repeated examinations,** especially during resuscitation, since shock may mask abdominal findings. Examinations should be performed frequently by the same individual until it can be ascertained definitely that significant visceral injury, peritonitis, or hemorrhage does not exist.

5. **Rupture of a hollow viscus** usually produces signs of peritoneal irritation and loss of bowel sounds. These signs may not be present on initial examination, and some patients with small-bowel and bladder injuries

may show surprisingly minimal early signs and must be reevaluated frequently.

6. **Injury of a solid viscus,** such as liver or spleen, usually presents with hemorrhage. Peritoneal irritation may occur when blood is present within the abdominal cavity. A trauma victim presenting with unexplained hypovolemic shock should be assumed to have an intra-abdominal injury.

7. Organ enlargement, particularly if secondary to other pathological conditions (e.g., lymphoma), makes the organ more susceptible to injury. A distended urinary bladder or pregnant uterus is at increased risk of injury from blunt trauma to the abdomen.

B. **Signs and symptoms of abdominal trauma**

1. **Pain** following abdominal trauma may be due to abdominal wall injury or to injury of underlying structures. Pain referred to the shoulder is seen with diaphragmatic irritation secondary to splenic or hepatic injury. Patients who have pain and other findings should not be given narcotics or other analgesics until a decision about the need for an operation has been made.

2. **Localized tenderness or abdominal wall rigidity** is a result of peritoneal irritation from blood or hollow viscus content and is usually an indication for exploration. Abdominal guarding during palpation makes evaluation of the abdomen difficult, particularly in anxious or uncooperative patients. This is particularly true if there is associated chest, spinal, or pelvic injury. Repeated gentle examinations are helpful. If rib fractures are present, intercostal nerve blocks will decrease pain and may help in evaluation of the abdomen. Absence of tenderness and rigidity is no assurance that intra-abdominal injury is absent.

3. **Abdominal distention** is always an ominous sign. If it occurs in a patient with a penetrating wound, injury of the liver, spleen, or a major vessel has probably occurred. In blunt trauma, abdominal distention may be due to ileus secondary to retroperitoneal injury, especially involving the pancreas, or to spinal injury.

4. The **absence of bowel sounds** (5 min), particularly in patients with seemingly shallow penetrating wounds, is an indication for exploratory laparotomy.

5. **Inability to resuscitate** from shock a hypovolemic patient with suspected abdominal injury is an indication for rapid operative intervention and direct control of the hemorrhage. If there are multiple fractures, the resuscitative effort must be vigorous before this decision is made. An abdominal tap is extremely useful in these situations.

C. **X-ray studies**

1. **Routine views**   At an appropriate time during the resuscitative effort, the following views should be obtained: flat and upright abdominal films and

chest film. Diagnostic features to look for include free air in the peritoneal cavity, retroperitoneal air (especially near the duodenum), elevation of the diaphragm, obliteration of the psoas shadows, displacement of the gastric air bubble, disturbances of normal bowel pattern, and the presence and location of foreign bodies.

2. **Intravenous pyelogram (IVP)**   An infusion IVP should be done on all patients suspected of having an intra-abdominal injury. The infusion of contrast material should be timed to permit obtaining an acceptable pyelogram along with the routine abdominal views. The IVP is useful in diagnosing kidney injury and is mandatory to assure the presence of a functioning contralateral kidney if nephrectomy is necessary.

3. **Other studies**   All patients with hematuria, especially those with pelvic fractures, should have cystography performed, preferably before the urinary bladder is catheterized. Selective angiography is useful in patients with blunt abdominal trauma whose initial diagnostic workup is inconclusive. Selective celiac angiography is particularly useful in demonstrating subcapsular splenic injuries. Upper gastrointestinal (GI) tract barium studies may be helpful in establishing gastric displacement by an enlarged spleen and in diagnosing a duodenal intramural hematoma. Occasionally sinography is performed in patients with penetrating injuries to ascertain whether the peritoneal cavity has been entered. Since false-negative sinograms can occur, it is preferable to explore the wound directly.

D. Laboratory examination

1. Although hemoglobin and hematocrit determinations are of little value in the initial appraisal of the patient with blood loss, they can be useful during the observation period to detect continued loss of blood.

2. A leukocyte count in excess of 15,000 in the absence of evidence of infection is suggestive of significant blood loss and is particularly useful in supporting an early diagnosis of delayed rupture of the spleen.

3. Elevation of serum amylase suggests pancreatic injury or bowel rupture. Elevation of transaminase suggests hepatic injury.

E. Other studies

1. **Abdominal paracentesis** is a helpful study in determining the presence of blood due to intra-abdominal injury. Peritoneal lavage is the preferred technique (see Chap. 25). If one can read newsprint through the effluent within the catheter, the lavage can be regarded as negative. A sample of the effluent is analyzed for red blood cells; greater than 100,000 cells/ mm^3 is an indication for exploratory laparotomy. The effluent can also be tested for bile, leukocytes, bacteria, and amylase. A negative test is never diagnostic and should be ignored—significant intra-abdominal injury can be present in spite of negative results.
   Lavage should not be done in patients with gaseous distention or in areas of old scars. In most instances, abdominal x-rays should be ob-

tained prior to lavage to avoid confusion about the origin of free intra-peritoneal air.

2. If rectal bleeding is seen or blood is present on the examining finger, the possibility of rectal injury should be evaluated by **proctosigmoidoscopy**. A nasogastric tube should be inserted in all patients suspected of having abdominal injury. The presence of blood in the aspirate may mean that an injury has occurred to the upper GI tract.

F. Emergency management of abdominal trauma

1. **Open wounds** caused by bullets, shotgun blasts, large knives, or similar means are an indication for abdominal exploration. If the injury is associated with shock or abdominal distention, the patient should be explored immediately. Otherwise, time is taken to perform the examinations listed above.

2. **Small open injuries** of the anterior abdominal wall in which penetration of the peritoneal cavity is unlikely can be treated expectantly. If there is any sign of peritoneal irritation, such as tenderness, rigidity, or absence of bowel sounds, the patient should be explored. The safest manner of caring for these patients is to explore the injury directly under local anesthesia in the operating room. If there is evidence that the peritoneal cavity has been entered, abdominal exploration under general anesthesia should be carried out.

3. Patients with **blunt trauma** to the abdomen are treated according to the symptoms, signs, and results of other examinations. A positive paracentesis is an explicit indication for laparotomy. If these patients have minimal findings at the time of initial examination but the suspicion of significant abdominal trauma is still present, the patient should be admitted to the hospital for observation. During this observation period, the patient should be examined frequently by the same examiner; repeated x-ray studies of the abdomen are performed. **Indications for exploratory laparotomy** in these patients include:

   a. Persistent abdominal wall tenderness or rigidity.

   b. Unexplained, even though minimal, persistent findings upon repeated examinations of the abdomen.

   c. Appearance of signs of shock or blood loss.

   d. Positive x-ray or laboratory findings.

G. Emergency exploratory laparotomy

1. **Steps prior to exploration**   In addition to the general principles applying to all patients undergoing an operation, the following should be done for patients being explored for possible intra-abdominal injury:

   a. Nasogastric suction.

    b. Placement of an indwelling urinary catheter.

    c. Parenteral administration of antibiotics in patients with signs of GI tract injury, severe shock, or massive trauma.

    d. Insertion of a chest tube in patients with even minimal pneumothorax or hemothorax.

2. The incision Exploratory laparotomy should be performed through a long midline incision. This incision has the advantages of speed of entry and access to the entire abdominal cavity.

3. The steps of an emergency exploratory laparotomy are:

    a. Rapid exploration of the entire abdomen to determine sites of hemorrhage.

    b. Immediate control of hemorrhage. If the hemorrhage is due to injury of solid organs, control can be achieved with use of packs. If the hemorrhage is from a major artery, the injury site should be controlled by vascular clamps. If the hemorrhage is due to injury to a major vein, initial control should be by direct pressure.

    c. After hemorrhage is initially controlled and before you continue an operative manipulation that is liable to be attended by further blood loss, allow the anesthesiologist to catch up with volume replacement.

    d. Control open injuries to the GI tract to prevent further contamination of the peritoneal cavity. If a retroperitoneal hematoma is present, this should be unroofed and sites of hemorrhage controlled.

    e. Definitive control of hemorrhage by vascular repair, ligation of vessels, removal of injured organs (spleen), or resection (liver).

    f. Repair open wounds in the GI tract as indicated. Repair wounds of solid viscera as indicated.

    g. If the peritoneal cavity has been contaminated by open wounds, lavage of the peritoneal cavity should be performed with copious amounts of normal saline solution. Consider the use of appropriate intraperitoneal instillation of antibiotic solution.

    h. A formal, complete exploration of the entire abdominal cavity should now be carried out. Included in this exploration should be entry into the lesser sac and visualization of the entire pancreas. If there is any evidence of hemorrhage or edema in this area, the pancreas should be totally mobilized and inspected for injury. A generous mobilization (Kocher's maneuver) of the duodenum should be carried out to inspect the entire posterior duodenal wall.

    i. Sites of previously repaired injuries should be reinspected, a final lavage of the peritoneal cavity performed, drains placed only for specific indications, and the abdominal wound closed in layers.

j. If peritoneal contamination has occurred, leave the skin and subcutaneous tissues open.

H. Management of specific injuries

1. **Abdominal wall**   Blunt trauma can cause injury to the abdominal wall without causing intra-abdominal injury. Musculature can be avulsed or major vessels transected. Rigidity, tenderness and a palpable mass can result, for example, from a rectus hematoma. Any mass within the anterior abdominal wall remains easily palpable when the patient raises his head, tensing the abdominal muscles, whereas this maneuver usually causes an intraperitoneal mass to become less palpable.

2. **Spleen**   The spleen is the most frequently injured intra-abdominal organ. A ruptured spleen is suspected if there has been trauma to the left side, especially if ribs are fractured. The clinical findings and evidence of hypovolemia vary from minimal to profound. Pain referred to the left shoulder is common. Other useful findings include leukocytosis, displacement of the gastric air bubble, and presence of blood on paracentesis. In doubtful cases, selective celiac arteriograms can be helpful. Contrast-filled splenic vessels should be seen out to the lateral edge of the abdominal cavity. In the presence of a subscapular splenic injury, a peripheral avascular rim will be seen on the arteriogram. Delayed rupture of the spleen should be suspected in a patient who has sudden abdominal pain and signs of hypovolemia occurring within 4 wk of an injury.

   Treatment is abdominal exploration and splenectomy. Control of hemorrhage at the time of exploration can be done with direct pressure with packs or rapid compression of the splenic pedicle. The essential step in the performance of splenectomy is incision of the splenic posterolateral peritoneal attachment. This allows delivery of the spleen into the wound so that the splenic pedicle can be secured without danger of injuring the tail of the pancreas. If there are no other injuries or specific indications for drainage, the splenic bed need not be drained.

3. **Liver**   The liver is the largest intra-abdominal organ, and the magnitude of parenchymal damage can range from minimal to almost total destruction.

   a. **Minimal injury**   Puncture wounds, lacerations, and low-velocity through-and-through missile injuries of the liver which are not bleeding at the time of exploration and which are in areas of the liver unlikely to lead to injury to major intrahepatic vessels are drained; the capsular wounds are not closed. Simple wounds that are bleeding should be explored and hemostasis attained by direct suture ligation of bleeding vessels followed by drainage; the capsule is not sutured. Implantation of foreign hemostatic materials should be avoided.

   b. **Major injury**   The key to success is total mobilization of the liver and control of the hepatic vasculature as follows:

      (1) Detach the falciform ligament from the anterior abdominal wall down to the anterior aspect of the suprahepatic vena cava.

(2) Incise the left triangular ligament from its left lateral margin to the suprahepatic vena cava.

(3) Retract the right lobe of the liver to the midline and incise the right triangular ligament, exposing the right lateral margin of the intrahepatic vena cava.

(4) Free the suprahepatic and infrahepatic vena cava adjacent to the liver; incision of the diaphragm usually is not necessary.

(5) Place a tape around the hepatoduodenal structures in the porta hepatis (Pringle's maneuver).

(6) Rapidly assess the extent of injury to ascertain if resection should be done. This decision is basically logistical, remembering that the amount of bleeding surface in a large, deep laceration may be more than the surface following resection. Resection must be done if avascular liver tissue is present.

(7) Large mattress sutures to control liver hemorrhage should be avoided since they create areas of necrotic tissue and may lead to abscess formation.

If hemorrhage is massive or if injury to the intrahepatic inferior vena cava has occurred, the liver can be totally isolated by placing vascular clamps on the suprahepatic and infrahepatic vena cava and using tape control of the porta hepatis. One can also insert a catheter within the vena cava to bypass the venous return from the lower body; this maneuver is somewhat difficult and uses valuable time, so that total vascular isolation of the liver is much preferred. Occasionally, massive arterial hemorrhage occurs in a through-and-through wound. Ligation of the involved lobar arterial supply is the preferred treatment.

When major hepatic resection, such as a right hepatic lobectomy or an extended right hepatic lobectomy, is to be carried out, it is wise to perform the resection through an anatomical plane after securing the lobar hepatic artery and portal vein inflow. If total mobilization of the liver has been carried out, one usually does not need to extend the midline incision into the right hemithorax. If, however, exposure and continued hemorrhage are problems, there should be no hesitancy in extending the incision.

Massive hemorrhage and hepatic trauma may lead to coagulation problems. Treatment should include administration of fresh blood, fresh frozen plasma, platelet concentrates, and specific clotting factors (see Chap. 16).

Following resection and control of hemorrhage, sump suction and soft rubber drains should be placed. The biliary tree is not drained routinely. There is controversy about biliary decompression. Proponents point out that insertion of a T-tube decreases the amount of bile loss through open surfaces of the liver and serves as a vehicle for postoperative detection of hematobilia. More recent evidence indicates that routine biliary decompression is associated with increased morbidity.

4. **Pancreas**   Unless there has been a significant rise in serum amylase noted prior to operation, injury of the pancreas is usually detected at the time of exploration. Minor contusions that do not involve the major ducts can be drained. Major injuries to the body and tail of the pancreas are treated by resection. Injuries to the pancreas on the right side of the superior mesenteric vessels that involve major ductal structures are treated by internal drainage into a Roux-en-Y jejunal loop. Massive injuries to the head of the pancreas may demand a pancreatoduodenectomy.

5. **Gallbladder and biliary tract**   Injuries to the biliary tract usually are caused by penetrating wounds, although the gallbladder can be injured by blunt trauma. An injured gallbladder must be excised. Injury to the extrahepatic biliary ductal system usually is detected at laparotomy by the presence of bile staining of tissues. Primary repair of biliary ductal injury is preferred; if the injury is extensive, a bypass such as a choledochojejunostomy must be performed.

6. **Stomach**   Gastric injuries should be suspected if nasogastric suction reveals the presence of blood. During laparotomy, particularly with penetrating injuries, the lesser sac should be opened, the entire stomach mobilized, and search made for sites of injury. Wounds of the stomach should be debrided widely and sutured.

7. **Duodenum**   Intraperitoneal duodenal injury may be suspected if bile or small-bowel content is recovered by paracentesis. Retroperitoneal injury to the duodenum is more frequent than intraperitoneal injury. Unless retroperitoneal air is seen on the preoperative abdominal x-ray, injury to the retroperitoneal duodenum will be discovered only when the duodenum is mobilized (Kocher's maneuver) during exploratory laparotomy.

The extent of the duodenal wall defect following debridement determines further treatment. Simple lacerations are closed in the direction of the wound. Extensive defects can be closed with a jejunal serosal patch onlay or isolated jejunal mucosal patch. All duodenal wounds are prone to breakdown. The duodenum should be decompressed internally with transgastric and transjejunal sump suction catheters. The operative area always is drained, and both internal and external drains remain in place for at least 10 days. Extensive injury to the duodenum and pancreas may require a pancreatoduodenectomy.

Intramural duodenal hematoma may occur following blunt trauma, particularly in children. The patient presents with vomiting; upper GI contrast studies may show the typical "corkscrew" deformity. Operative evacuation of the hematoma is curative.

8. **Small intestine**   Small-bowel injury should be suspected in any patient with penetrating abdominal injury. In blunt trauma, small-intestinal injury usually occurs at or near sites of mesenteric fixation. Signs of peritoneal irritation usually are present and small-bowel content some-

times is recovered on paracentesis. Treatment consists of debridement and primary closure. If many individual perforations occur within a short segment of bowel, the entire involved segment is resected. A meticulous search for perforations should be made, with particular attention to the mesenteric border.

9. **Colon**　Patients with colon injury may present with signs of peritonitis, or upright x-rays may show free air. Barium enema should never be done in patients suspected of having colon injury. Preoperatively vigorous fluid replacement and systemic antibiotics are required. The choice of operative treatment is:

   a. Primary repair only if injury is minimal, there are no other significant injuries, no peritoneal contamination has occurred, and treatment is instituted within 3 hr of injury.

   b. Resection is the safest procedure. This is especially true if there is extensive colon injury, significant fecal contamination has occurred, operative treatment has been delayed, or there are associated organ injuries. The ends of the colon are converted to a colostomy and a mucous fistula; continuity is restored at a second operation when peritonitis has resolved.

   Copious peritoneal lavage should be carried out. Septic complications are frequent and should be anticipated.

10. **Female reproductive organs**　Injuries to the female reproductive organs usually occur in pregnant women and may cause sudden vaginal hemorrhage following blunt trauma. Hysterectomy or removal of injured adnexa may be necessary. Salvage of a pregnancy depends on gestational age and degree of fetal injury.

VI. UROLOGICAL INJURY

A. General considerations

1. Genitourinary injury from either blunt or penetrating trauma is most common in young adults and is **rarely an isolated lesion.** The objective of management of genitourinary trauma is preservation of renal tissue and function.

2. **Urinalysis** provides baseline information, but is negative for hematuria in 20% of genitourinary injuries. The presence of gross or microscopic hematuria suggests genitourinary injury and requires further investigation. Each voided specimen should be retained for comparison with previous specimens to follow the course of hematuria.

3. **Complications** of genitourinary trauma are hemorrhagic shock, urinary extravasation leading to sepsis or abscess formation, acute tubular necrosis, and devascularization and necrosis of renal parenchyma resulting in uremia if the patient has a solitary kidney or preexisting renal disease.

B. Diagnosis

1. The **history** may direct attention to specific injuries; for example, pelvic fractures frequently are the cause of a ruptured bladder or prostatic urethra.

2. **Physical examination** should be directed to discover the presence of an expanding flank mass, fractured ribs, a suprapubic mass, tenderness of pubic rami on pelvic compression, a mass or tenderness in the perineum or scrotum, and blood at the urethral meatus. Rectal examination will provide evidence of injury to the prostatic urethra and the presence or absence of a pelvic hematoma.

3. **Plain abdominal films (KUB** [kidney, ureter, and bladder]) should be carefully evaluated for loss of psoas shadows, fractures impinging on urinary structures, foreign bodies lying in proximity to the genitourinary system, loss of radiolucent fat lines, and free air or fluid in the abdomen.

4. **An infusion IVP** should be done in all patients suspected of having genitourinary injury. Excretory urograms (IVP) should be performed through the IV started when the patient entered the emergency room. In shock, the kidneys may fail to be visualized, but despite this fact the IVP remains the single most important roentgenographic examination of the urinary tract in cases of trauma. To facilitate IVP, shock should be corrected with fluid or blood replacement rather than vasopressors, as the latter will diminish renal blood flow while maintaining an adequate central blood pressure. Drip infusion pyelography using 50-100 ml of contrast medium will provide information regarding the size, shape, and position of the kidneys, may demonstrate urinary extravasation, and, most importantly, will determine the status of the contralateral kidney and ureter. In the presence of renal injury, the contrast medium may not be excreted into the renal pelvis, but if the main renal artery is intact and not occluded by hematoma, a nephrogram of the injured kidney almost always will be visualized. Nonvisualization of the kidney suggests occlusion or transection of the main renal artery and is an indication for **renal arteriography.** Especially in children, the initial IVP may not reveal the collecting system of an injured kidney, but a pyelogram 12-24 hr later may reveal the site and degree of renal trauma.

5. **Retrograde urethrograms** are essential in defining urethral injuries. Retrograde injection of 15-30 ml of sterile contrast medium permits localization of urethral extravasation or obstruction and should precede instrumentation of the urethra.

6. The **urethral catheter** has been **recommended** as a diagnostic and therapeutic instrument to (a) assess patency and continuity of the urethra, (b) facilitate accurate measurement of urinary output, and (c) splint the injured urethra. However, it has been **condemned** because it may (a) complete a partial laceration of the urethra, (b) introduce bacteria into a pelvic hematoma, or (c) lead to a false diagnosis.

Assessment of a potentially injured urethra by retrograde (injection) urethrography is essential before attempting to introduce a catheter. If a catheter is necessary and if the urethra is intact, a Foley-type indwelling catheter should be inserted aseptically and attached to a closed drainage system. Frequent urinalysis will indicate the need for urine culture. When infection occurs, the drainage system should be changed and antibiotics initiated if appropriate (see Chap. 14).

7. **Cystograms** may be obtained by catheterization if the urethra is found to be normal. Contrast material (150–300 ml) is instilled by gravity into the bladder through the catheter. Oblique, lateral, AP, and postvoiding views are all essential as the full bladder may obscure anterior or posterior extravasations.

8. **IV bolus tomography** will outline the renal arterial architecture and serves the same purpose as arteriography if cardiac output is adequate.

9. **Percutaneous retrograde femoral renal arteriograms** are indicated if the IVP fails to visualize the kidneys, and whenever penetrating renal trauma has occurred.

C. **Assessment and management of genitourinary injuries**

1. Injuries of the **penis** are diagnosed by physical examination. Contusions require no specific treatment. Lacerations of the penis are debrided and repaired primarily. Amputation of a part of the penis is treated by debridement followed by closure of the stump using a "fish-mouth" technique to form a urethral meatus. Avulsion of penile skin requires coverage by a split-thickness skin graft or by burying the penis in a subcutaneous abdominal or scrotal tunnel. If urinary diversion is needed because of trauma to the penile urethra, a suprapubic cystostomy is used.

2. The **anterior urethra** consists of the bulbous urethra in the perineum and pendulous urethra in the penis. Injuries are caused by straddle or sporting trauma to the perineum and by torsion, foreign body, and toilet seat trauma to the penis. Iatrogenic instrumentation also is a common cause of urethral injury. Urethral injury may be suspected if there is blood at the urethral meatus, and is confirmed by a retrograde urethrogram. Suprapubic cystostomy for 10 days will allow healing, generally without stricture, of injuries to the pendulous (penile) urethra. Adequate perineal drainage in addition to suprapubic cystostomy is required in cases of injury of the bulbous urethra. Secondary urethroplasty is done later if required.

3. The **posterior urethra** consists of the prostatic and supramembranous urethras. Partial or complete urethral laceration occurs in 10% of pelvic fractures. The symptoms are minimal or no urethral bleeding, inability to void, a symmetrical midline expanding suprapubic mass, and a boggy pelvic mass on rectal examination. The prostate may be obscured by the pelvic hematoma. The diagnosis is confirmed by retrograde urethrogra-

phy. Treatment consists of suprapubic cystostomy; the pelvic hematoma resolves without drainage. Urethral catheterization is avoided for fear of introducing infection or converting a partial laceration to a complete urethral transection. A partial laceration heals in 10-14 days; complete laceration is repaired by posterior urethroplasty after 3-4 mo.

4. **Laceration or avulsion of scrotal skin** is common in farm and industrial accidents and frequently is seen in association with penile amputation. The testes usually are not injured. Treatment consists of debridement, transfer of the testes to subcutaneous pockets in the thigh or inguinal canal, and adequate dressing of the scrotal area. Because regeneration of the scrotum will occur in 2-3 wk, debridement should not remove all scrotal skin. If a testicle has ruptured, a rapidly enlarging mass will be noted in the scrotum. The scrotum should be opened and drained, and the tunica albuginea of the testicle reconstituted.

5. In the **female perineum,** avulsion, transection, contusion, or laceration of the urethra is uncommon but may occur with direct trauma, as in straddle-type injuries. If there has been a perineal injury with laceration or hematoma, passage of a catheter may be required to facilitate voiding. A voiding cystourethrogram should be done to confirm the integrity of the urethra.

6. The **bladder** is most commonly injured in automobile accidents involving young adults. Approximately 6% of pelvic fractures have an associated bladder injury. About 80% of bladder ruptures occur extraperitoneally; 20% are intraperitoneal. The signs of bladder injury are inability to void; midline, irregular, tender suprapubic mass; pubic ramus fracture or diastasis of symphysis pubis; and ileus if there is intraperitoneal extravasation of urine. The diagnosis is established with a cystogram after confirmation of the integrity of the urethra by urethrography. For anterior ruptures, treatment consists of suprapubic cystostomy and drainage of the space of Retzius; for posterior (intraperitoneal) ruptures, abdominal exploration and repair of the vesical tear are necessary.

7. Injury of the **ureter** usually results from an iatrogenic mishap; more rarely, external violence or a penetrating missile causes injury. Retrograde pyelography to confirm a suspected injury should only be done immediately prior to surgical repair. Some important considerations in ureteral injuries are:

   a. If at least one third of the ureteral wall is intact, the ureter will re-epithelialize satisfactorily over a splint.

   b. Splinting is indicated if there has been previous ureteral injury or if infection is present.

   c. Absorbable sutures should be used to achieve a watertight closure. Injuries of the upper third of the ureter are treated by ureteropyeloplasty; in the middle third, oblique ureteroureterostomy is carried out; when injury involves the lower third or pelvic ureter, reimplantation into the bladder is done.

8. **Blunt kidney injury** results in renal contusion or a parenchymal laceration, with or without extravasation. The diagnosis is established with an IVP. Tomograms or an arteriogram may reveal a parenchymal defect or extravasation. Treatment of blunt trauma begins with close observation and bed rest. As hematuria due to contusion subsides, ambulation is begun, usually after 3–7 days. In cases of more severe parenchymal laceration an expanding flank mass may be present; if the patient demonstrates cardiovascular instability, an arteriogram is indicated to determine parenchymal viability before surgical repair or heminephrectomy. Urinary extravasation is best treated by early restoration of urinary tract continuity.

9. **Penetrating kidney injuries** usually are caused by sharp objects (knife) or a missile (bullet). The diagnosis is established by an IVP in the same manner as with blunt trauma. Delayed extravasation often is seen with bullet wounds. In general, debridement and early surgical repair are indicated. Arteriovenous fistulas, common with knife wounds, may close spontaneously, but usually require operative repair. Because of the possibility of delayed renovascular hypertension, an IVP and measurement of blood pressure are obtained every 6 mo for 2 yr.

10. **Interruption of spinal cord function** by vertebral displacement or compression, hematoma, or cord edema usually is followed by bladder paralysis. Paralysis is often temporary, but may last up to 4 mo. The primary concern is preservation of the muscular wall of the bladder during this period, and this is best accomplished by intermittent catheterization of the bladder under strict aseptic technique. Watch for return of anal sphincter tone and bulbocavernosus reflex. The bladder then will need to be assessed by cystometry. If properly cared for, most of these bladders will function satisfactorily after spinal shock has subsided.

VII. VASCULAR AND EXTREMITY INJURY

A. **General comments** Except for hemorrhage from a major vascular wound, trauma to an extremity rarely is immediately life-threatening. Temporary measures, such as control of hemorrhage by pressure, application of dressings to prevent further contamination, and temporary immobilization of fractures or dislocations, are sufficient initial therapy while attention is being directed to treatment of life-threatening injuries elsewhere in the body.

1. As soon as possible, check to make certain **all peripheral pulses are present.** Injury to major arterial or venous vessels may constitute a threat to viability of the limb. Once life-threatening injuries elsewhere in the body are controlled, the nature of vascular injuries should be defined by appropriate examinations, including arteriography, and the injured vessel repaired.

2. Careful **examination should be made for nerve and tendon injuries** associated with any laceration, contusion, or fracture.

3. Examination of an extremity wound in the emergency room should be made with **aseptic precautions.** Careful and complete debridement of devitalized tissue should be done and, if the injury is not further complicated, the wound should be repaired. In the event of extensive injury to a nerve, tendon, or major blood vessel, exploration and repair should be done in the operating room.

B. Fractures

1. **Simple fractures** are the most obvious consequence of trauma but are *not a threat to life and limb.* They should be promptly immobilized (a pillow makes a good temporary splint) to prevent further soft tissue injury. When other injuries have been treated and the patient's condition is stable, manipulation and reduction can be carried out. Detailed x-ray studies of fracture fragment position can be deferred until the patient is ready for definitive reduction.

2. **Fractures or dislocations associated with vascular injury or nerve compression** (usually involving the knee, hip, elbow, or shoulder) should be manipulated promptly to restore pulses and eliminate nerve stretch or compression. The principle of initial treatment is to restore vascular and neural integrity.

2. **Compound fractures** are those in which a skin wound communicates directly or indirectly with the fracture. They should be treated as soon as possible with systemic antibiotics, debridement of nonviable tissue, removal of devitalized bone fragments, and copious cleansing irrigation. Primary wound closure usually is possible, but should be deferred if viability of deep tissues is questionable or contamination has been massive. Definitive reduction, if convenient and not requiring internal fixation, often can be accomplished immediately. When this is not feasible, temporary splinting and definitive reduction (with or without internal fixation) can be delayed until the immediate threat of infection has passed.

4. **Pelvic fracture** is frequently accompanied by large loss of blood owing to the vascularity of the marrow of pelvic bones, the inability to splint pelvic fractures effectively, and the fact that surrounding tissues do little to tamponade bleeding. Prompt blood transfusion is essential. Lacerations of the bladder, urethra, and rectum should be sought and treated appropriately. Shock persisting after adequate volume replacement requires immediate abdominal and pelvic exploration to control the hemorrhage. Selective angiography of the aorta and pelvic vessels should be considered if bleeding is persistent. The bleeding point often can be defined and sometimes can be controlled by embolizing autogenous clots selectively into the bleeding branch.

C. Clinical manifestations of vascular injuries

1. **External hemorrhage**   Blind clamping of a hemorrhaging vessel is never done. Such clamping frequently fails to control bleeding, may damage

adjacent nerves, and may increase the arterial injury and complicate repair. Pressure applied at or proximal to the arterial wound will control hemorrhage while preparations to repair the vascular injury are in progress.

2. **Decreased or absent pulses** indicate partial or complete obstruction of flow due to arterial interruption or spasm. Decreased or absent pulses are accompanied by pallor, altered sensation, and severe pain in the distal portion of the extremity; the pain is due to ischemia and often is more severe than the pain associated with other body injuries. Pulses may be absent in elderly patients owing to atherosclerosis; a clue may be the symmetrical absence of pulses in the contralateral uninjured extremity. *Absence of pulses and persistence of ischemia in the injured extremity after relief of shock indicates arterial obstruction rather than spasm.*

Initial treatment measures in patients with absent or decreased pulses are:

   a. Correction of shock.

   b. Search for and manipulation of any fracture or dislocation which may be causing arterial occlusion.

   c. Angiography if the pulse deficit persists.

   d. Immediate arterial exploration if obstruction is identified.

If reflex vasoconstriction is demonstrated on angiography, it may be observed for spontaneous resolution. Sympathetic block may be helpful. Observation must not be prolonged. If reduced pulses and diminished arterial perfusion persist, or if pulses disappear, the involved artery must be promptly explored.

3. **Bruit** indicates the presence of an abnormal arteriovenous (AV) connection. The vessels should be explored as soon as the situation is recognized, and primary repair undertaken. Angiography may be helpful, but usually it is not mandatory prior to operation. Exploration may be delayed if there is no threat to viability of the extremity and if other injuries or their consequences demand priority in treatment.

4. **Expanding hematoma** indicates continuing hemorrhage from an artery. Prompt exploration and repair are indicated. Delay may result in shock, nerve compression, or formation of a false aneurysm.

5. **Swollen extremity**

   a. Swelling indicating the onset of **acute myofascitis** is delayed in onset and associated with diminished pulses, decreased capillary perfusion, hypoesthesia (in the absence of evidence of primary nerve injury), and muscle paresis. Immediate treatment by extensive fasciotomy to decompress completely the involved musculofascial compartments is urgent. Extensive incision of skin, as well as the underlying fascia constricting each of the muscular compartments, may be necessary. Prophylactic fasciotomy often is wise upon completion of a delayed arterial repair.

   b. Soft, diffuse edema may follow revascularization or may be due to major venous thrombosis. Doppler venous flow evaluation or phlebography will confirm the presence of venous thrombosis. Moderate elevation of the limb and toe-to-knee elastic support usually are sufficient treatment for revascularization edema. Anticoagulation with heparin should be employed in addition when venous thrombosis is demonstrated.

D. Angiography demonstrates the site and defines the nature of the arterial lesion and also defines the status of the distal arterial bed. Direct needle injection into a major vessel proximal to the site of injury is most convenient; elective catheter angiography from a remote site is the alternative. Angiography should be performed preoperatively to evaluate diminished or absent pulses at or distal to an injury, with a bruit or thrill suggesting an AV fistula and a pulsating hematoma suggesting false aneurysm. However, when the site and nature of a vascular injury is obvious from clinical examination, angiography is not necessary and may delay treatment. Penetrating injuries in the vicinity of major vessels, without other evidence of vascular injury, should be studied by angiography. Occasionally arterial injury may be present even though pulses are palpable, evidence of significant hemorrhage is lacking, and arteriograms are apparently normal. It is sometimes best to explore penetrating wounds with potential vascular injury if logistics and the patient's condition permit. After completion of vascular repair, operative angiography should be carried out to define the lumen in the area of repair and the distal bed.

E. Arterial injuries and their consequences   Extremity ischemia is the invariable consequence of major arterial interruption. Nerve and muscle are the tissues most sensitive to ischemia. Prompt restoration of perfusion is required to prevent gangrene or severe functional impairment.

   1. Laceration   A tear or irregular incision in a vessel is the result of external penetration by a knife, bullet, or protruding metal or glass object in an automobile accident, or internal penetration by a bone fragment. Arterial lacerations continue to bleed because the intact portion of the vessel wall prevents retraction closure of the arterial wound. If the wound communicates externally, progressive hemorrhage ensues. If not, an expanding hematoma develops which may (a) continue to enlarge and require urgent intervention or (b) become tamponaded by surrounding tissues. In such a contained hematoma, a fibrous capsule eventually forms. Liquefaction of the center of the clot occurs. Communication with the arterial lumen through the laceration produces a pulsating hematoma or false aneurysm which continues to expand at a variable rate (weeks or months) causing progressive deformity, pain, and nerve compression. Eventually the hematoma disrupts, with further internal hemorrhage, or external hemorrhage if there is compression necrosis of the overlying skin.

2. **Transection** is a completed laceration, usually accompanied by moderate or insignificant bleeding owing to symmetrical retraction of the circumference of the transected ends of the artery followed by thrombus formation. Delayed hemorrhage may occur owing to relaxation of spasm of the transected vessel, liquefaction of the thrombus, or dislodgment of the thrombus by arterial pressure. Severe ischemia usually is present, but may be variable depending on the availability of collaterals and the degree to which associated soft tissue damage may have compromised collaterals. Thrombosis proximal and distal to the injury further obstructs collaterals, often converting mild or moderate ischemia to severe, limb-threatening ischemia within a short time.

3. **Perforating or penetrating injuries** from small objects or small-caliber missiles may produce arterial occlusion, internal hemorrhage with false aneurysm formation, or, if in proximity to a major venous channel, an A V fistula. External hemorrhage usually is minimal or absent owing to the repositioning of skin and fascia, with obliteration of the injury tract.

4. An **AV fistula** produces a variable degree of peripheral ischemia depending on (a) its size, (b) the degree of reversal of flow from the distal arterial limb into the low-resistance venous system, and (c) whether acute or delayed occlusion of the artery distal to the injury develops. A thrill or bruit becomes evident over a fistula, cardiac output is invariably increased, and, with large fistulas, progressive cardiomegaly and high-output cardiac failure ensue. Secondary varicose veins become evident in the extremity. The proximal arterial limb feeding the fistula gradually enlarges and becomes tortuous and aneurysmal over a period of a few years. Temporary occlusion of flow through an AV fistula by external pressure produces an immediate reduction in pulse rate (Nicoladoni-Branham sign).

5. **Blunt injury (contusion)** may produce partial or complete **intimal transection** without disruption of the outer media and adventitia. Dissection of the distal intima by arterial flow leads to progressive obstruction and thrombosis. The contused segment, though intact externally, has a characteristic bluish discoloration owing to the subintimal dissection. Severe ischemia with a cool, pale, pulseless extremity usually is evident, although arterial occlusion may not become complete until later. The common femoral and distal brachial arteries are prone to this form of vascular injury owing to absence of protection by overlying tissue.

6. **Reflex vasoconstriction** accompanies injuries adjacent to or directly involving blood vessels and is accompanied by mild to moderate peripheral ischemia. In the absence of arterial disruption or intimal injury, the outcome is spontaneous resolution.

7. **Acute myofascitis and ischemic contracture** may involve the forearm, calf, or anterior tibial compartment of the leg. It is seen most frequently in association with fractures in or about the elbow and knee and is characterized by intense, firm edema, pain, and progressive anesthesia of the hand or foot. The process appears to be related to massive muscle swell-

ing and local venous thrombosis secondary to prolonged ischemia followed by restoration of arterial flow. Outflow of blood from the involved muscles encased in an unyielding fascial envelope is blocked. If this is not promptly decompressed by fasciotomy, necrosis of nerve and muscle ensues, with late fibrosis, contracture, and neurological deficit. Involvement of the forearm in this process after supracondylar fracture of the humerus is called Volkmann's contracture.

F. **Venous injuries and their consequences**   Obstruction may be the result of traumatic thrombosis, compression due to arterial hemorrhage into a confined musculofascial space, or distortion by bone or ligament injury. Marked edema and superficial venous congestion usually develop. If venous return is massively obstructed, gangrene may ensue. Obstruction of venous outflow will reduce arterial inflow. As a consequence, in the presence of venous injury, repair of a concomitant arterial injury, especially of the popliteal artery, is prone to thrombosis.

G. **Conduct of vascular exploration**   The objective is to restore unimpeded blood flow to and from tissues peripheral to the injury. Incomplete repair may result in delayed functional ischemia or early thrombosis, threaten limb loss, and require reoperation through a potentially infected field.

1. Prepare and drape the entire involved extremity and adjacent portions of the trunk to permit adequate exposure and effective control of the injured vessels proximal and distal to the point of injury. Temporary manual compression of the common femoral or upper brachial artery usually affords sufficient control of hemorrhage to facilitate direct exposure of a more distal injured vessel.

2. A temporary shunt is useful to maintain flow through a functioning carotid artery which must be temporarily clamped to control hemorrhage and permit vascular repair.

3. After vascular control has been achieved, debride all traumatized and devitalized tissue and thoroughly irrigate the wound.

4. Remove distal propagated thrombus with a Fogarty balloon catheter.

5. Autogenous vein grafts and patches are preferable to prosthetic material. The latter is prone to infection in a contaminated wound. Venous grafts should be obtained from the saphenous system of the noninjured leg to avoid venous compromise in the event of subsequent venous thrombosis of the injured extremity. Arm veins may be employed if the saphenous is unavailable.

6. Simple arterial lacerations, whether partial or complete, can be managed by debridement of the vascular wound edges and restoration of vascular continuity by primary suture, patch angioplasty, or end-to-end anastomosis. The choice of technique depends on the nature of the vascular wound and the size of the injured vessel.

7. Low-velocity missile injuries require somewhat wider debridement. Vessel continuity can often be restored by direct anastomosis. High-velocity missile injury is deceptive; there is considerable damage beyond that grossly apparent. Wide debridement and restoration of continuity by vein graft almost invariably are required.

8. Contused vessels with intimal dissection and thrombosis over a short segment can be managed by thrombointimectomy and vein patch angioplasty.

9. Extensive arterial injury of any type is best treated by end-to-side vein graft bypass from the healthy vessel proximally to a healthy vessel distal to the site of injury.

10. Repair of an AV fistula is accomplished by interruption of the fistula tract and restoration of both arterial and venous continuity. Management of the arterial injury will depend on its extent and nature, although minor debridement and direct suture are frequently satisfactory. The venous side also should be repaired; avoid ligation unless there is an adjacent and unobstructed collateral vessel to carry the venous outflow.

11. Major venous injuries (caval, iliac, femoral, popliteal, subclavian, axillary) should be repaired by suture or graft interposition, employing the same principles and techniques outlined for arterial debridement and repair. Technique must be infinitely meticulous. Low molecular weight dextran should be given during and immediately after operation. Anticoagulation with heparin should be instituted 24 hr postoperatively.

12. Coverage of a vascular repair must be achieved with viable tissue (skin or muscle) to prevent suture line infection and secondary hemorrhage. When soft tissue destruction is massive, this may not be possible. Temporary coverage under these circumstances can be accomplished with skin autografts.

SUGGESTED READING

Ledgerwood, A. M., and Lucas, C. E. Massive thigh injuries with vascular disruption. *Arch. Surg.* 197:201, 1973.

Rich, N. M., and Hobson, R. W. *Venous Surgery in the Lower Extremity.* St. Louis: Green, 1973.

Slaney, G., and Ashton, F. Arterial injuries and their management. *Postgrad. Med. J.* 47:257, 1971.

2. PROBLEMS ENCOUNTERED IN THE EMERGENCY ROOM

I. THE COMATOSE PATIENT

A. General comments

1. **Coma** is a state of unconsciousness in which the patient is incapable of sensing or responding adequately to either external stimuli or homeostatic mechanisms.

2. In contrast, **stupor** is a state of consciousness in which the patient will respond to strong stimuli, i.e., open his eyes or move on command, although overall behavior responses are not normal. Psychotropic drugs such as marijuana, mescaline, and lysergic acid diethylamide (LSD) may produce profound behavioral disturbances and delirium but rarely coma.

3. When a patient in coma is first seen, the airway should be cleared, and an oral airway placed or an endotracheal tube passed. A respirator should be used to assist ventilation if spontaneous respirations are inadequate. Oxygen should be administered if the patient is cyanotic or there is other evidence of hypoxia. Blood pressure should be checked to be sure the patient is not in shock. Any obvious bleeding from traumatic injuries should be stopped. Care should be exercised in moving the patient until it is certain that there is no spinal cord or head injury. A history should be obtained from anyone who comes to the hospital with the patient.

B. Etiology of coma An easy mnemonic to remember is: **A, E, I, O, U** (the vowels) + **T, I, P, P, S.**
   A = Alcoholism—60% of admissions for coma
   E = Epilepsy—2.4% of admissions for coma
   I = Insulin—too much or too little
   O = Opium—look for narcotic injection sites; tachypnea may indicate respiratory insufficiency due to pulmonary or fat embolus
   U = Uremia—also other metabolic causes of coma (e.g., hepatic failure, nonketotic hyperglycemia)
   T = Trauma—includes spontaneous cerebrovascular accidents—23% of admissions for coma
   I = Infection—meningitis, encephalitis, pneumonia
   P = Poison—barbiturates, lead
   P = Psychogenic unresponsiveness
   S = Shock—myocardial, bacterial, hypovolemic (blood loss)

C. Physical examination

1. First, note the pulse, blood pressure, temperature, and respiratory rate. Fever denotes bacterial infection (meningitis, pneumonia, or septicemia). Hyperthermia is seen in heat stroke. Hypothermia is seen in peripheral circulatory collapse (barbiturate intoxication, phenothiazine overdose, or alcoholism). The pulse rate is helpful in diagnosing patients in coma secondary to complete heart block (very slow pulse), whereas those with a pulse above 160 may be in coma secondary to an ectopic arrhythmia causing cerebrovascular insufficiency. The respiratory rate and rhythm are helpful. Tachypnea may indicate respiratory insufficiency due to pulmonary or fat embolus. Those in diabetic, uremic, or lactic acidosis (anoxic or spontaneous) or those who have ingested poisons (ethylene glycol, methyl alcohol, or decomposed paraldehyde) have very rapid, deep (Kussmaul's) respirations. In strokes, tumors, and other diseases of the CNS, breathing is slowed and often irregular (Cheyne-Stokes respiration). The blood pressure may be elevated with strokes and hypertensive encephalopathy. Obviously, blood pressure is low or unrecordable in shock.

2. The whole patient should be examined. It is possible that one might see a patient with a gunshot wound in his chest and presume this to be the cause of his coma, only to find later that there is another, less obvious gunshot wound in his head.

3. The skin should be checked for color (cyanosis in hypoxia, cherry red in carbon monoxide poisoning), edema, vascular spiders (cirrhosis, hepatic coma), and evidence of injection sites. A hot, dry skin may be seen in high-output gram-negative sepsis or heat stroke.

4. The head should be checked for trauma, especially in patients who have a history of convulsions. The neck should be checked for rigidity.

5. The eyes may show nystagmus, ocular palsy, or conjunctival ecchymoses. The pupils may be small but reactive in narcotic or barbiturate overdosage. The pupils are normal with overdosage of glutethimide (Doriden). The pupils may be unequal with CNS lesions. They may be dilated in alcoholism. Beware of the malingerer who may instill mydriatics. Examine the fundi for papilledema, hemorrhages, or microaneurysms.

In psychogenic unresponsiveness often there is active resistance to opening of eyelids and they usually close rapidly when released. The steady, slower closure of passively opened eyelids and the roving eye movements which occur in comatose patients cannot be voluntarily mimicked. Doll's eye movements (oculocephalic reflex—eyes deviating opposite to the rotational direction of the head) are not seen and caloric testing (oculovestibular reflex) will produce the normal response of nystagmus toward the irrigated ear in psychogenic unresponsiveness.

6. The breath is very important to observe; odors of certain diseases are very characteristic. Diabetic acidosis characteristically produces the odor of acetone, uremia of urine, hepatic coma of mustiness. Alcoholics have a characteristic ethanolic smell. In ingestion of hydrocarbons, there is a gasolinelike odor.

7. The chest should be checked for findings of pneumonia. The heart may show murmurs of bacterial valvular disease, or a rub in uremic pericarditis.

8. The abdomen should be examined for evidence of trauma, tenderness, rigidity, ascites, caput medusae, and organomegaly.

9. The extremities may be flaccid or spastic, or they may demonstrate unequal reflexes, clonus, or Babinski's reflex, all indicative of a CNS disorder.

D. Laboratory examinations

1. When the diagnosis is not obvious from the history or physical examination, a series of laboratory tests must be done to determine the cause of the coma.

2. When poisoning is suspected, a nasogastric or Ewald tube should be passed with the patient in a semiupright position to avoid aspiration. In coma, no matter what the cause, pharyngeal reflexes are virtually absent. The gastric specimen should be sent for chemical analysis.

3. A retention catheter should be passed into the bladder to obtain a urine specimen and to monitor urine output, which should be maintained at around 50 ml/hr. The urine should be tested for sugar, acetone, protein, and specific gravity. A high specific gravity, 4+ glucose, and positive acetone typify diabetic coma. A low specific gravity with large amounts of protein in the urine is characteristic of uremia.

4. If barbiturate or aspirin overdose is suspected, venous blood should be drawn for those determinations. Venous blood also should be examined for glucose, blood urea nitrogen (BUN), carbon dioxide, sodium, potassium, chloride, and calcium. Urine and serum osmolarities are helpful to rule out hypo-osmolar and hyperosmolar states. Elevated serum calcium levels may indicate that the coma is caused by metastatic disease. Arterial blood gas determinations help rule out acid-base disorders and pulmonary dysfunction.

5. A spinal tap should be done if a primary CNS lesion is suspected. When there is papilledema or high pressure is suspected, precautions should be taken to prevent shift of CSF (see Chaps. 1 and 25). When the pressure is found to be elevated, only small amounts of fluid should be withdrawn slowly, at a rate of less than 1 ml/min to a maximum volume of 5 ml. Jugular compression tests are obviously contraindicated. The spinal fluid should be examined for leukocytes and erythrocytes, and sugar and protein levels determined. Some fluid should be smeared and Gram-stained for bacteria if the leukocyte count is high. Fluid should always be sent for bacterial culture and sensitivity tests.

6. An electroencephalogram (EEG) should be performed to rule out brain death. However, patients with deep barbiturate poisoning or metabolic

brain disease, particularly with hypothermia, may appear dead and have isoelectric EEGs.

SUGGESTED READING

Plum, F., and Posner, J. B.   *The Diagnosis of Stupor and Coma* (2nd ed.). Philadelphia: Davis, 1972.

II. OCULAR EMERGENCIES   The definitive treatment and follow-up care of eye problems are best undertaken by an ophthalmologist. However, there are two situations, chemical burns and central retinal artery occlusion, in which treatment must be started at once, as minutes count, and many situations in which the physician first contacted by the patient must initiate protective treatment measures.

A. Minutes count

1. **Chemical burns**   Eyes exposed to acid or alkali must be irrigated immediately with copious amounts of saline solution or tap water. The lids should be everted and the cul-de-sacs cleaned with a cotton swab to remove any residual particulate material. No attempt should be made to neutralize the chemical, as heat of neutralization may cause additional damage. Subsequent treatment depends on the amount and nature of the ocular damage.

2. **Central retinal artery occlusion**

   a. **Signs and symptoms**   There is abrupt, painless loss of vision in one eye due to blockage of the central retinal artery by an embolus or thrombus. When viewed, the fundic arterioles are extremely attenuated. After a short period of time there is edema of the retina due to ischemia. The fovea maintains its normal color, producing, in contrast to the whitened retina, a cherry red fovea. A major branch of the central retinal artery may be blocked individually; in this case, only the portion of the retina supplied by that branch is altered.

   b. **Treatment**   The objective is to move the blockage to a more peripheral and, hopefully, less vital portion of the arterial tree. This is accomplished by:

      (1) Carry out digital massage on the eye through closed lids to lower the intraocular pressure. The finger pressure should be removed every 10–15 sec.

      (2) Decrease aqueous humor production, which also lowers intraocular pressure, by administering acetazolamide (Diamox), 500 mg IV and 500 mg by mouth.

      (3) Dilate the retinal arterioles by having the patient breathe into a paper bag to increase his P_{CO_2}.

      (4) If these measures are not successful within a short period of time, carry out drainage of aqueous humor from the anterior chamber. Topical anesthesia and topical antibiotic drops are applied and a

30-gauge needle inserted into the anterior chamber. Extreme caution should be used to avoid damage to the lens. Only a portion of the aqueous humor should be drained.

B. **Hours count**

1. **Laceration of the globe** is often obvious but may be missed if the lids are swollen shut or care is not used in exploring lid and brow lacerations. A seemingly innocent brow laceration may penetrate the globe. The involved eye should be covered with a patch and protected with a shield. No attempt should be made to investigate the details of the injury, as intraocular contents may be lost during any manipulation. The detailed evaluation can be best made with the patient under general anesthesia for definitive repair by an ophthalmologist.

2. **Orbital cellulitis** Periocular infection is potentially very dangerous, as an extension of the infective thrombophlebitis may lead to cavernous sinus thrombosis. The stage of the infection can be assessed further by evaluating such signs as proptosis, retinal venous engorgement, and papilledema. Most cases of orbital cellulitis result from ethmoidal or frontal sinus disease. Broad-spectrum IV antibiotics, warm soaks, and drainage of any sinus abscess are indicated; the patient should be hospitalized.

C. **Red eyes** A number of conditions cause a red eye. They must be differentiated one from another as their treatment is entirely different.

1. **Acute angle closure glaucoma** is a relatively infrequent cause of decreased vision, but its onset is abrupt, often at night, and immediate diagnosis and treatment are essential. There is usually extreme pain, blurred vision, diffuse redness of the eye, and little or no discharge. The cornea is "steamy," and the anterior chamber is virtually absent. The pupil is usually in a middilated position. The intraocular pressure is elevated, often to a very high degree. The pupil must be constricted with 2% pilocarpine drops given every 5 min for 30 min and then hourly until a response is noted. Diamox should be used to reduce intraocular pressure which, in turn, allows pilocarpine to constrict the pupil more readily. The usual dose of Diamox is 500 mg by mouth plus, in certain cases, 500 mg IV. An operative procedure to place a hole in the iris to allow normal aqueous flow is necessary after the acute attack has been brought under control.

2. **Acute iritis** is a relatively common cause of a red eye which may be difficult to distinguish from acute conjunctivitis. Vision is usually somewhat blurred and there may be light sensitivity. Associated pain is not generally as intense as with angle closure glaucoma. An important feature is the pupil, which is often smaller than that on the uninvolved side. The conjunctival injection is most marked around the edge of the cornea. The cornea is clear. There is little or no discharge. The anterior chamber is generally of normal depth. There are inflammatory cells in the anterior chamber, but the magnification of a slit lamp may be necessary to observe

them. The intraocular pressure is normal or even somewhat low unless the condition has been present for a significant period of time, in which case secondary glaucoma may ensue. Prompt and vigorous dilation of the pupil is essential to prevent adhesions of the iris to the lens, with subsequent cataract formation or glaucoma. Topical steroid drops are used to decrease the inflammatory response.

3. **Acute conjunctivitis** is the most common cause of a red eye. It may be allergic, bacterial, or viral in origin. There is usually a discharge which varies with the different causative agents. A smear often is useful in making the diagnosis. Vision is essentially normal, and there is burning and itching rather than true pain. The conjunctiva is diffusely red, while the cornea, anterior chamber, and pupil are unremarkable. Most cases of acute conjunctivitis are treated as a bacterial infection, with broad-spectrum antibiotic drops. This is generally a safe practice as long as the cornea is not ulcerated.

D. **Foreign bodies and ocular trauma**

1. **Conjunctival foreign bodies** often cause a great deal of pain, especially if the cornea is abraded. The foreign body may be lodged under the lids, in which case the lid must be everted to identify the offending material. A topical anesthetic is useful to allow an adequate examination. Topical fluorescein should be applied to the cornea to identify any corneal abrasion. The fluorescein stains areas of denuded cornea green, while normal epithelium is unstained. The fluorescence can be viewed best using a Wood lamp or a slit lamp with a cobalt blue filter.

2. **Corneal foreign bodies** embedded in the cornea usually can be removed with a cotton swab after application of a topical anesthetic. If this is unsuccessful, a spud or 25-gauge needle may be used to lift the foreign body and remove it. Magnification with a loupe or slit lamp generally is necessary and this treatment is best carried out by an ophthalmologist. The eye should then be treated with a topical antibiotic ointment and an intermediate-acting dilating drop, such as 5% homatropine solution, to relieve ciliary spasm. The eye is then covered with a tight patch with two eye pads and rechecked in 48 hr. Topical anesthetics should never be given the patient to use at home as they retard corneal healing and a bacterial ulcer may result.

3. **Corneal abrasions**   The surface epithelium of the cornea may become abraded, resulting in exquisite pain and lacrimation. The diagnosis is made with fluorescein (see paragraph **1**, above) and treated as after the removal of a corneal foreign body (see paragraph **2**, above). Abrasions, especially with vegetable matter, may lead to fungal ulcers of the cornea.

4. **Blunt trauma**   Many types of intraocular injuries may be caused by blunt trauma, and their recognition is important. Among the more common ones are:

a. Hyphema, or blood in the anterior chamber. The patient should be sedated and placed on absolute bed rest.

b. Traumatic iritis.

c. Iridodialysis. The iris is torn at its insertion into the ciliary body.

d. Glaucoma.

e. Dislocated lens or cataract.

f. Vitreous hemorrhage.

g. Retinal edema and hemorrhages.

h. Retinal tears and subsequent detachment of the retina.

i. Choroidal or scleral rupture often occurs under one of the recti muscles and may be overlooked. The conjunctiva may need to be reflected and the muscle mobilized to rule out a rupture. The intraocular pressure usually is low as determined by a tonometer. Hyphema is often present. An unusually deep anterior chamber should alert the examiner to the possibility of scleral rupture.

j. Papilledema.

k. Optic nerve injury.

5. Intraocular foreign body There should always be a high level of suspicion regarding the possibility of an intraocular foreign body as they are occasionally overlooked, with unfortunate results. When the history affords even the vague possibility of an intraocular foreign body, further investigation is indicated, including a thorough ophthalmological examination as well as radiological views of the orbit. If the foreign body is believed to be lodged in the anterior portion of the eye, a bone-free radiologic examination with dental film often is useful. Many objects capable of penetrating the globe unfortunately are not radiopaque and a negative x-ray does not necessarily rule out an intraocular foreign body. Once an intraocular foreign body is diagnosed, the patient should be placed on IV antibiotics, and topical antibiotic drops should be applied to the eye.

III. EPISTAXIS

A. General comments

1. Reluctance on the part of the physician to initiate appropriate therapy in epistaxis is due to lack of understanding of nasal anatomy and the probable sources of bleeding.

2. Trauma, hypertension, and arteriosclerosis are the common systemic causes of nosebleed Blood dyscrasias, tumors, inflammation, foreign bodies, etc., are causes listed in texts, but it is unusual to identify any of them in patients with epistaxis.

3. Bleeding may arise from the anterior nose or from the posterior nose. The clinical signs and the details of required treatment of these two types of hemorrhage are outlined below.

4. In general, treatment of epistaxis involves the use of packing, cautery, or vessel ligation. Systemic drugs (Adrenosem, Koagamin, Premarin, vitamin K) are not of value.

B. Anterior nasal hemorrhage

1. An intermittent or continuous flow of blood is noted from one side of the nose.

2. The most frequent (90%) site of bleeding is on the medial side of the naris in the anteroinferior portion of the nasal septum known as Little's area. Here a confluence of blood vessels called *Kiesselbach's plexus* lies beneath the mucous membrane.

3. Continuous venous bleeding is more common, but at times a pulsating eroded arterial vessel is seen.

4. Anterior nasal bleeding is first temporarily controlled by packing and pressure. A compressed dental roll moistened with 5% cocaine or 1:1,000 epinephrine solution is inserted well into the inferior nasal vestibule and external pressure is applied to the lateral walls of the anterior nose ("pinch") for 5 min.

5. If the bleeding continues, an injection of 1–2 ml of 1% lidocaine containing 1:100,000 epinephrine is indicated. The anesthetic is infiltrated with a 25-gauge hypodermic needle into the mucosa around the bleeding point. The vestibule is then packed again.

6. Cautery of the bleeding point is carried out once bleeding is under control. The mucosal ulceration is exposed with the aid of a headlight or mirror and nasal speculum. Chemical cautery can be applied with a silver nitrate stick or a small cotton-tipped applicator moistened with 50% trichloracetic acid. The bleeding point is circumferentially cauterized. If bleeding recurs, packing is repeated, withdrawn, and cautery is applied again. Chemical cautery is ineffective unless the bleeding is controlled before application. Electric cautery is more effective and, if a suction-tip electrode is used, can be applied during active bleeding.

7. The treated area is then covered for 24 hr with petrolatum (Vaseline) or iodoform gauze impregnated with antibiotic ointment.

C. Posterior nasal hemorrhage

1. Blood flows posteriorly into the pharynx and also may flow anteriorly out the naris. With profuse posterior hemorrhage, blood may issue from both

nares. The patient may expectorate blood, aspirate and cough up blood, or swallow blood and later expel it by emesis.

2. The posterolateral nasal fossa, beneath the inferior turbinate, is the second most frequent site of origin of nasal hemorrhage. The vessels in this area are known as the nasopalatine plexus of Woodruff. The bleeding is often profuse and difficult to manage.

3. In posterior nasal hemorrhage an initial injection of 2-3 ml of 1% lidocaine with 1:100,000 epinephrine into the greater palatine foramen is recommended. The foramen lies just medial and posterior to the last molar tooth and can be palpated as a dimple in the hard palate. Bleeding will subside or diminish in 75% of patients and facilitate postnasal packing.

4. Balloon tamponade is the second step in treating posterior nasal bleeding. A #14 or 16 Foley catheter is passed along the nasal floor on the bleeding side until the tip is visible on the posterior pharyngeal wall below the soft palate. The balloon is partially inflated with 10 ml of air or saline and the catheter is withdrawn until resistance is noted. Then another 5 ml of air or saline is added to the balloon, the catheter is withdrawn further until taut, and the posterior choana is occluded. The nose anterior to the balloon is then packed. Finally, gauze or an ophthalmic patch is draped over the catheter and an umbilical clamp is applied to it, occluding the anterior nose. A vaginal tampon can be substituted for the balloon to occlude the posterior choana. In profuse nasal hemorrhage, bilateral posterior nasal packs may be necessary to control the bleeding. The patient is admitted to the hospital, sedated, and carefully observed for signs of hypoxia and for recurrent bleeding. The obstruction of the nose by the pack, enforcing mouth breathing, combined with the palatal edema which often develops, leads to hypoventilation and decreased Pa_{O_2}. Supplemental oxygen is administered as required. Posterior nasal packs should be removed in 24-48 hr. Prophylactic antibiotics are recommended to prevent sinusitis and otitis media.

5. Major vessel ligation is required for recurrent or intractable posterior nasal hemorrhage. For posteroinferior nasal bleeding, the branches of the internal maxillary artery are interrupted via an approach through the posterior wall of the maxillary sinus. Alternatively, the external carotid artery can be ligated above the level of the superior thyroid artery. External carotid ligation is less likely to control bleeding because of extensive collateral circulation.

For persistent hemorrhage from above the level of the middle turbinate, the anterior and posterior ethmoidal arteries are ligated. These vessels are approached through a curvilinear incision on the medial orbital rim; by a subperiosteal dissection they are located on the superior medial wall at the junction of the orbital plate of the frontal bone with the lamina papyracea of the ethmoid bone.

In post-traumatic nasal hemorrhage with intracranial rupture of the internal carotid artery, neurosurgical intervention is occasionally necessary.

IV. ACUTE UROLOGICAL PROBLEMS

A. Hematuria

1. Hematuria is the presence of blood in the urine. It may be macroscopic or microscopic; initial, terminal, or total; and may or may not be accompanied by pain. The presence of hematuria demands a full investigation of the urine and the urinary tract.

2. The **age of the patient** has some bearing on the diagnosis.

   a. In infants under 1 yr of age, an ulcerated meatus is the most common cause of hematuria.

   b. In children, acute glomerulonephritis is the most likely cause of hematuria. Microscopic hematuria may accompany pyelonephritis.

   c. In young adults, a stone, glomerulonephritis, tuberculosis, urethritis, or hydronephrosis is often the cause.

   d. In the elderly, prostatic disease and neoplasm of the kidney or bladder are most likely.

3. Etiology

   a. Hematuria from the **lower urinary tract**

      (1) Infections (cystitis, prostatitis, urethritis).

      (2) Specific infections such as tuberculosis.

      (3) Parasitosis (schistosomiasis).

      (4) Calculus in the bladder or ureter.

      (5) Tumor, benign or malignant.

      (6) Foreign body in the bladder.

      (7) Trauma.

      (8) Hypertrophy or carcinoma of the prostate.

   b. **Renal and pelvicalyceal lesions**

      (1) Nephritis, acute, subacute or chronic.

      (2) Nephropathies.

      (3) Specific infections such as tuberculosis.

(4) Stone, nephrocalcinosis, oxalosis, gout.

(5) Tumor, benign or malignant.

(6) Polycystic disease of the kidney.

(7) Hydronephrosis and various congenital anomalies.

(8) Renal infarction.

(9) Thrombosis of renal vein.

(10) Trauma.

c. Systemic diseases

(1) Hemorrhagic diseases and coagulation defects.

(2) Leukemia, polycythemia, sickle cell anemia, cirrhosis of the liver, drug-induced hematuria.

4. **Diagnosis** of hematuria starts with an adequate **history** which should record the presence or absence of edema, pyrexia, headache, malaise, sore throat, urinary frequency, and dysuria. The presence of pain suggests cystitis or calculus. *Painless hematuria is very suggestive of a malignancy.* The duration and incidence of the hematuria should be determined. Does it occur at the commencement of micturition (common in urethral conditions), throughout (common in upper urinary tract conditions), or at the end of micturition (common in prostatic or vesical conditions)?

5. The **physical examination** is directed to the presence or absence of pallor of the mucous membranes, edema, puffiness of the eyelids, and tenderness over the kidneys, in the suprapubic area, or in the area of the liver or spleen. Cardiac murmurs, if present, are described and the blood pressure is recorded.

6. A **urinalysis** should be performed on fresh urine. Brownish urine suggests a renal origin of hematuria, while bright red bleeding suggests the lower tract as the origin. Microscopic examination may reveal casts, suggesting nephritis, or white blood cells, suggesting cystitis, pyelonephritis, or tuberculosis.

7. The **radiological evaluation** of hematuria begins with an excretory urogram. Distortion of the calyces and pelvis is seen in granulomas, cysts, and tumors, while alteration of normal cupping of the calyces is seen in pyelonephritis and papillary necrosis. Radiopaque densities observed in the parenchyma, calyces, pelvis, or ureter are characteristic of stone, nephrocalcinosis, oxalosis, or cystinuria. Radiolucent filling defects are characteristic of tumor, blood clot, or gouty calculi. A dilated collecting system suggests obstruction either by stone or tumor. Delayed IVP films

often will demonstrate the ureter down to the point of obstruction. In the case of stone, there is a tapered ureter to the point of obstruction, while in ureteral tumor there often is a filling defect, with distal dilation of the ureter. Nephrotomography may be indicated to help differentiate a solid from a cystic mass in the kidney. A cystogram is indicated when a filling defect in the bladder has been noted on the excretory urogram or when there is terminal hematuria. In the presence of a tumor there will be a filling defect and, if the bladder wall has been penetrated by the tumor, there will be decreased mobility of the involved vesical wall. A cystogram will also visualize stone or bladder diverticula. A voiding cystourethrogram delineates the urethra. The post-voiding cystogram demonstrates any significant residual urine. A retrograde pyelogram is indicated in the presence of hematuria when the entire collecting system has not been visualized adequately by excretory pyelography. Aortography and selective renal arteriography demonstrate the integrity of the renal arterial tree, identify AV malformations, and demonstrate abnormal vessels seen with granulomas or neoplasms.

8. **Endoscopy**   Evaluation of the patient by endoscopy should be performed while blood is being excreted with the urine. In most cases, this will permit the examiner to identify the anatomical site of lower tract bleeding or to determine if bleeding is unilateral or bilateral when it arises from the upper urinary tract. Generally, in the very young patient, endoscopy is the last procedure to be performed after a negative workup, while in the elderly patient it is utilized early; in the young the cause of hematuria is most commonly nephritis, while in the elderly it is a neoplasm.

9. Exfoliative **cytology** of the urinary sediment is valuable in identifying urothelial tumors. Aspiration cytology can be utilized to differentiate between malignant and benign lesions of the kidney. In hematuria without a suspected renal mass lesion, aspiration cytology is of relatively little value in establishing a diagnosis.

10. **Biopsy** of most of the genitourinary tract can be performed. When hematuria originates in the upper tract, needle or open biopsy of the kidney often is the most definitive diagnostic maneuver available. The bladder is biopsied endoscopically, while the prostate gland is biopsied transurethrally, transperineally, or transrectally.

11. **Sonograms** of the kidney can differentiate between solid and cystic masses associated with hematuria.

12. **Bleeding from the urinary tract is not an acute emergency**   A proper diagnostic workup must be completed. Acute symptomatic measures include evacuation of clots from the bladder, relief of pain, relief of obstruction, bedrest, and, rarely, transfusion. Definitive treatment will depend on the ultimate diagnosis.

B. **Torsion of the testis** is likely when a boy or young man experiences acute testicular pain without obvious trauma. He may have lower abdominal pain, with nausea and vomiting, and he may have had similar episodes with spontaneous resolution. Frequently the disorder has been treated as an acute epididymitis by another physician.

1. **Findings**

   a. The testicle and soon the scrotum are swollen and tender.

   b. A fever may be present.

   c. No urinary symptoms or evidence of urethritis is present; urinalysis is normal.

   d. Prostatic secretions are normal.

   e. The testis on the contralateral side may be lower. Elevating the ipsilateral testis may cause the pain to increase.

2. **Etiology** Torsion occurs when a congenital anomaly of the mesorchium allows the testis and epididymis to twist on a pedicle inside the tunica vaginalis, resulting in venous occlusion and thrombosis. The initiating factor seems to be spasm of the cremaster muscle, which inserts obliquely on the cord.

3. **Differential diagnoses**

   a. Mumps orchitis is usually associated with parotitis and is rare before puberty.

   b. Epididymitis is uncommon before puberty and usually is associated with pyuria.

   c. Traumatic orchitis is elicited by the history.

4. **Treatment** Manual detorsion is attempted if the patient is seen before induration makes palpation of the abnormally positioned testis impossible. If detorsion is successful, bilateral orchiopexy can be done electively. Immediate operation is indicated if the testis cannot be rotated into normal position. The testis is rotated and sutured to the tunica vaginalis. The contralateral side is also sutured at the same time to prevent its torsion and subsequent sterility. If torsion is corrected within 4-6 hr, the entire testis survives. Between 6-10 hr, the seminiferous tubules may necrose but the interstitial cells survive, allowing continued androgen production. After 10-12 hr of torsion, it is rare that any part of the testis survives.

C. **Torsion of the appendix testis** The small pedunculated appendages at the upper pole of testis may undergo torsion spontaneously, resulting in pain and induration. If seen early, the isolated area of induration is easily felt, the diagnosis is made, and operation is unnecessary. If seen later, after the entire testicle and epididymis have swollen, it is necessary to explore the scrotum to rule out testicular torsion. The twisted appendix is simply excised.

V. VAGINAL BLEEDING AND OTHER GYNECOLOGICAL PROBLEMS

An understanding of the physiological process of menstruation is helpful in managing patients with vaginal bleeding. Every physician who works in an emergency room should be capable of performing an adequate examination; a female nurse or attendant should be present at all times. The differential diagnosis of the acute abdomen (see Chap. 5) requires that the physician be constantly aware of pelvic pathology.

Abnormal uterine bleeding usually is an early symptom of cervical cancer. Every patient having a pelvic examination must have a Papanicolaou smear even if there is bleeding. All patients with perimenopausal or postmenopausal bleeding must have a dilation and curettage to exclude endometrial carcinoma.

A. Traumatic lesions

1. **Perineal or vaginal lacerations** are the result of direct trauma. Hymenal tears may bleed profusely and require suture under local anesthesia. Coital vaginal injuries are uncommon in premenopausal women, but are more common after the menopause owing to atrophy of vaginal mucosa. Vaginal lacerations bleed profusely and require initial control with a tight vaginal pack, replacement of blood loss, and suture under general anesthesia. If the lacerations are in the periurethral region, an indwelling catheter should be placed.

2. **Perineal or vaginal hematoma** occurs as the result of blunt trauma or a straddle-type fall. Usually the hematoma involves the vulva and perineum; rarely does it extend into the vagina. Rarely, avulsion, transection, contusion, or laceration of the urethra occurs. These injuries result in excruciating pain. Most cases may be treated by bedrest, ice packs to the perineum and vulva, and an indwelling catheter if urinary retention occurs. If the hematoma extends rapidly, it may require evacuation and placement of drains under general anesthesia.

3. **Foreign bodies** in the vagina or in the urethra are most commonly seen in young children. Rarely, a foreign body such as a tampon may be forgotten in adult females. The foreign body results in vaginitis and an offensive and malodorous discharge which occasionally is bloodstained. Often the foreign body can be identified and gently removed in the examining room.

B. Rape is labial penetration by the penis without consent, using force, fear, or fraud.

1. **Immediate care of physical injuries**   Victims of rape may experience a variety of traumatic injuries ranging from laceration of the hymen, vulva, or vagina to rupture of the cul-de-sac.

2. **Prevention of venereal disease**   Perform a serological test for syphilis. Cultures for gonorrhea are taken from the cervical canal, urethra, and rectum. If indicated, a throat culture is taken. Smears should be stained and examined for gram-negative intracellular diplococci. Antibiotic prophylaxis of venereal disease is undertaken by administering procaine

penicillin, 4.8 million units IM, and probenecid, 1 gm orally. If the patient is allergic to penicillin, an appropriate alternative antibiotic should be prescribed. Follow-up is mandatory to evaluate the gonococcal cultures and serology and to provide any additional needed treatment.

3. **Prevention and alleviation of psychological damage** requires tact and gentleness on the part of the examining physician. Rape is a particularly demoralizing kind of assault. Psychiatric referral and careful follow-up of the patient often are indicated.

4. **Medicolegal examination** involves recording:

   a. History of events surrounding the assault.

   b. Patient's emotional state.

   c. Menstrual history, including use of contraception.

   d. Coital history other than the rape incident.

   e. Condition of the patient's clothing; look for blood or seminal stains. Collect any hairs or foreign fibers as evidence.

   f. Physical examination, including inspection of all body surfaces. Describe in detail any evidence of trauma such as bruises, abrasions, or lacerations.

   g. Pelvic examination, including examination of any dried secretion from the perineum and thighs. Record any evidence of trauma, especially to the introitus. Take carefully labeled smears for spermatozoa from the vulva, vagina, and cervix. A Papanicolaou smear is also taken. Examine a fresh drop of vaginal aspirate for motile spermatozoa. Seminal fluid in the vaginal aspirate may be tested for acid phosphatase (Phosphatabs Acid). Perform a careful bimanual examination.

5. **Prevention of pregnancy** may be offered as Premarin (the "morning after" pill), 20-25 mg daily, or ethinyl estradiol, 1-5 mg daily, for 5 days. All patients should be checked after 21 days for possible pregnancy if no menstrual bleeding has occurred. The option of therapeutic abortion also may be offered to these patients.

C. **Bleeding due to abortion**   Abortion is the termination of pregnancy prior to 20 wk of gestation or when the fetus weighs less than 500 gm. The incidence of spontaneous abortion is between 10-15% of all pregnancies. The exact incidence of induced abortion is not known. Induced abortions may be therapeutic or criminal.

1. **Threatened abortion** is associated with vaginal bleeding or bloody vaginal discharge and may be accompanied by cramps and backache. The cervix is closed and not effaced. Speculum and vaginal examinations are made to exclude any local cause of bleeding. Bed rest and avoidance of coitus

are advised. In most cases the bleeding will cease and the pregnancy continue. If bleeding persists, the patient should be advised that she may abort. The effectiveness of progestational agents in preventing abortion is controversial.

2. **Inevitable abortion** is associated with rupture of the membranes and the presence of cervical dilation. Rarely, the membranes seal, but the usual course is progression of the abortion, accompanied by bleeding. The patient should be hospitalized, have blood typed and crossmatched and an IV infusion of oxytocin (10-20 units per liter IV fluids) started to aid completion of the abortion. If the passage of tissue seems to be incomplete, the products of conception should be evacuated by sharp or suction curettage under anesthesia.

3. **Incomplete abortion** is the most common disorder of early pregnancy requiring treatment. Surgical intervention nearly always is necessary. The history is one of severe uterine cramps accompanied by considerable bleeding and, frequently, by the passage of the products of conception. On pelvic examination the cervical os is found dilated and effaced and tissue is found in the cervical canal or vagina. Blood is typed and crossmatched, an IV infusion with oxytocin is started, and evacuation of the products of conception by sharp or suction curettage is done when the patient's condition is stable. Ergonovine, 0.2 mg IM or IV, is administered after curettage to maintain the uterus firmly contracted.

4. **Complete abortion** occurs in early pregnancy, prior to 10 wk, when the fetus and the placenta are passed as an intact conceptus. The patient has contractions and bleeding, and when examined the uterus feels firm and contracted, with a tightly closed cervix. If cramps and bleeding persist, this type of abortion is managed by dilation and curettage and evacuation of any residual products of conception from the uterine cavity.

5. **Septic abortion** The gravid uterus and adjacent parametria are extremely vulnerable to infection. On sterile pelvic examination, if the tenderness is limited to the uterus, the infection probably is contained within the uterine cavity. Parametrial thickening or tenderness associated with lower abdominal tenderness, guarding, rigidity, or rebound indicates pelvic peritonitis.

   The patient should be hospitalized. Cervical specimens should be taken for aerobic and anaerobic culture and a Gram stain examined. If there is fever above 38.3°C (101°F), blood for culture should be drawn. Blood should be typed and cross matched and IV fluids started. A central venous catheter is mandatory in severe infections. An indwelling catheter is required to monitor urine output. Appropriate antibiotics should be started, preferably by the IV route (see Chap. 14). Unless massive hemorrhage dictates the need for immediate evacuation of the uterus, it is best to prevent and control the spread of infection by an intensive 24-hr antibiotic treatment prior to dilation and curettage. If there is suspicion of prior intrauterine manipulation, an x-ray of the abdomen should be obtained to look for evidence of uterine perforation (presence of subdiaphragmatic air) or the presence of a foreign body or gas in the subcutaneous tissue. If the diagnosis of perforated uterus is made, exploratory laparotomy is required to exclude traumatic injury to the bowel and other viscera. In the presence of extensive pelvic infection or uncontrollable hemorrhage, hysterectomy may be a life-saving procedure.

D. Ectopic pregnancy means implantation of a pregnancy outside the uterine cavity. Almost all ectopic pregnancies (95%) occur within the fallopian tube. The clinical picture of ectopic pregnancy is rarely typical. The physician must "think ectopic" when faced with the triad of amenorrhea and pain followed by abnormal uterine bleeding.

1. **Signs and symptoms** The patient is in the childbearing years. The first symptom usually is a delay in menstruation lasting a week or two, followed by vaginal spotting. Amenorrhea of longer duration may be followed by frank vaginal bleeding. Passage of a decidual cast may occur as a result of a falling hormonal level. Cramplike pain occurs in the pelvis or lower abdomen on the affected side. With rupture of the tube, pain is severe and steady, associated with a feeling of faintness or actual syncope. Pallor, sweating, tachycardia, and hypotension are due to intra-abdominal bleeding. There is diffuse abdominal tenderness, with guarding. Percussion reveals shifting dullness and crown tympany. Pelvic examination may reveal a tender adnexal mass and fullness in the cul-de-sac. There is pain on moving the cervix, which may be softened and blue, and there may be slight uterine enlargement.

There is a mild leukocytosis and there may be anemia. Pregnancy tests have not been of value in suspected ectopic pregnancy. A negative pregnancy test does not exclude an ectopic pregnancy. The diagnosis may be supported by the free flow of blood at culdocentesis when hemoperitoneum is present. Confirmation of the diagnosis usually requires evaluation of the adnexa by laparoscopy, culdotomy, or laparotomy.

2. **Treatment** of an ectopic pregnancy is aimed at controlling the intra-abdominal hemorrhage. Usually a salpingectomy is performed, with excision of the cornual portion of the involved tube.

3. **Differential diagnosis** Conditions that may be confused with an ectopic pregnancy are:

   a. Intrauterine pregnancy with threatened or incomplete abortion.

   b. Pelvic inflammatory disease.

   c. Torsion of an ovarian cyst or fallopian tube.

   d. Corpus luteum cyst.

E. Acute pelvic inflammatory disease

1. There are two **types** of acute pelvic inflammatory disease:

   a. Gonorrheal infection ascends from the cervix along the endometrium to produce an acute salpingitis; pelvic peritonitis follows when purulent exudate escapes.

b. Pyogenic infection occurs in puerperal and postabortive states as well as in postoperative infections of the genital tract.

2. **Signs and symptoms**   Acute symptoms usually appear during or after a menstrual period. Fever, leukocytosis, and tachycardia are present. There is severe pain in the pelvis and lower abdomen accompanied by tenderness, guarding, and abdominal distention. Urinary frequency and dysuria may occur. On pelvic examination there is leukorrhea and marked tenderness bilaterally, especially on motion of the cervix. Tubo-ovarian masses (abscesses) may be palpated in some cases. There may be infection also of the urethra and Skene's glands. A culture should be taken, streaking the material directly onto Thayer-Martin medium, and a smear examined for gram-negative intracellular diplococci.

3. **Treatment**   The patient is kept at bed rest. Fluids are given IV. Vigorous parenteral antibiotic therapy is instituted. Usually the infection subsides. If rupture of a tubo-ovarian abscess occurs, generalized peritonitis and septic shock may ensue. An immediate operation then is essential; almost always hysterectomy and bilateral adnexectomy are necessary.

VI. HAND INJURIES AND INFECTIONS

A. **Functional anatomy**   In order to make an accurate diagnosis of a hand injury, a knowledge of the functional anatomy of the hand is mandatory.

1. **Volar surface of wrist**

   a. The volar surface of the wrist (Fig. 2-1) is divided into radial and ulnar portions by the centrally placed flexor carpi radialis and palmaris longus tendons. The median nerve lies beneath these central tendons. Approximately 15% of patients do not have a palmaris longus tendon of one wrist.

   b. The ulnar border of the wrist is bounded by the flexor carpi ulnaris. Directly beneath it lie the ulnar artery and nerve.

   c. Between the flexors carpi radialis and ulnaris lie all the superficialis and profundus flexor tendons to the fingers.

   d. Radial and deep to the flexor carpi radialis lie the flexor pollicis longus (thumb) and the radial artery.

2. **Palm of hand**

   a. The transverse carpal ligament forms the roof of the carpal tunnel (Fig. 2-2). This space contains nine tendons and one nerve: the superficialis and profundus tendons to each finger, the flexor pollicis longus, and the median nerve.

   b. The ulnar artery and nerve have a separate, more superficial compartment just lateral to the pisiform bone, through which they enter the

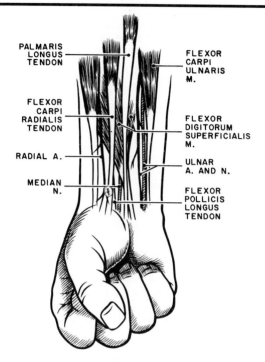

Figure 2-1. The volar aspect of the wrist.

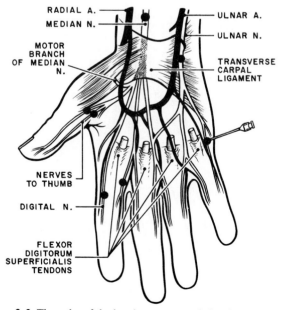

Figure 2-2. The palm of the hand: anatomy and sites for nerve blocks.

hand. The motor branches of the ulnar nerve at this level innervate the hypothenar muscles, all the interossei, two ulnar lumbricals, and usually both heads of the adductor pollicis.

c. The motor branch of the median nerve leaves the main trunk at the distal edge of the transverse carpal ligament to innervate the thenar muscles and the two radial lumbrical muscles.

d. The superficialis tendons divide to embrace the profundus and insert laterally into the base of the middle phalanges. The profundus tendons insert into the distal phalanges.

3. Dorsum of hand and wrist

a. Because structures of this area are superficial, they are frequently injured in "minor" injuries (Fig. 2-3).

b. There are six separate tendon compartments at the wrist.

c. There are two tendons to the index finger and frequently two tendons to the little finger; the central two digits have a single extensor.

d. The long extensor to the thumb angles obliquely across the two radial wrist extensors.

e. The sensory branch of the radial nerve is frequently overlooked and when injured can produce painful neuromas.

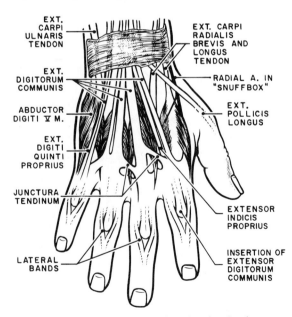

Figure 2-3. The dorsum of the hand and wrist.

B. Examination of the injured hand

1. Preliminary steps

    a. Obtain a **history** of the injury: How? When? Where? Reconstruct the position of the hand at the time of injury. Details of the patient's general health and how he normally uses his hand (musician, mechanic, monk) are essential.

    b. The **type of injury** should be classified as follows:

        (1) Tidy laceration (i.e., clean laceration sustained from a sharp knife).

        (2) Untidy laceration (i.e., crushing injury of digit or hand).

        (3) Severe **crushing injury** and mangling of hand.

        (4) Burn.

        (5) Traumatic amputation.

        (6) There are many variants of the injuries listed, such as shearing lacerations, oblique amputations, and avulsing injuries of the skin.

    c. It is best to put the patient supine on a cart or table with the arm at right angles to the body supported by a sturdy arm board. A Mayo stand or table also should be provided and covered with sterile towels.

    d. The examination should be done with sterile technique, including cap and mask. A basic instrument set and ample dressings must be ready.

    e. The initial examination determines the general condition of the hand and the need for further procedures. All but the simplest procedures should be performed in an operating room with adequate assistance. Observe the hand for variations of normal posture, with and without passive movement. Inspect the arm and hand for injury to specific component parts as described below.

2. Vascular injuries

    a. A cold, pale, pulseless, painful hand indicates severe arterial damage. Circulation must be restored promptly.

    b. A compression bandage ordinarily will control bleeding. If arterial bleeding makes examination impossible, a blood pressure cuff applied to the upper arm and inflated above systolic blood pressure will stop or slow bleeding. At no time should vessels be clamped blindly, endangering nearby structures.

    c. If both radial and ulnar arteries at the wrist have been severed, the hand will survive in most cases because of the collateral circulation via the volar and dorsal interosseous arteries. However, the skin nutrition may be significantly impaired. At least one of the main arteries should be repaired in the operating room.

3. Tendon injuries

a. Location of the wound is a valuable guide to the possibility of tendon injury; the diagnosis of tendon injury is simple applied anatomy.

b. Inability to flex the distal phalanx when the middle phalanx is immobilized suggests division of the flexor digitorum profundus.

c. Holding all digits except the one being tested in extension, and attempting to flex the digit being tested, check function of the flexor digitorum superficialis tendon.

d. A laceration over the dorsal surface associated with inability fully to extend the digit suggests severance of the common extensor tendons or of the extensor indicis proprius (index finger) or extensor digiti quinti (fifth digit).

e. Lacerations near the distal phalangeal joint and a droop of the distal phalanx indicate injury of the extensor complex in this region (mallet finger deformity).

f. Inability to extend fully the distal phalanx of the thumb indicates laceration of the extensor pollicis longus tendon.

g. Injuries over the thumb metacarpal and radial aspect of the wrist, with inability to extend and abduct the thumb, suggest injuries to the short extensor and long abductor tendons. The long extensor also may be divided.

h. All active movement tests are subjective and are of no use in the young or uncooperative. All other joints except the one involved should be controlled by the examiner to reduce "trick" movements. Only complete lack of movement is diagnostic; impaired movement is only suggestive.

4. Bone injuries

a. Suspect a bone injury if the appearance of the normal architecture of the hand is distorted.

b. Light palpation may reveal fracture through excessive tenderness or crepitation.

c. X-ray examination is required to define the precise extent of bone injury. PA, oblique, and lateral views should be ordered. In children with incomplete epiphyseal growth, the normal hand also should be x-rayed for comparison.

5. Nerve injuries

a. Anesthesia distal to an injury suggests damage to sensory nerves (Fig. 2-4). Examination must be careful, with repeated measuring of light touch with a hair or wisp of cotton, without the patient's looking.

b. The dorsal sensory branch of the ulnar nerve is given off about 5 cm proximal to the distal wrist crease. In injury occurring distal to this division, motor function may be absent but dorsal sensory function may be present.

c. Tests for ulnar motor function include:

(1) Ability of the patient to deviate the long finger in ulnar or radial abduction with the palm flat on a table (interosseous function).

(2) Strong pinch between volar surfaces of the thumb and index without hyperflexion of the interphalangeal joint of the thumb (Froment's paper sign).

d. Median nerve injury can cause sensory loss (Fig. 2-4). Motor injury can accompany sensory loss or be isolated following injury to the motor nerve alone distal to its division in the thenar area (see Fig. 2-2).

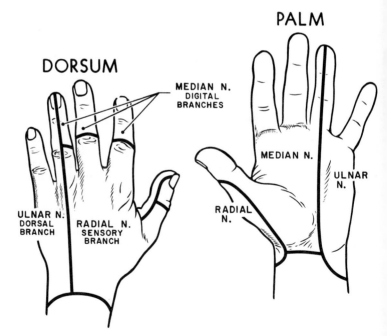

Figure 2-4. Sensory innervation of the hand.

e. Tests for median motor function include:

(1) Abduction of thumb at right angles to the palm of the hand.

(2) Opposition of the thumb to the base of the fifth digit.

(3) Observation and palpation of the thenar muscles during function.

C. Treatment of hand injuries

1. General considerations

a. The **primary objective** in treating hand injuries is to insure that the patient is no worse off after treatment than before treatment.

b. Prompt healing of all skin wounds and restoration of bone architecture is of fundamental importance because of the inverse relationship between wound healing and disability from joint stiffness and scar formation.

c. Achievement of prompt healing of any laceration is directly related to the care taken in wound preparation and tissue handling. Excessive scar formation results in part from insufficient debridement, repeated tissue manipulation, and sutures which are too heavy, include too much tissue, are tied too tightly, and removed too late.

d. **The injured hand should not be subjected to repeated examinations,** as this increases the chance of introducing infection. An initial examination followed by definitive examination in the operating room should suffice.

e. Simple lacerations, i.e., those which involve only skin and muscle with no additional injury to bone, tendon, nerve, or major blood vessels, can be repaired in the emergency room if facilities are adequate.

f. Most injuries—particularly any injury involving bone, tendon, nerves, or major blood vessels—require the full facilities of an operating room for repair. **Do not attempt to treat complicated hand injuries in the emergency room.**

g. Complicated wounds should be managed by a surgeon with experience and skill in the treatment of hand injuries. *The obligations of the physician who first sees a patient with a major hand injury are to cleanse the wound, apply an immobilizing and protective dressing, and obtain consultation.*

2. Preparation and anesthesia

a. Surgical preparation of the injured hand begins with the removal of any clothing that may interfere with ready access to the hand and arm. Also remove any watches and rings.

b. Unless there is severe hemorrhage, the entire hand should be immersed in a basin of soap and warm water or antiseptic and allowed to soak for 10 min. The advantages of soaking are that dirt and debris are loosened and the patient is more comfortable.

c. Children should be put in mummy wraps to restrain them, and someone should be in constant attendance with the injured child. Unattended children may wriggle out of any restraint and injure themselves.

d. Following the initial soak, anesthesia should be established prior to definitive preparation of the hand for repair. The great advantage is that anesthesia makes preparation much less painful to the patient.

e. Once anesthesia has been established, the entire hand and forearm should be scrubbed gently with soap and water for 10 min. The scrub should be done by a surgeon or nurse wearing sterile gloves as well as a cap and mask. The patient should be wearing a mask as well. Dirt and debris ground into the wound should be removed by gentle scrubbing. Any bits of stone or glass should be picked out. The wound and extremity should be irrigated repeatedly with sterile saline solution.

f. Next, an antiseptic solution should be applied to the skin around the wound; it should not be applied in the wound itself. Finally, the arm and hand should be carefully draped.

g. Hemostatic tourniquet

(1) It is debatable whether an arm tourniquet should be used in an emergency room. These machines are far from infallible and exceedingly high pressures may be applied unknowingly. On the other hand, there is no doubt that any procedure in the hand is greatly facilitated by the use of a tourniquet. Any major procedure must be done under tourniquet control in the operating room.

(2) For repair of lacerations of the digits, a small tourniquet may be used. An 8 Fr catheter or a $\frac{1}{4}$-in. Penrose drain is placed tightly around the base of the finger and held with a medium-sized hemostat. **Rubber bands are never used for tourniquets** as they may be forgotten and incorporated in the bandage, resulting in gangrene and necessitating amputation of the digit. It is almost impossible to overlook a long rubber tourniquet held in place with a hemostat.

(3) For other procedures, an arm-cuff tourniquet (applied prior to preparation of the extremity) is inflated to 250 mm Hg. The pressure of a tourniquet becomes increasingly painful to the patient unless the entire extremity is anesthestized. However, adults usually can tolerate a tourniquet for 30 min.

(4) A tourniquet used on a child often increases anxiety and restlessness and probably should be used only for repair of complex injuries.

(5) A hemostatic tourniquet should not be left in place for longer than 20 min on a digit or 1½ hr on the arm.

3. General and regional anesthesia

a. **General anesthesia** is required for severe hand injuries requiring extensive reconstruction, abdominal or cross-arm flaps, or procurement of tissue from other parts of the body.

b. **Regional anesthesia** of the entire upper extremity is the procedure of choice, particularly if the patient has eaten recently or if a tourniquet is needed for repair of hand injuries when extensive exposure is anticipated. It is often necessary to supplement a regional block with general anesthesia or dissociative tranquilizing agents. Therefore, regional anesthesia is best done in the operating room with the assistance of an anesthesiologist. Techniques include brachial plexus block using a scalene, a supraclavicular, or an axillary approach, and IV regional anesthesia.

c. Any method of local or regional anesthesia requires a careful history of possible systemic reaction to anesthetic agents and preparation for treatment of such reactions.

d. **Digital nerve block** (see Fig. 2-2)

(1) Anesthetic solutions containing **epinephrine should never be used in digital nerve blocks,** since the resulting vasoconstriction may produce gangrene and necessitate amputation.

(2) A preliminary preparation of the hand is made consisting of a gentle soap and water wash and the use of an alcohol-iodine solution to prepare the skin. The surgeon dons sterile gloves and the patient's hand is placed on a sterile towel with the palm up.

(3) A syringe is filled with 10 ml of 1 or 2% lidocaine hydrochloride (Xylocaine) solution. Other anesthetic agents may be used. A #25 hypodermic needle, ¾ in. long, is fitted on the syringe.

(4) The needle point is placed slightly proximal to the palmar edge of the interdigital cleft, pointed toward the palm, angled 20 degrees from the long axis of the digit being anesthetized, and slowly inserted until it encounters the proximal phalanx. It is then withdrawn slightly and the plunger is pulled back to be sure that the needle point is not in a vessel.

(5) A "ballooning" of the dorsum of the web space is produced with an injection of 3 ml of anesthetic solution. Greater volumes are not used because mechanical vascular constriction is as disastrous as pharmacological constriction. The injection is then repeated on the other side of the digit through a separate needle puncture.

(6) For the ulnar side of the fifth digit, the solution is placed proximal to the base of the digit and 5 mm from the ulnar border of the hand.

(7) For the radial side of the index finger, the solution is placed proximal to the flexion crease and 5 mm from the radial border of the hand.

(8) The digital nerves of the thumb flank the flexor pollicis longus tendon. This tendon is easily palpated on the flexor surface of the metacarpophalangeal joint of the thumb. From 2-3 ml of solution is placed on each side of the tendon at the base of the thumb.

(9) If an injury affects the dorsum or the lateral borders of the finger, it is advisable to supplement the digital blocks with a field block across the dorsum of the digit above the interdigital cleft; 2 ml of anesthetic solution is placed transversely across the dorsum of the digit just beyond the knuckle.

e. **Median nerve block** (see Fig. 2-2)

(1) The needle is placed 1 cm from the ulnar side of the flexor carpi radialis tendon and 1 cm proximal to the distal flexion crease of the wrist. It is angled slightly toward the ulna; often a slight "give" can be felt as the needle penetrates the fascia. [See (3).]

(2) Paresthesias in the distribution of the median nerve are often elicited as the needle point contacts the nerve. It is preferable to inject the anesthetic around the nerve; intraneural injections may result in troublesome neuritis.

(3) A syringe is filled with 10 ml of anesthetic solution. Half of this volume (five milliliters) is injected around the nerve, making certain that intravascular injection does not occur. The needle is then withdrawn to a subcutaneous position and the volar aspect of the wrist infiltrated.

f. **Ulnar nerve block at the wrist** (see Fig. 2-2)

(1) The ulnar nerve lies superficially just to the radial side of the pisiform bone, which is easily palpated.

(2) The needle is directed to this location and 5 ml of anesthetic solution is injected.

g. **Ulnar nerve block for the dorsum of the hand**

(1) The sensory branch of the ulnar nerve which innervates the dorsum of the hand, the dorsum of the fifth digit, and ulnar side of the ring digit leaves the main branch of the ulnar nerve 5 cm proximal

to the distal flexion crease of the wrist. An ulnar nerve block at the wrist will not give anesthesia to the dorsum.

(2) If anesthesia of the dorsum is desired, a field block of the dorsum and ulnar side of the wrist is effective.

(3) Inject 5 ml of anesthetic solution subcutaneously from the midportion of the dorsum of the wrist to well down on the ulnar side of the wrist just distal to the ulna.

h. Ulnar nerve block at the elbow

(1) The ulnar nerve lies superficially in the epicondylar notch at the ulnar aspect of the elbow.

(2) A satisfactory and complete ulnar nerve block can be obtained with injection of 5 ml of solution in this area.

i. Radial nerve block at the wrist

(1) The radial nerve lies near the cephalic vein in the proximal portion of the anatomical snuffbox.

(2) Injection of 5 ml solution into this area will give anesthesia in the distribution of the sensory branch of the radial nerve.

4. General aspects of repair

a. The **cardinal principles** of management are:

(1) Strict asepsis.

(2) Removal of all foreign material.

(3) Careful debridement of all devitalized tissue.

(4) Conversion to a "surgically sterile" wound by excision, where possible, of contaminated tissues.

(5) Primary closure without tension.

b. Certain factors may make primary skin closure impossible or unwise:

(1) Inability to obtain asepsis because of interval between injury and treatment or because of type of injury [see human bites, paragraph **5.h(1),** below] where "cardinal principle 4" (above) cannot be achieved.

(2) Inability to determine extent of devitalized tissue. Time often is necessary for full demarcation of injury.

(3) Inability to obtain primary skin closure because of extent of skin and soft tissue loss.

c. Where primary skin healing cannot be achieved without tension it is necessary to provide coverage using **local flaps** or tissue from other areas. It is beyond the scope of this section to discuss indications and techniques of skin grafts, advancement of flaps, or pedicle flaps which may be needed to achieve wound closure. Treatment involving such procedures should be done in the operating room by a surgeon skilled in the management of hand injuries.

d. **Suture material recommended** is as follows:

(1) Muscle: 4-0 chromic catgut.

(2) Subcuticular ligatures: 4-0 synthetic absorbable suture (Dexon).

(3) Subcutaneous sutures (4-0 absorbable) are not recommended in repair of hand injuries but should be used in injuries of the arm and forearm.

(4) Skin: 5-0 or 6-0 nylon.

5. **Specific injuries**

a. **Simple lacerations** should be closed with simple or mattress sutures (see Chap. 25).

b. **Slicing wounds** with beveled edges or "trap door" lacerations often heal poorly, resulting in unsightly scar or functional impairment. The management of these wounds involves careful debridement of devitalized tissue and primary coverage.

c. **Untidy lacerations,** following debridement of irregular and traumatized wound margins, nearly always need both simple as well as mattress sutures for closure.

d. **Stellate lacerations** often present difficult problems; adequate undermining and closure without tension are mandatory. The use of a tip stitch to approximate a triangular wound is important in preserving blood supply to the tip (see Chap. 25).

e. **Tendon or bone exposure** requires early wound closure. If a bone or tendon remains exposed, it becomes necrotic. Primary or early delayed closure of such injuries may be associated with a subsequent wound infection, but frequent inspection, proper dressings, immobilization, and systemic antibiotics will control sepsis in most cases.

f. **Nerve and tendon injuries** are cared for using the principles summarized in Figure 2-5.

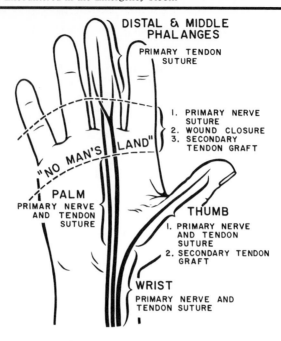

Figure 2-5. Principles of management of acute nerve and tendon injuries of the hand.

   g. In **avulsion injuries,** a considerable amount of skin and soft tissue is present but has been torn from deeper structures. Repair of such wounds requires precise judgment, especially when the pedicle is based distally. Even though the arterial supply is adequate, venous outflow may be compromised.

   h. Bites and puncture wounds

      (1) Human bites are among the most dangerous and difficult injuries seen in the hand. They are usually sustained over the dorsal surface of the metacarpophalangeal joint and are caused by a clenched fist smashing into a tooth of an adversary. They frequently involve the extensor tendon mechanism and the metacarpophalangeal joint.

      (2) Bite wounds should not be closed unless the "cardinal principles" can be fulfilled   The skin around the wound is carefully cleaned, a resilient dressing is applied, and broad-spectrum antibiotics are started. The hand and forearm should be immobilized and elevated.

      (3) Dog bites, especially if large and deforming, may be closed primarily. Impeccable wound preparation and antibiotics are indicated. Puncture wounds should be left open.

i. Wringer and roller injuries

(1) This type of trauma varies from trivial to mangling and crushing injuries, especially if the extremity remains between the turning rollers, resulting in an abrasive and shearing effect on the skin.

(2) Severe injury is obvious. The danger is in underestimating what appears to be a trivial wringer injury. If neglected, considerable swelling of the hand and arm may result and in a very few hours cause ischemia, necrosis, hemorrhage, and Volkmann's contracture, resulting in a permanently disabled extremity.

(3) Wringer injuries should be wrapped in a resilient compression dressing and the extremity kept elevated. X-rays should be obtained early to determine whether there are fractures.

(4) Most patients, especially children, should be admitted to the hospital for observation.

j. Traumatic amputations may be partial or complete.

(1) Survival of partially amputated fingertips and digits depends on the presence of at least one intact neurovascular pedicle.

(2) Patients with complete fingertip amputations may bring the fingertip with them to the hospital. Ordinarily replacement is not recommended because of almost universal failure to survive. In rare instances (e.g., a clean, sharp amputation of a child's fingertip), replacement may be attempted.

(3) Skin from the amputated tissue, if not traumatized, can be used as graft coverage for the open wound.

(4) New techniques in microsurgery make reimplantation possible, even of distally amputated digits. The amputated part should be thoroughly cleansed, placed in a sterile wrapper, then placed in a plastic bag and immersed in ice. The proximal stump should be cleansed, a compression dressing applied, and a surgeon experienced in microsurgical techniques notified. With proper cooling of the amputated digit, successful reimplantation has been performed up to 33 hr after injury.

6. Dressings and splints

a. Wounds of the palm, dorsum of the hand, or wrist

(1) After wound closure, a piece of sterile nylon or fine-mesh gauze should be placed over the wound, followed by the application of several sterile gauze squares.

(2) Additional gauze squares are opened and placed in each interdigital cleft to absorb perspiration and prevent compression of the digital neurovascular bundles. More gauze squares are fluffed and applied around all sides of the hand and forearm to form a bulky dressing.

(3) If the injury does not involve the tips of the digits, they are left exposed in order to assay postoperatively the state of circulation and sensation.

(4) The gauze squares are held in place by a Kling bandage. If additional padding is necessary, 3-in. Webril is applied.

(5) The hand is then splinted in functional position: the wrist in 30 degrees of dorsiflexion, each digit in a gentle, semiflexed position, the thumb in abduction and opposition. It may be necessary to splint the hand to relieve tension on skin closure, tendon repair, or nerve anastomosis.

(6) A plaster splint of 12–14 thicknesses of 4-in. wide plaster strips is then applied and molded to the volar aspect of the palm and forearm. Cohesive works very well in holding the plaster splint and dressing in place; the 3-in. width is preferable.

b. **Wounds of the digits** The same general principles apply to dressing of individual digits. Immobilization promotes wound healing. If a laceration is confined to a digit, a foam-rubber aluminum splint should be applied with the digit in semiflexion.

c. **Follow-up care**

(1) If a wound has been prepared properly, debrided, and sutured with meticulous technique, the initial dressing ordinarily may be left in place for 7–10 days. If there is risk of infection or other complication, an inspection of the wound should be made earlier.

(2) **Sutures should not be removed too quickly** Palmar skin is thick and heals slowly. Sutures should be left in the palm for 2–3 wk. The skin of the dorsum of the hand and forearm heals more quickly, and sutures may be removed in 10–14 days.

D. **Infections in the hand**

1. **General principles**

a. **Examination** of the digits, hand, and forearm may reveal local or generalized swelling due to cellulitis (the diffuse stage of infection), discoloration, obvious abscess, red streaks of lymphangitis, or enlarged epitrochlear or axillary lymph glands.

b. The patient often complains of **throbbing pain** in the area of infection. The pain is accentuated when the hand is dependent. Pain is worse at night and may prevent the patient from sleeping.

c. Pitting **edema of the dorsum** of the hand is characteristic of all serious or deep infections of the hand. Swelling involves only the dorsum, since the skin there is loose, whereas the skin of the palm is anchored to the underlying fascia. This dorsal swelling has trapped more than one unwary surgeon into making an incision for drainage on the dorsum, only to find that no pus is present.

d. Infections should be examined and treated in a room adequately equipped and used only for treatment of infections. The room should be thoroughly cleansed after treatment of every infection.

e. One must decide whether the infected hand can be treated in the emergency room or in the main operating room. In general, infections confined to the digits can be treated in the emergency room if adequate equipment is available. Deep abscesses of the hand, forearm, and upper arm are best treated in an operating room.

f. Brief, accurate, and complete records must be kept. A simple diagram of an infected digit tells much more than a lengthy description in writing.

g. **Treatment of an infected hand is based on seven principles:**

(1) Immobilization to ensure rest of the part.

(2) Elevation to prevent or reduce swelling.

(3) Smear and culture of pus or exudate to determine bacterial sensitivities.

(4) Antibiotics as indicated by smear, culture, and sensitivity testing.

(5) Tetanus prophylaxis.

(6) Drainage of abscesses through properly placed incisions.

(7) Removal of all foreign material.

2. Management of early infections

a. In early, nonlocalized infections, there is a tender, red, swollen area in the hand. There is no fluctuance or other evidence of abscess formation. A wound of entry may be present. Lymphangitis and lymphadenopathy may or may not be found. The important feature in this type of infection is the absence of localized pus.

b. Treatment of an early infection in the absence of abscess is limited to **immobilization to enforce rest, elevation, antibiotic therapy, and tetanus prophylaxis** if indicated.

c. Hot, wet soaks have been an accepted and standard form of treatment of this type of infection. There are several disadvantages of this method, however. Frequent soaks militate against proper immobilization, may macerate the skin, and (if too hot) may cause serious burns. Neither hot or cold soaks are recommended.

d. The entire hand and forearm should be immobilized in the position of function using dry, bulky dressing, a splint, and a sling.

e. In the presence of an early infection without pus, it still may be possible to obtain material for smear, culture, and sensitivity testing. Sterile saline is carefully injected into the infected area and reaspirated. A small amount of the material is used to make a Gram-stained smear; the rest of the solution and the tip of the needle are dipped into a sterile broth culture tube.

f. Antibiotics are definitely indicated in early diffuse infections. Penicillin G is the drug of choice for most infections unless the patient gives a history of sensitivity to this drug. If a resistant staphylococcal infection is suspected, an appropriate penicillinase-resistant synthetic penicillin should be prescribed. If the patient gives a history of sensitivity to penicillin or is a highly allergic individual, erythromycin may be prescribed.

3. Diagnosis and management of **established infections and abscesses**

a. If pus is present, it must be evacuated immediately   Needle aspiration may be useful for diagnosis.

b. Differentiation must be made between the infected hand with pain, tenderness, cellulitis, and lymphangitis but without localized pus as opposed to the infected hand where pus is present. *If localized pus is not present and an incision is made, the infection will be aggravated, and septicemia may result.*

c. Give antibiotics 1 hr prior to incision and drainage. The purpose is to obtain an effective blood level to help prevent sepsis during operative manipulation of the abscess.

d. Felon (pulp abscess)

  (1) This is an **infection of the pulp tissues on the volar aspect of the fingertip** and often follows a minor penetrating wound. Do not confuse a felon with an intradermal blister or infection which may be simply debrided.

(2) As the infection progresses, the pulp area becomes indurated, swollen, discolored, and very tender.

(3) If pus is present, prompt drainage is best accomplished through a lateral incision after adequate anesthesia.

(4) Specimens of pus must be taken for smear, culture, and sensitivity testing. After drainage has been established, further care involves dressings, immobilization, elevation, and continuation of antibiotics.

e. Paronychia

(1) Paronychia is an **infection in the skin around the fingernail.** It is caused most frequently by the patient's picking and tearing at a hangnail.

(2) Paronychia may be acute or chronic. In the acute form, there may be subungual extension of the infection, with pus present under the fingernail.

(3) This infection is characterized by a red, swollen, and tender nail fold. There may be a droplet of pus visible along the cuticle or the pus may be present only in the tissues around the nail.

(4) Following digital block, the abscess is unroofed. If pus is present beneath the nail base, the eponychium is pushed proximally to expose the entire base of the nail. No incisions are required during this procedure. The nail base is elevated bluntly and the proximal portion of the nail removed with a sharp scissors.

(5) It is important to inspect the nail daily to prevent early adhesion of the nail fold to the nail. When signs of infection have subsided, soapy, warm water soaks several times daily should be encouraged.

f. Infection of the volar digital subcutaneous space

(1) This infection usually follows minor penetrating trauma to the digit on the volar aspect of the middle and proximal phalanges.

(2) One of the **common errors** in the diagnosis of hand infections is mistaking a volar subcutaneous space infection of a digit for a flexor tendon sheath infection (acute tenosynovitis). Inasmuch as methods of treatment of these two lesions are radically different, this differentiation must be made (see paragraph **g**, below).

(3) Examination of the infected finger will show the skin in the affected area to be red and warm. There is localized swelling, but usually not a fusiform enlargement of the entire digit as is seen in tenosynovitis. Light palpation over the course of the flexor tendon with the tip of a hemostat is helpful. The incision for drainage of pus is placed directly over the abscess and should follow the direction of Langer's lines. Incisions vertical to flexion creases on the digit must not be made. It is permissible, however, to design transverse or curving incisions. Extreme care must be taken to avoid puncture of the tendon sheath at the time of drainage.

g. **Acute suppurative tenosynovitis**

(1) These infections may result in a completely useless digit because of destruction of the tendon and surrounding structures. Tenderness localized over the tendon sheath is elicited by light pressure with a closed hemostat.

(2) A suppurative infection involving the tendons of the three central digits may burst through the tendon sheath into the palmar space. Infections of the thumb flexor tendon follow the tendon through the carpal tunnel into the radial bursa in the forearm. Infections of the fifth digit may follow the tendon sheath into the ulnar bursa of the forearm or may involve the tendon sheath of the thumb.

(3) **Diagnostic criteria of acute tenosynovitis are:**

(a) The skin of the involved digit may be hot and red.

(b) The digit is held in flexion.

(c) There is fusiform swelling of the infected digit.

(d) Exquisite pain is elicited by passive flexion and extension of the digit.

(4) If acute suppurative tenosynovitis is seen early, a thin, seropurulent exudate frequently is present. It may be possible to abort the infection with immobilization, elevation, and large doses of antibiotics. Careful, frequent reexamination of the digit must be performed.

(5) If surgical drainage is indicated by the presence of pus in the tendon sheath, general anesthesia or a brachial plexus or axillary block is necessary. Antibiotics should be given at least 1 hr before operation. Expose the distal and proximal portions of the tendon sheath and irrigate with an antibiotic solution.

h. **Web space infections**

(1) These infections are situated in the fatty tissue of the distal palm in the interdigital clefts. They may be the result of penetrating trauma or a blister which has opened and become infected.

(2) Examination reveals erythema, pain, swelling, and tenderness. The involved digits may be held in abduction but can be flexed and extended without exquisite tenderness.

(3) It may be quite difficult to tell whether or not localized pus has formed in a web space infection.

(4) If pus is present, immediate incision and drainage of the web space are indicated.

(5) A longitudinal incision is made over the infection just proximal to the digital cleft. These infections may burrow to the dorsum of the hand. The entire cavity must be unroofed.

i. Abscesses of the palm

(1) These infections are situated deep to the palmar fascia. They may occur in conjunction with a suppurative tenosynovitis. Sometimes the abscess may be confined to either the thenar or middle palmar space, but most commonly pus is spread diffusely throughout the palm.

(2) Examination of the hand will show marked swelling, with the digits held relatively immobile in a flexed position. The skin color may be normal but usually is red or purple and hot to the touch. The palm is extremely tender to palpation. Pitting edema of the dorsum is practically always present. Fever and lymph gland enlargement are common.

(3) Treatment of a deep palmar abscess is a serious matter and requires full operating room facilities, including the hemostatic tourniquet, adequate light, instruments, dressings, and assistants.

(4) Neglected palmar abscesses may cause compression of the median nerve; decompression of the median nerve by incising the transverse carpal ligament then is indicated, with concomitant drainage of the abscess.

SUGGESTED READING

De Jong, R. E.   Modified axillary block with block of the lateral antibrachial cutaneous nerve. *Anesthesiology* 26:615, 1965.

Rank, B. K., Wakefield, A. R., and Hueston, J. T.   *Surgery of Repair as Applied to Hand Injuries* (4th ed.). Baltimore: Williams & Wilkins, 1973.

Winnie, A. P.   Interscaline brachial block. *Anesth. Analg.* (Cleve.) 49:455, 1970.

3. CARDIAC ARRHYTHMIAS

I. GENERAL COMMENTS   An ECG, preferably displayed on both a monitoring oscilloscope and a direct writing recorder, is necessary for the diagnosis and treatment of an arrhythmia. The significance of an arrhythmia depends on the specific type of abnormal rhythm and its effect on the state of the entire circulatory system. Dangerous arrhythmias may:

A. Decrease myocardial contractility and cardiac output, thus leading to ischemia of major organs, i.e., brain, liver, and kidney.

B. Result in congestive heart failure and pulmonary edema.

C. Lead to cardiac arrest.

D. Predispose to intracardiac thrombosis with subsequent embolization.

E. Be the first indication of underlying cardiac pathological disorder, i.e., silent myocardial infarction or preinfarction syndrome.

II. ETIOLOGY

A. Coronary artery disease leading to myocardial ischemia and infarction.

B. Hypertensive heart disease.

C. Rheumatic heart disease predisposing to myocarditis and valvular heart disease.

D. Cardiomyopathy.

E. Hypoxemia secondary to inadequate respiratory exchange, e.g., pneumothorax, atelectasis, airway obstruction, and pleural effusion.

F. Acid-base and electrolyte disturbances, e.g., hypokalemia due to prolonged gastrointestinal fluid loss, and hyperkalemia associated with renal shutdown.

G. Septicemia, particularly gram-negative.

H. Drugs, especially digitalis, diuretics, quinidine, and catecholamines.

I. Congenital heart disease, e.g., atrial septal defect, Ebstein's disease, and congenital heart block.

J. Trauma, e.g., myocardial contusion and postoperative conduction defect.

K. Neoplasm or inflammation of the myocardium or pericardium.

L. Operative procedures such as endoscopy, pneumonectomy, and open cardiotomy.

III. TYPES OF ARRHYTHMIA (Fig. 3-1)

A. Sinus arrhythmia is due to changes in vagal tone during the respiratory cycle, resulting in an increase in heart rate during inspiration (short R-R interval) and a slowing during expiration (long R-R interval). It is common in children and young adults and has no clinical significance.

B. Sinus tachycardia presents as a **rate of 100–165/min in adults** with a normal sinus mechanism and **up to 210/min in children.** It may be initiated by emotional stress, exercise, fever, anoxia, hypotension, hyperthyroidism, anemia, heart failure, catecholamines, or atropine. If it is allowed to persist, congestive heart failure may ensue.

C. Supraventricular tachycardia of infancy presents as a **rate greater than 210/min** (often 240-260/min) and will result in cardiac failure if the arrhythmia persists over 24 hr. After reversion to a normal mechanism, ischemic changes may be visible on the ECG for several days.

D. Sinus bradycardia is due to increased vagal tone. There is a normal sinus mechanism with a **rate of 45-60/min.** It may occur with increased intracra-

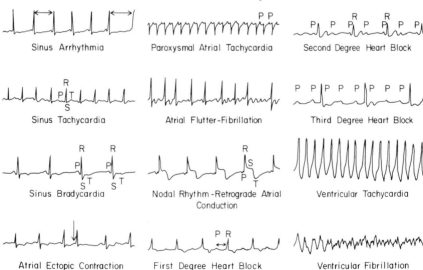

Sinus Arrhythmia   Paroxysmal Atrial Tachycardia   Second Degree Heart Block

Sinus Tachycardia   Atrial Flutter-Fibrillation   Third Degree Heart Block

Sinus Bradycardia   Nodal Rhythm -Retrograde Atrial Conduction   Ventricular Tachycardia

Atrial Ectopic Contraction   First Degree Heart Block   Ventricular Fibrillation

Figure 3-1. Typical electrocardiograms (lead II) of cardiac arrhythmias.

nial pressure, myxedema, traction on the intestinal mesentery, and during general anesthesia, and is seen without other pathological disorders in athletes, elderly patients, and during sleep. If cardiac output is impaired, hypotension will result.

E. **Sick sinus syndrome** presents as an apparent bradycardia, often just after a period of exercise or other activity which has induced a sinus tachycardia. The rate of 25-55/min does not respond to usual doses of atropine or isoproterenol. Attacks of syncope or dizziness occur as a result of the bradycardia itself or as a result of episodes of sinus arrest during which there is a delayed appearance of atrial, nodal, or ventricular escape rhythm.

F. **Ectopic (premature) contraction** is the most frequent type of arrhythmia and arises from ectopic foci in the atrium, atrioventricular (AV) node, or ventricle. This arrhythmia is recognized by the **compensatory pause** following the extrasystole.

G. **Paroxysmal atrial tachycardia (PAT)** presents as an **atrial rate of 150-220/ min** with a 1:1 ventricular response. This arrhythmia may be seen in the absence of other cardiac disease and usually responds to vagal stimulation (carotid massage or Valsalva's maneuver). When associated with second degree AV block, PAT may be a manifestation of digitalis intoxication or hypokalemia. ECG diagnosis may be difficult since the nonconducted P-wave may be buried in the T-wave. Helpful diagnostic procedures include carotid sinus pressure, an esophageal ECG lead, or direct recording from an atrial pacing wire previously placed during surgery.

H. **Atrial flutter and fibrillation**   The **atrial rate is 250-350/min in flutter and 400-700/min in fibrillation.** The ventricular rate (60-180/min) varies with the degree of AV block and may be regular or irregular with flutter but always is irregular with atrial fibrillation. In atrial fibrillation, there is a discrepancy between the precordial rate and the radial pulse rate. This **pulse deficit** is secondary to the variations in ventricular volume and filling time. These arrhythmias are associated with acquired mitral valvular disease, coronary artery disease, pneumonectomy, pneumonia, and hyperthyroidism. Symptoms are present when the ventricular rate is very rapid (exceeding 130/min), resulting in decreased diastolic filling and cardiac output, and may be manifest as congestive heart failure, syncope, focal neurological deficit, or hepatic or renal insufficiency. Atrial fibrillation often is associated with atrial stasis and thrombosis. Emboli to the brain, kidney, extremities, spleen, or GI tract occur in 30% of fibrillating patients.

I. **Nodal rhythm** results from sinoatrial node inhibition and failure of the atrium to take over the pacemaker function of the heart. It may result from reflex vagal stimulation (bronchoscopy, tension on bowel mesentery), posterior wall myocardial infarction, or digitalis intoxication.

J. **Heart block** is associated with **prolongation of AV nodal conduction time.** It may result from interruption of the conduction pathway (infarction, surgery) or from a prolonged nodal refractory period secondary to increased vagal tone. Drugs that prolong AV conduction time include digitalis, potassium, quinidine, and procainamide.

1. **First degree heart block** is present if the P-R interval exceeds 0.2 sec in adults but is rarely responsible for symptoms or significant alteration in cardiac function.

2. **Second degree heart block** occurs when there is intermittent failure of AV conduction so that every second or third impulse (2:1 or 3:1 block) from the atrium is conducted to the ventricle. In Wenckebach's phenomenon, a form of second degree block, there is a gradual, progressive increase of the P-R interval until one P-wave is not conducted to the ventricles (dropped beat). The next subsequent P-wave is conducted and the entire sequence repeats. Patients with second degree block due to a myocardial infarction should be monitored continuously since they may suddenly develop complete heart block with asystole.

3. **Complete (third degree) heart block** occurs when the AV node is completely refractory and fails to conduct any impulses from the atrium to the ventricle. There is an idioventricular rate of 30-50/min. A few patients are asymptomatic, but most have symptoms of cerebral ischemia (dizziness, loss of memory), syncopal episodes or convulsions associated with asystole (Adams-Stokes attacks—failure of the ventricles to initiate an impulse), and congestive heart failure due to a failure of the chronotropic demand response for increased myocardial contractility during activity.

4. **Implantation of an artificial pacemaker** is indicated in all patients with symptomatic heart block. Temporary myocardial pacing wires usually are placed in patients with evidence of conduction abnormalities following open-heart surgery. In fact, pacing wires probably should be placed in all patients undergoing cardiac surgery. If there is persistence of the conduction defect for more than 3 wk postoperatively, a permanent pacemaker is implanted.

5. Complete heart block associated with an acute myocardial infarction carries a high mortality and should be treated by the immediate placement of a temporary transvenous endocardial catheter electrode.

K. **Wolff-Parkinson-White syndrome** is a conduction abnormality found more frequently in young adults and is due to an increase in impulse conduction time between the atrium and the ventricle. It may result in an abnormal site of ventricular activation secondary to an aberrant conduction pathway. The P-R interval is less than 0.12 sec and a distorted QRS complex is present with a delta wave. Symptoms occur during episodes of tachycardia and may lead to sudden death from a ventricular arrhythmia.

L. **Ventricular tachycardia** is a **rapid (150-250/min), slightly irregular rhythm arising in an irritable ectopic ventricular focus** which constitutes a life-threatening emergency because of impaired cardiac output, decreased coronary perfusion, and a tendency to progress to ventricular fibrillation. The ECG reveals bizarre, slightly irregular QRS complexes. Carotid massage does not decrease the heart rate. Ventricular tachycardia is due to severe myocardial ischemia (70% of cases), digitalis intoxication, electrolyte disturbances, hypoxia, heart block during Adams-Stokes attacks, or excessive catecholamine administration. Patients who have undergone prolonged anoxic cardiac arrest or inadequate coronary perfusion during cardiac surgery may exhibit multifocal premature ventricular contractions which may progress to ventricular tachycardia and fibrillation.

M. **Ventricular fibrillation** (see Chap. 4) is characterized by irregular, uncoordinated movements of the ventricular muscle and is accompanied by complete cessation of ventricular ejection and peripheral organ perfusion. It is usually caused by myocardial ischemia, but also may be due to drug toxicity (digitalis, quinidine, procainamide), exposure to high voltage electricity, hypoxemia, trauma, and renal and hepatic failure. Ventricular fibrillation probably is the terminal event in adult cases of sudden unexplained death in which no anatomical cause can be found. Treatment must be instituted within 3-4 min to avoid permanent brain damage.

IV. TREATMENT

A. During arrhythmia conversion, the **ECG should be monitored** continuously. Treatment of specific arrhythmias is outlined in Table 3-1.

TABLE 3-1. Treatment of Arrhythmia

Arrhythmia	Treatments (in order of preference)	Comment
Sinus tachycardia	Correct underlying cause	Digitalis only for heart failure
Sinus bradycardia	Atropine, isoproterenol, cardiac pacing	
Supraventricular tachycardia of childhood	Digitalis, carotid sinus pressure	If untreated, will result in cardiac failure within 24 hr
Sick sinus syndrome	Ventricular pacemaker	Cardiac arrest due to sinus arrest with absent escape rhythm
Premature atrial ectopic beats	Sedation, quinidine, atropine	
Premature ventricular ectopic beats	Lidocaine, treat digitalis intoxication, procainamide, diphenylhydantoin, quinidine	If multifocal, may lead to ventricular fibrillation
Paroxysmal atrial tachycardia	Sedation, vagal stimulation, vasopressors, digitalis, cardioversion, propranolol, atrial pacing	If associated with block, may be secondary to digitalis intoxication
Atrial flutter	Digitalis, cardioversion	
Atrial fibrillation	Digitalis, cardioversion	Administer quinidine before elective cardioversion
Complete heart block	Isoproterenol, cardiac pacing	Prepare for insertion of a permanent pacemaker
Wolff-Parkinson-White syndrome	Digitalis, quinidine, cardioversion, atrial pacing	In refractory cases, surgical transection of anomalous pathway may be indicated
Ventricular tachycardia	Sedation, lidocaine, procainamide, cardioversion, diphenylhydantoin	May lead to ventricular fibrillation

TABLE 3-2. Drugs Used in Arrhythmia Therapy

Drug	Dosage	Comment
Lanatoside C	**Adult, IV:** 0.8 mg, then 0.2 mg every 2 hr	
Digoxin	**Adult, IV:** 0.75 mg initially, then 0.25 mg every 4-6 hr to effect or total of 1.5 mg **Adult, oral:** total digitalizing dose 2-3 mg over 48 hr; maintenance, 0.25-0.50 mg/day **Children over age 2:** digitalizing dose, up to 40 μg/kg orally in divided doses over 24 hr; maintenance is ¼ the total digitalizing dose **Children under age 2:** digitalizing dose, up to 100 μg/kg IM in divided doses over 24 hr; start with ¼ total dose, give remainder in divided doses over next 12-18 hr; maintenance is ¼ the total digitalizing dose	Digitalize with ECG control to note effect. Suspect toxicity if nausea, vomiting, diarrhea, yellow vision, or arrhythmia occurs. Up to 12 hr after cardiac surgery, the heart is extremely sensitive to digitalis. Treat toxicity with 40-60 mEq of potassium chloride plus 5 units of regular insulin in 500 ml 10% dextrose in water infused over 2-4 hr. Monitor ECG to avoid hyperkalemia (tented T-waves)
Digitoxin	**Oral:** 1.0-1.5 mg over 48 hr; maintenance, 0.1 mg/day	
Diphenylhydantoin (Dilantin)	**IV or oral:** 100 mg every 8 hr	May produce hypotension
Isoproterenol	**IV:** dilute 1 mg in 250 ml 5% dextrose in water	Maintain heart rate below 120/min by adjusting dose; may cause ventricular irritability
Lidocaine	**IV:** 40-60 mg, may be repeated in 15 min	Can cause convulsions and myocardial depression
Procainamide	**Oral:** 0.5-1.0 gm initially, then 500 mg every 2-4 hr until toxicity occurs or arrhythmia is interrupted; maintenance, 500 mg every 4-6 hr **IM:** 200-500 mg every 6 hr **IV:** 200-500 mg (not to exceed 25 mg/min)	Toxicity indicated by widening of QRS complex and prolongation of P-R and Q-T intervals; can decrease blood pressure by peripheral vasodilation; not to be used in the presence of complete AV block
Propranolol	**Oral:** 5-20 mg every 6 hr **IV:** 0.5 mg increments to a maximum of 6 mg	Use with great caution in patients with low cardiac output; may potentiate congestive heart failure
Quinidine sulfate	**Oral:** 200-300 mg every 4-6 hr	Toxicity manifested by blurred vision, hypotension, paradoxical tachycardia (prevented by prior digitalization), or increase in Q-T interval; contraindicated in heart block; therapeutic blood levels 3-8 mg/liter

B. A functioning **defibrillator** with paddles, laryngoscope, endotracheal tube, and anesthesia bag connected to oxygen should be at the bedside. **Drug actions** are summarized in Table 3-2.

C. **Vagal stimulation** can be initiated by the Valsalva maneuver (have the patient inhale deeply, hold his breath, and bear down hard against the closed glottis as he slowly counts to 10) or by unilateral carotid sinus massage (the carotid bifurcation is compressed with the fingers against the posterior cervical vertebrae for not more than 3–5 sec). Carotid sinus massage should not be performed on patients with cerebral vascular disease or a carotid bruit.

D. **Electrical defibrillation** with a direct current instrument that can deliver a shock of up to 400 watt-sec.

E. **Cardioversion** with an instrument capable of delivering a direct current shock of 50–400 watt-sec that can be synchronized to follow the R-wave by exactly 20 msec.

F. **Cardiac pacing** may be instituted by passing a transvenous endocardial catheter under fluoroscopic control into the right ventricle. Flow-directed (balloon-tipped) pacing catheters can be used in emergency situations when fluoroscopic facilities are not immediately available. The safest method of pacing the heart is with a battery-operated electrical stimulator.

SUGGESTED READING

Ferrer, M. I.   The sick sinus syndrome. *Circulation* 47:635, 1973.

Levitsky, S., and Hastreiter, A.   Cardiovascular surgical emergencies in the first year of life. *Surg. Clin. North Am.* 52:61, 1971.

Sealy, W. C., Boineau, J. P., and Wallace, A. G.   The identification and division of the bundle of Kent for premature ventricular excitation and supraventricular tachycardia. *Surgery* 68:1009, 1970.

4. CARDIAC ARREST

I. DEFINITION AND GENERAL COMMENTS Cardiorespiratory arrest is the **sudden cessation of effective circulation or respiration.** Either one may be the primary event but failure of the other quickly follows, and both must be restored for survival. In the interval between these events and the onset of cellular death, resuscitation may be performed without irreversible sequelae. The extent of the grace period depends on the degree of preexisting cellular hypoxia and whether circulatory or respiratory failure occurs first. The brain, being almost totally dependent on aerobic metabolism, is the organ least able to withstand hypoxia. Following circulatory arrest the pupils begin to dilate in 30-40 sec, respiration ceases within 60 sec because of medullary depression, and in the normothermic adult, serious brain damage ensues within 2-4 min, depending on the level of cerebral oxygenation at the moment of arrest. If respiratory failure occurs first, the circulation may continue for up to 5 min with diminishing effect, and brain damage may not become irreversible for 4-6 min or even longer.

    A. Cardiac arrest may be manifest as:

        1. Mechanical asystole, which accounts for 80% of cardiac arrests occurring in the operating and recovery rooms. Fortunately, this type of arrest is the most amenable to reversal.

        2. Ventricular fibrillation, which accounts for 75% of arrests in intensive care units and is the most common form of arrest following myocardial infarction.

        3. Ineffective ventricular contraction, which produces an inadequate cardiac output and may be caused by hypoxia or arrhythmia.

    B. Respiratory arrest may be manifest as:

    1. Cessation of effective mechanical breathing.

    2. Ineffective gas exchange or transport.

II. ETIOLOGY The mechanisms of sudden cardiac and respiratory arrest are multiple, complex, and interrelated. In nearly all patients the **common denominator is hypoxia,** alone or in conjunction with other factors.

A. **Usual causes of respiratory arrest**

   1. **Airway obstruction** by foreign body, vomitus, blood, mucus, or laryngeal or bronchial spasm.

   2. **CNS depression** by head trauma, stroke, hypercapnia, or overdosage of a barbiturate, narcotic, tranquilizer, or anesthetic agent.

   3. **Neuromuscular failure** secondary to poliomyelitis, muscular dystrophy, myasthenia, or curare-like drug overdosage.

B. **Usual causes of either cardiac or respiratory arrest** (all result in ineffective gas exchange)

   1. **Flail chest.**

   2. **Pneumothorax.**

   3. **Massive atelectasis.**

   4. **Acute pulmonary embolization.**

   5. **Alveolar-capillary block** from congestive failure, overwhelming pneumonia, lung burn, gram-negative septicemia, or heavy metal poisoning.

   6. **Carbon monoxide poisoning.**

C. **Usual causes of cardiac arrest**

   1. **Low cardiac output** resulting from cardiac tamponade, shock, sudden arrhythmia, or toxic myocarditis.

   2. **Hypercapnia** secondary to asthenia, obesity, chronic lung disease, or faulty anesthetic technique (especially unrecognized postoperative muscle paralysis).

   3. **Hyperkalemia** following rapid transfusion of cold banked blood or excessive potassium replacement therapy in the presence of low urine output.

   4. **Vagal stimulation and hypoxia** associated with drowning, intubation or aspiration, traction on abdominal viscera, cor pulmonale, or pain.

   5. **Direct stimulation of the heart** by an intracardiac catheter or electrode or during operative displacement or manipulation of the heart.

   6. **Coronary occlusion** by embolus, thrombus, or ligature, or replacement of coronary blood flow by contrast medium.

   7. **Drug sensitivity or overdosage** of cardiac glycosides, catecholamines, or anesthetic agents, especially cyclopropane, trichloroethylene, or halothane.

8. Uncontrolled hypothermia from exposure, rapid transfusion of cold banked blood, or use of an ineffective heat exchanger.

9. Hyperthermia, especially in children.

10. Acidosis secondary to diabetes mellitus, inefficient extracorporeal circulation, pancreatic fistula, renal failure, or starvation.

11. Electric shock.

12. Hypocalcemia or hypercalcemia, especially in infants.

III. PREVENTION   Conditions tending to promote cardiorespiratory arrest are usually preventable. Errors most often are those of omission. There are **three cardinal rules:**

A. Identify the high-risk patient by careful attention to a history of cardiac, renal, or pulmonary disease, diabetes, drug allergy, alcohol or opiate addiction, and bleeding tendencies. Patients receiving steroids, digitalis, diuretics, or anticoagulants need particular attention.

B. Obtain adequate data to detect and correct serious aberrations. Particular attention should be paid to the following points:

1. Maintenance of adequate circulating blood volume and normal concentrations of electrolytes.

2. Judicious choice of preoperative medication, particularly in patients with respiratory insufficiency and in anxious and apprehensive patients.

3. Vagal stimulation by intubation or other maneuvers during induction of anesthesia should be carried out only when the patient is well oxygenated.

4. Blood loss during operation should be measured and replaced as it occurs. Interference with venous return (e.g., pressure on the inferior vena cava) must be avoided.

5. Arterial blood gases and pH must be monitored frequently, especially in the early postoperative period.

6. Respiratory insufficiency must be expected and watched for closely, postoperatively. During recovery from anesthesia, respiratory drive often is depressed and oxygen supplementation or mechanical assistance with a ventilator may be needed. A patient who is well oxygenated immediately after operation may still develop progressive hypercapnia and hypoxia in the early postoperative period, triggering an irritable myocardium into ventricular fibrillation.

C. Avoid dangerous maneuvers known to have a high risk of cardiac arrest. Tracheal suctioning in a hypoxic patient often is the setting for arrest in the postoperative period. Electronic monitors may be a source of small leakage currents, which may lead to ventricular fibrillation.

IV. DIAGNOSIS

   A. Early (prodromal, prearrest) symptoms and signs

      1. CNS: restlessness, anxiety, disorientation, combativeness. A previously cooperative patient who becomes difficult to manage postoperatively is much more likely to be hypoxemic than psychotic.

      2. Respiratory: dyspnea, tachypnea, gasping, gurgling, laryngeal stridor, wheezing, pallor, cyanosis.

      3. Cardiovascular: mottling, cyanosis, peripheral venous distension, weak or irregular pulse, hypotension, profuse sweating.

   B. Late symptoms and signs indicating that cardiorespiratory arrest is present

      1. Absence of pulse in major arteries.

      2. Absence of audible or visible breathing or the presence of gasping respirations; respiratory arrest usually follows circulatory arrest by 45-60 sec.

      3. Dilation of pupils is seen 1-2 min after complete arrest and indicates beginning of damage to the anoxic brain.

      4. Sluggish, dark-colored bleeding at operative site.

      5. Flaccidity.

      6. Convulsions.

V. TREATMENT   The aims are the earliest possible **restoration of effective circulation** and recognition and **correction of the cause** of the arrest. Resuscitation alone is not sufficient. The grave threat of recurrent arrest can be averted only by correcting the physiological derangements precipitating arrest and by appreciating and correcting the damage caused by the arrest itself. Every arrest results in serious functional derangements. Ventilation-perfusion relationships are altered by creation of a functional AV shunt which results in hypoxia despite ventilation with pure oxygen. Increased physiological dead space produces hypercapnia. Cardiac output is markedly reduced; peripheral arterial flow often is 30-50% of normal. Tricuspid and mitral regurgitation resulting from cardiac compression during resuscitation elevates venous pressure and produces venous stasis. Mean arterial pressure is reduced and low tissue perfusion pressure results. Severe and progressive metabolic acidosis causes peripheral vasodilation, pooling of blood, and further impairment of circulation. Adequate provision must be made to cope with these events.

   A. Steps in cardiorespiratory resuscitation (Fig. 4-1)
      A—Airway.
      B—Breathing.
      C—Circulation.
      D—Definitive therapy: diagnosis, defibrillation, drugs, disposition.

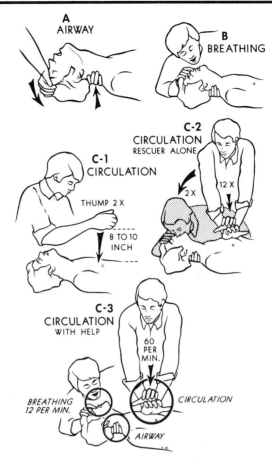

Figure 4-1. The essential steps in cardiopulmonary resuscitation are establish an airway (A), restore breathing (B), and restore circulation (C).

B. Respiratory resuscitation

1. **Airway**   Establishing a patent airway is the most important single step in successful resuscitation. Put one hand under the back of the shoulders, lift the head and neck slightly upward, and push down on the forehead, thus hyperextending the head. Next, shift the tongue forward to open the airway by lifting the vertical rami of the mandible. Foreign material in the mouth or pharynx is manually removed.

2. **Breathing**   Ventilation of the lungs is the crucial prerequisite to cardiac massage. If the patient does not spontaneously begin to breathe as his airway is opened, mouth-to-mouth ventilation is begun immediately. Cover the patient's mouth tightly with your own (a single-thickness hand-kerchief may be interposed) and pinch the patient's nose. Take a deep

breath and blow until the patient's chest rises. Remove your mouth and allow passive expiration to occur. Repeat 12 times/min. The patient's chest must rise, his lungs must produce resistance as they inflate, and air must be felt to escape during expiration, otherwise ventilation is not adequate. The exhaled air of the rescuer, who doubles his own ventilation, is about 18% oxygen and 2% carbon dioxide, an adequate composition for resuscitation. In infants and children, both the nose and mouth can be covered by the resuscitator's mouth. Care must be taken not to overinflate the lungs. The lungs are inflated 20-30 times/min in infants.

3. A portable self-filling, nonrebreathing bag and tight-fitting mask may be used as soon as they are available. Tracheal intubation minimizes the danger of regurgitation and aspiration but should not be attempted except by a skilled person, and then not until the patient is well oxygenated by external ventilation and circulation has been restored.

C. Cardiac resuscitation

1. **Circulation**   After four or five effective lung inflations, feel for the carotid pulse. If it is absent, place the patient on the floor unless a bed board is immediately at hand. Strike the sternum sharply with the fist; this may stimulate the heart to beat, especially in cardiac asystole. If a carotid pulse is not felt in 2 or 3 sec, begin external cardiac compression. Even in the operating room, external compression should be tried before thoracotomy is considered. Apply pressure with the heel of one hand covered by the second hand over the lower fourth of the sternum in the midline. Do not apply pressure over the xiphoid, as laceration of the liver may result. Do not touch the chest wall with the fingers. Hold the elbows straight to minimize fatigue. Lean the weight of your torso toward the patient until the sternum in the adult is compressed 1.5-2 in. Extra pressure does not produce greater blood flow and may fracture the sternum. Compression time of $\frac{1}{2}$ sec is followed by sudden release for an interval of 1 sec accomplished by shifting your weight backward. Release of pressure should be complete but the hands should remain in position in contact with the lower fourth of the sternum, lest the hands shift and ribs or underlying viscera be injured. Compression should be at the rate of 60/min and should never be interrupted for more than 5 sec. In small children only the heel of one hand is used. In infants, encircle the chest with both hands and exert midsternal pressure with the thumbs; compression rate should be 100/min and displacement only $\frac{1}{2}$-$\frac{3}{4}$ in. If you are alone, hold the infant's head hyperextended with one hand and compress the sternum with the other, holding your thumb on the spine and two fingers over the sternum. In children and adults, if only one rescuer is available, he should ventilate the patient two times, then compress the sternum 12 times at the rate of 1/sec. Carotid pulses should be checked repeatedly. The pupils are the best means of judging results. Maintenance of pupillary constriction, following previous dilation, is evidence that oxygenated blood is reaching the brain.

2. **Diagnosis and definitive therapy**   As soon as help is available and both ventilation and effective massage have been started, then:

   a. **Start an IV,** preferably in a large vein, using an IV catheter.

b. Inject sodium bicarbonate (NaHCO$_3$), one ampule (4.75 gm or 44.6 mEq) in adults; use half this dose in children. Repeat every 8 min until arterial blood gas and pH values are available to guide treatment. Acidosis, always present and usually severe, inhibits cardiac resuscitation. Moderate overcorrection is transitory and seldom harmful.

c. Begin ECG monitoring. Placement of lead II is sufficient.

d. If the ECG shows fibrillation, carry out **external defibrillation.** Apply two well-pasted electrodes firmly on the chest wall over the long axis of the heart. Start with an external direct current stimulus of 200 watt-sec in an adult; if ineffective, progress stepwise to 500 watt-sec. If unsuccessful, resume massage, and:

(1) Improve myocardial oxygenation by improving ventilatory resuscitation.

(2) Warm the patient with hot water bags, heating pads, or a hyperthermia blanket if body temperature is below 34°C (93.2°F).

(3) Give epinephrine, 0.5 ml of a 1:1,000 concentration diluted in 10 ml of saline, slowly IV. The fibrillatory status of the heart is enhanced by cardiotonic drugs. Weak, fine fibrillations are converted into coarse, stronger ones.

(4) Isoproterenol HCl, 0.1-0.3 mg IV every 3-5 min, also may be used and has a positive inotropic effect but causes peripheral vasodilation, decreasing effective perfusion pressure. If used, it should be given with a vasoconstrictor, e.g., phenylephrine HCl, 3-5 mg.

(5) Repeat NaHCO$_3$ unless pH is normal.

(6) Eliminate irritable foci by giving a myocardial depressant such as procainamide, 200 mg, or lidocaine, 50 mg. The concomitant use of cardiotonic and cardioplegic drugs poses no paradox; each has its specific purposes.

e. When **fibrillation ceases or is converted** and the heart is beating too slowly, too weakly, or not at all:

(1) Give calcium chloride (CaCl$_2$), 0.5-1.0 gm IV and repeat every 8 min. The cardiotonic effect of calcium results from correction of the imbalance of potassium ions across the myocardial cell membrane.

(2) Give atropine, 0.4-0.6 mg IV, for marked bradycardia with supraventricular rhythm. If effective, repeat in 15 min.

(3) Give isoproterenol HCl, 8.0 mg in 500 ml of 5% dextrose in water by IV drip, to control bradycardia resulting from heart block. The rate of drip is determined by the patient's response.

(4) Start external cardiac pacing by transvenous (cephalic or external jugular) transthoracic myocardial or epicardial electrodes if complete or progressive heart block is present or if there is refractory bradycardia or myocardial irritability.

f. Closed or open cardiac resuscitation   External cardiac compression with closed chest offers the best chance of successful resuscitation, even in arrest which occurs in the operating room. The following are the rare indications for open resuscitation:

(1) The cause of arrest is within the chest, e.g., cardiac tamponade.

(2) Only an internal defibrillator is available.

(3) The chest is already open in the course of a thoracic operation.

(4) There is tension pneumothorax or a flail chest.

(5) The patient is very obese or barrel-chested, so that external cardiac compression is ineffective.

VI. POSTRESUSCITATION CARE   Underlying conditions leading to the cardiorespiratory arrest must be corrected or arrest will recur.

A. All or nearly all patients should be intubated and ventilation should be assisted or controlled by a respirator. Scrupulous attention to removal of airway secretions is always required. Hyperventilation with mild alkalosis produces a tractable patient who does not fight the respirator, helps compensate for residual or recurrent metabolic acidosis, and reduces the danger of interrupting ventilation for suctioning.

B. Arterial pressure, pulmonary artery pressure (Swan-Ganz catheter), and ECG are monitored constantly.

C. Arterial blood gases, pH, and serum electrolytes are determined frequently enough to permit maintenance of normal values.

D. IV vasopressors, cardiotonic drugs, antacids, and antiarrhythmic agents should be used as indicated.

E. Patients not already digitalized should receive lanatoside C or digoxin.

F. The osmotic diuretic agents urea and mannitol may help prevent renal failure. Do not use furosemide or ethacrynic acid unless fluid overload is present. Do not use any diuretic until some spontaneous urine output is assured.

SUMMARY OF MANAGEMENT OF CARDIAC ARREST

1. Despite philosophical discussions of selection of patients for resuscitation, most surgical patients are salvageable and merit an all-out effort.

2. Confirm diagnosis (apneic, pulseless) and suitability for resuscitation. Summon help. Note time. TIME IS CRITICAL. You have 2-4 min to reestablish ventilation and cardiac output.

3. Rotate patient's mandible forward, clear airway, and give 3 or 4 rapid mouth-to-mouth ventilations.

4. Thump chest sharply 1 or 2 times; this occasionally will reestablish heartbeat.

5. Place patient on hard surface and begin external massage, 60 compressions/min. Use steady firm compression to depress lower sternum 1 in. Avoid jabbing blows. Mouth-to-mouth ventilation should continue at 12-16 cycles/min. If alone, perform 12 compressions followed by two ventilations, and repeat this sequence continuously. **Do not stop massage longer than 30 sec until effective spontaneous heartbeat is restored.** Have an assistant monitor pupils and carotid pulses for effectiveness of compression.

6. Insert oral airway and provide 100% oxygen ventilation via tight-fitting mask. Insert endotracheal tube if skilled at doing so, but do not waste time attempting endotracheal intubation if not immediately successful. Ventilation via mask and oral airway is adequate for resuscitation.

7. Give sodium bicarbonate, 44.6 mEq (1 ampule) IV, and repeat bicarbonate administration every 5-10 min until spontaneous cardiac function is restored and the pH is normal.

8. Monitor ECG and determine if arrest is caused by fibrillation or asystole.

9. If fibrillating, after oxygenation is restored by ventilation and cardiac massage, defibrillate with direct current countershock, 200-500 watt-sec. Repeat if not immediately effective.

10. If unable to defibrillate, give epinephrine. In certain instances, 10% calcium chloride or 50% glucose may also be effective. Repeat defibrillation countershock.

11. For excessive ventricular irritability, lidocaine, 50 mg IV, is of value but only after restoration of cardiac function.

12. If asystole exists and does not respond to ventilation and massage, 10% calcium chloride is often effective. Epinephrine, glucose, and isoproterenol also may be helpful.

13. Dexamethasone may be useful for reduction of cerebral edema and for its cardiotonic effect if the period of arrest has been prolonged.

14. Diagnose and treat the cause of arrest. A common cause of arrest after open-heart operations is cardiac tamponade. In such cases, closed massage may be mechanically ineffective. Should tamponade be suspected, the chest should be reopened immediately and open massage instituted, taking care to avoid direct myocardial damage consequent to overzealous squeezing. Morbidity from reopening the chest is of considerably less danger than is refractory arrest from tamponade.

15. Monitor vital signs, pH and blood gases, ECG, and fluid intake and output. BE READY FOR SUBSEQUENT EPISODES OF ARREST IN THIS PATIENT.

G. Dexamethasone or other steroids will minimize cerebral edema.

H. Selected patients may benefit from prolonged moderate hypothermia 30–31°C (86–87.8°F).

SUGGESTED READING

American Heart Association and National Academy of Sciences, National Research Council Standards for Cardiopulmonary Resuscitation (CPR) and Emergency Cardiac Care (ECC). *J.A.M.A.* 227 (Suppl. Feb. 18), 1974.

Goldberg, A. H. Current concepts: Cardiopulmonary arrest. *N. Engl. J. Med.* 290:381, 1974.

5. ACUTE ABDOMINAL PAIN

Pain, along with hemorrhage, represents a catastrophe of great moment in the life of any patient. Abdominal pain is among the most frightening of all, since the connotation to the patient experiencing it encompasses the entire gamut of catastrophes. Abdominal pain is the most common presenting complaint in patients with acute surgical disease of the abdomen (Table 5-1). It is incumbent upon the surgeon first to decide what is the most likely diagnosis; second, to prove that diagnosis to be correct; and then to undertake treatment indicated for that diagnosis. In the course of investigating a patient with abdominal pain, it is extremely important that no analgesics or sedatives ever be given until a decision is made as to a proper working diagnosis or until operation is obviously indicated.

I. **THE HISTORY** In surgical disease, perhaps more than in any other area of medicine, the history assumes overwhelming importance. The primary points that assist in making a diagnosis are:

A. **Localization of pain** Certain viscera provide reasonably good localization of the pain which they generate, whereas others afford little information in this regard. The stomach and duodenum, for example, are quite reliable, and pain localization is invariably in the vicinity of the epigastrium, either to the right or the left of the midline. The pain in pancreatitis likewise localizes reasonably well in the upper abdomen (see Table 5-2). The appendix classically causes pain in the right lower quadrant. The tube and ovary yield pain to the right or the left of the suprapubic area. Other organs, such as the small intestine, have poor pain localization; the pain may be perceived anywhere in the abdomen, although periumbilical pain is most commonly observed.

B. **Radiation and referral of pain** Although a great deal is written about the diagnostic value of radiation of pain, it may not be helpful and can be confusing. Biliary tract pain traditionally radiates around the right side of the back to the angle of the scapula, whereas pain of pancreatic origin frequently radiates directly through to the back. Appendiceal pain, for an entirely different reason, occasionally commences in the epigastrium and ultimately migrates to the right lower quadrant. Pain referred to remote areas can be highly suggestive of specific organ involvement, e.g., perihepatic inflammation referred to the right shoulder, and uterine and rectal disease to the low back.

C. **Quality of pain** Acute abdominal pain is characterized in one of two ways. It is **constant,** more or less, or it is **cramping (colicky)** in character. Constant pain frequently waxes and wanes, but is not rhythmical or cyclical and does not appear in successive waves, as is the case with abdominal cramps. Constant abdominal pain is usually caused by inflammatory or neoplastic involvement of a solid viscus. Cramping abdominal pain is always caused by obstruction of a hollow viscus, e.g., intestinal obstruction, ureteral calculus, dysmenorrhea (blood clot obstructing the cervical os), or by increased intra-

TABLE 5-1. Differential Diagnosis of Acute Abdominal Pain by Location

Right upper quadrant
  Acute cholecystitis
  Perforated duodenal ulcer (forme fruste)
  Acute pancreatitis (bilateral pain)
  Acute hepatitis
  Acute congestive hepatomegaly
  Pneumonia with pleural reaction
  Acute pyelonephritis
  Angina pectoris

Left upper quadrant
  Ruptured spleen
  Perforated gastric or marginal ulcer
  Acute pancreatitis (bilateral pain)
  Ruptured aortic aneurysm
  Perforated colon (tumor, foreign body)
  Pneumonia with pleural reaction
  Acute pyelonephritis
  Acute myocardial infarction

Central (periumbilical)
  Intestinal obstruction
  Appendicitis
  Acute pancreatitis
  Mesenteric thrombosis
  Strangulated groin hernia
  Dissecting or rupturing aortic aneurysm
  Diverticulitis (small intestine or colon)
  Uremia

Right lower quadrant
  Appendicitis
  Acute salpingitis, tubo-ovarian abscess
  Ruptured ectopic pregnancy
  Twisted ovarian cyst
  Mesenteric adenitis
  Incarcerated, strangulated groin hernia
  Meckel's diverticulitis
  Cecal diverticulitis
  Regional ileitis
  Perforated cecum (tumor, foreign body)
  Psoas abscess
  Ureteral calculus

Left lower quadrant
  Sigmoid diverticulitis
  Acute salpingitis, tubo-ovarian abscess
  Ruptured ectopic pregnancy
  Twisted ovarian cyst
  Incarcerated, strangulated groin hernia
  Perforated descending colon (tumor, foreign body)
  Regional ileitis
  Psoas abscess
  Ureteral calculus

TABLE 5-2. Differential Diagnosis of Severe Epigastric Pain

Diagnostic Features	Perforated Peptic Ulcer	Acute Pancreatitis	Acute Cholecystitis
Onset	Sudden, sharp	Gradual	Gradual
Location	Epigastric→generalized rapidly	Epigastric→slowly spreading	Right upper quadrant only (early)
Radiation	Diffuse	Through to back	Around to back and angle of scapula
Vomiting	Absent to few times	Multiple episodes, persistent	Few to many times
Alcoholic intake	Variable	Usually heavy preceding attack	Occasional, not heavy
Previous attacks	Ulcer history (45%)	Frequently similar to current episode	Frequently similar to current episode
Dietary intolerance	Spices, alcohol	Fatty foods	Fatty foods, cabbage
Shock, prostration	Common early	Seen late	Unusual
Tenderness	Diffuse	Epigastric→diffuse	Right upper quadrant
Rebound tenderness	Early (first 4 hr)	Late (after 24 hr)	Rare
Rigidity	Boardlike	Moderate to severe	Unilateral rectus guarding
Peristaltic sounds	Absent	Hypoactive	Normal to hypoactive
Costovertebral angle tenderness	Bilateral	Left-sided	Right-sided
Position	Flat (supine)	Lying on side, hips flexed	Flat (supine) or on side
X-ray	Free air (70%), ileus	Ileus, sentinel loop, colon cutoff sign	Ileus, calculus in right upper quadrant (10%)
Laboratory	Moderate amylase elevation, elevated hematocrit, high leukocyte count	Marked amylase elevation, modest hematocrit elevation, low calcium (after 5 days), glycosuria	Minimal amylase elevation, moderate rise in leukocyte count

luminal pressure in a hollow viscus without obstruction, e.g., subsiding ileus after operation or enteritis with hyperperistalsis and increased intraluminal fluid volume.

D. Duration of pain The duration of abdominal pain is of great significance. Acute appendicitis will not persist as a local process for more than 72–96 hr; acute cholecystitis may not presist for more than 36–48 hr before a complication ensues. As a rule, acute inflammation persists as an acute process for 5 days or less. In contradistinction, regional enteritis may cause abdominal pain for several weeks, neoplasm of the intestinal tract may cause pain for weeks or months, and metabolic disease (diabetes mellitus, porphyria, etc.) may cause abdominal pain in recurrent attacks over long periods of time.

E. Intensity of pain Although not invariably the case, the most acute surgical entities usually cause the most intense or severe pain. A perforated peptic ulcer characteristically results in very severe pain resulting from the highly irritating nature of duodenal and gastric content. On the other hand, the pain of acute pancreatitis is a result of retroperitoneal and intraperitoneal dissemination of enzyme-laden fluid which does not cause pain of as great intensity as is experienced in perforated ulcer. Colon perforation (diverticulitis, perforated carcinoma, trauma) is also marked by pain of moderate intensity at first, but the amount of pain increases with time until the patient develops findings which are quite similar to those of the perforated ulcer patient.

F. Nature of onset of pain Some surgical diseases are characterized by a very sudden and abrupt onset, such as acute perforation of a hollow viscus. The patient frequently likens this to being struck a severe blow. In patients with intestinal obstruction, appendicitis, or diverticulitis, the pain is much more likely to be gradual in onset. One can differentiate the pain of pancreatitis, with its gradual onset, from the pain of perforated peptic ulcer, with its sudden, abrupt onset, by questioning the patient about the manner in which pain began.

G. Associated vomiting In some diseases, vomiting is frequent and persistent, whereas in others it is infrequent or absent. Frequent vomiting at the onset of symptoms is seen in patients with irritation or inflammation of the pancreas and biliary tract. It is extremely unusual to observe individuals with acute pancreatitis without vomiting, and it is relatively uncommon to see acute cholecystitis with no vomiting whatsoever. Of patients with intestinal obstruction and distention, those with colon obstruction are less likely to vomit. In patients with high intestinal obstruction, vomiting is persistent and characteristic of the lesions causing the obstruction (carcinoma of the pancreas, stenosing duodenal ulcer, etc.). The character of the vomitus is of little help unless no bile is observed, suggesting a preampullar lesion, or unless the vomitus is feculent, indicating distal intestinal obstruction.

H. Other diagnostic points

   1. The **age** of the patient is of considerable consequence, since certain diseases are largely limited to certain age groups. Appendicitis is generally a disease of patients between 5 and 50 yr, intussusception is seen primarily under the age of 2, cholecystitis is unusual under the age of 20, and colon obstruction is uncommon under the age of 35.

2. The **position** which the patient assumes in order to obtain relief from pain can also be extremely helpful in diagnosis. The victim of pancreatitis characteristically lies on his side with the vertebral column, knees, and hips flexed. This position relaxes the psoas muscle, which is irritated and in spasm because of retroperitoneal inflammation. Patients with retrocecal appendicitis occasionally flex the right hip and knee in order to relax the right psoas muscle. The patient with diffuse peritonitis of any etiology commonly prefers to lie in bed in an immobile state; motion or position change is resisted because of the exquisite pain occasioned by movement of the parietal peritoneum.

3. Certain **drugs** are associated with acute surgical diseases. For example, if the patient is known to have been on steroids, this would lead one to think of perforation of a peptic ulcer; the chronic use of salicylate or other antirheumatic agents would lead to the same conclusion. A history of antacid ingestion suggests esophagitis, ulcer, or biliary-pancreatic disease. If the patient had ever used potassium chloride in tablet form, ulceration and subsequent stenosis of the small intestine may occur, with the acute abdominal pain based on intestinal obstruction due to a stricture.

4. It is helpful to know whether the patient has taken any **medication to relieve pain.** Vomiting (frequently digitally induced) which produces relief from pain is indicative of ulcer or high obstruction. Relief from pain with passage of flatus or after an enema could indicate incomplete left colon obstruction.

II. **THE PHYSICAL EXAMINATION**   A careful physical examination is absolutely essential in the intelligent evaluation of a patient with acute abdominal pain. Thoroughness and a systematic approach are important; errors of omission far outnumber errors of commission. An examination pattern rigidly adhered to will pay handsome dividends in these patients.

A. **General considerations, vital signs**

1. The **appearance** of the patient will frequently give some general clues as to the severity of the illness. The detection of pallor, cyanosis, or simply a facial expression contorted by pain supports the supposition that a grave abdominal catastrophe has occurred.

2. **Tachycardia** is common in patients with profound illness such as ruptured viscus, gangrenous intestinal obstruction, or diffuse peritonitis. The initial pulse rate has less value than serial observation of this sign. A rising pulse rate in a patient undergoing active but nonoperative treatment for acute abdominal pain is an ominous sign, and usually means that an operation is required.

3. **Tachypnea** has somewhat the same connotation, although very rapid respiratory rates are observed in patients with peritonitis from pancreatitis, hemorrhagic shock, and similar lesions. The relative value of the respira-

tory rate as a physical finding is largely comparative; if the respiratory rate increases under management, this is an ominous sign and may herald the need for an operation.

4. **Fever** is common in patients with acute abdominal disease, although the temperature is likely to be normal or only slightly elevated early in the course of the disease. It is essential that the temperature in patients on surgical services be obtained rectally. The initial temperature is not as valuable as the constant observation of this sign during the course of expectant management. As a rule, the temperature in patients with acute appendicitis, uncomplicated intestinal obstruction, ruptured ectopic pregnancy, and other acute surgical emergencies may be close to normal; the initial temperature will rarely exceed 101°F rectally. When perforation occurs or intestinal gangrene supervenes, the temperature will increase to 39.4-40.0°C (103-104°F), but will then fall if shock ensues. With an initial temperature over 103°F it is far more likely that one is dealing with pulmonary or urinary tract infection than with an intra-abdominal process as the cause of the fever. Temperature over 104°F at any time means abscess, fulminant systemic infection, or infection involving the CNS, lung, or urinary tract.

B. **Examination of the abdomen**   The astute physical diagnostician is made, not born. Meticulous attention to small details will frequently spell the difference between diagnostic success and failure. The principles to be emphasized include the following:

1. **Always examine the area remote from the site of maximal pain first**   It is important to examine both sides of the abdomen with both hands, the examiner's right hand examining the left side of the patient's abdomen, his left the right side of the patient's abdomen. The assessment of rigidity can be enhanced by placing a pillow under the patient's knees and having the patient breathe gently, but deeply, through the mouth. The finding of unilateral rectus spasm is indicative of an acute inflammatory process beneath that rectus muscle, as the patient is unable voluntarily to contract one rectus to a greater degree than the other.

2. **True rigidity or intense bilateral guarding is suggestive of diffuse peritonitis**   This impression can be substantiated by the finding of rebound tenderness, in which gentle manual pressure elicits somewhat less tenderness than the sudden release of that pressure. It is important not to cause excessive or intense pain by injudicious eliciting of tenderness or rebound tenderness. Only one examiner should attempt to detect this finding. As a rule, such a finding requires operative treatment.

3. **Cutaneous hyperesthesia** can be demonstrated by stroking the skin with the fingernail or a needle. The patient is requested to tell the examiner if any area of skin-stroking causes pain; this will indicate the spinal segment innervating the area of parietal peritoneum irritated by the acute inflammatory disease.

4. **Palpation of solid viscera** is important, but rarely diagnostic. Of greater value is the finding of referred tenderness, in which pressure at a distance

from the inflamed viscus will cause acute tenderness over that viscus (Rovsing's sign in acute appendicitis). This suggests parietal peritoneal involvement by an inflammatory lesion. Also of importance is the physical finding of iliopsoas spasm (psoas sign) reflected in persistent flexion of the hip or by severe pain on passive hyperextension of the hip with the patient lying on the contralateral side, suggestive of an inflammatory retroperitoneal lesion on the affected side. The psoas sign is seen, on the right side, in acute retrocecal appendicitis, in perinephric abscess, and in posterior perforation of cecal carcinoma. Left-sided psoas spasm can be observed with perinephric abscess, perforated sigmoid diverticulitis, and perforated sigmoid carcinoma.

5. Of considerable importance is the assessment of the **frequency of peristaltic sounds.** In patients with diffuse peritonitis or intense localized inflammatory disease, the bowel sounds disappear or become markedly hypoactive. Normal activity in the fasting state is 10–20 sounds/min. With localized peritonitis, such as appendicitis or diverticulitis, the intestinal sounds are somewhat hypoactive but they usually are present. The bowel sounds are hyperactive in diffuse inflammatory disease of the intestinal tract, early intestinal obstruction, or subsiding paralytic ileus. It must be remembered that an acute inflammatory process anywhere in the body, severe metabolic disease (diabetic coma, uremia), or acute trauma can cause moderate to severe ileus with nearly total (but rarely complete) loss of peristaltic sounds.

6. The **pitch of intestinal peristaltic sounds** is difficult to describe, and can only be learned by repeated auscultation of the abdomen. It is imperative that the house officer and student auscultate the abdomen with the same care with which auscultation of the chest is practiced. The pitch of bowel sounds is dependent on the tension of the wall of the intestinal tract and the length of the air-fluid interface in that particular section of intestine. Just as the pitch of a drum is raised by increasing the tension of the drum head, so the pitch of bowel sounds is increased by increased intraluminal tension. As paralytic ileus subsides, the large amount of air and fluid which has accumulated during the period of intestinal inactivity is subjected to ever-increasing pressure by the contracting smooth muscle; this situation is identical to that which exists early in a mechanical intestinal obstruction while active peristalsis proximal to the obstruction continues. High-pitched bowel sounds are not always indicative of intestinal obstruction, unless the other three prime findings of intestinal obstruction are observed: distention, cramping abdominal pain, and obstipation.

7. **Abdominal distention** is best assessed by measuring the abdominal girth at the umbilicus and by viewing the lateral contour of the anterior surface of the abdomen in relation to an imaginary line between the symphysis pubis and the xiphoid. In patients without distention, the anterior abdominal border usually will be observed to lie below the xiphipubic line. Even in the very obese patient, when the individual lies flat in bed, the normal abdominal contour is scaphoid or flat. When the abdomen is moderately distended, lateral inspection will demonstrate the abdominal wall to be at or slightly above the xiphipubic line. As distention increases,

the abdominal contour becomes grossly rounded, accompanied by increased tension of the abdominal wall and tightness of the skin.

8. In addition to determining the presence of distention, the examiner must decide whether the distention is gaseous or fluid by careful **percussion** of the abdomen. Distinguishing ascites from ileus or obstruction is a matter of determining the percussion note as well as the presence or absence of **shifting dullness.** The presence of fluid, with its dull note, may signify carcinomatous ascites, portal hypertension, congestive heart failure, hemoperitoneum, or inflammatory ascites. With tympany to percussion, the presence of mechanical or paralytic ileus is apparent; massive pneumoperitoneum will also produce this finding.

C. **Rectovaginal examination** (pelvic examination)

1. The rectovaginal or pelvic examination is one which is frequently done in a cursory fashion or is not attempted at all. This omission can be disastrous in the assessment of patients with acute abdominal pain. The **lower third of the abdomen** is hidden in the lower false and true pelvis by bone and soft tissue, and **can be evaluated only by digital rectal or rectovaginal examination.** The presence of a pelvic abscess will be detected by finding severe tenderness and cul-de-sac fullness on digital examination. Fullness may be apparent in intestinal obstruction or paralytic ileus when it is caused by markedly distended and edematous loops of intestine impinging on pelvic structures.

2. Of great importance is the finding of a **unilateral mass or extreme tenderness on one side** of the pelvis or other, most frequently suggesting appendicitis or appendiceal abscess on the right or tubo-ovarian abscess on the left. It can be difficult to distinguish right-sided tubo-ovarian disease from appendiceal inflammatory disease, but **tenderness on manipulation of the cervix** will be extreme in patients with pelvic inflammatory disease. It should be remembered that rectal or rectovaginal examination is relatively unsatisfactory unless the bladder is empty; furthermore, the simplest approach to cul-de-sac disease from a diagnostic standpoint is the rectovaginal route (digital examination, colpocentesis, culdoscopy). The use of the cervical smear to detect gonococcal disease of the genital tract is not particularly rewarding. Finding intracellular gram-negative diplococci is difficult and infrequent. On the other hand, in the male patient acute or chronic prostatic inflammation can be detected readily by the bogginess, extreme tenderness, and enlargement of the prostate on rectal examination.

3. If possible the female patient should be examined on a firm table during this part of the evaluation. If the patient is too ill to be moved from her bed, a board or serving tray covered with a bath towel and placed under the patient's sacrum will provide a firm surface for a reasonably satisfactory rectovaginal examination in bed. Little or nothing will be learned if the patient is examined on her side, as it is impossible to utilize bimanual examination, which is extremely helpful and a key part of this examina-

tion. Twisted ovarian cyst, twisted pedunculated uterine myomas, presacral tumors, and other ballotable or fixed pelvic masses are much easier to detect via bimanual examination.

III. **LABORATORY TESTS** The laboratory provides little help in the differential diagnosis of acute abdominal pain. Routine tests, such as complete blood count, urinalysis with microscopic examination, BUN, creatinine, blood sugar, and serology are usually drawn on admission.

 A. **Urinalysis** The presence of proteinuria and the finding of erythrocytes or leukocytes in the urine on a clean or catheterized specimen can be significant; pyonephrosis, perinephric abscess, retrocecal appendicitis, or retroperitoneal abscess from rupture of the duodenum or colon can lead to these findings. Pancreatitis characteristically causes slight proteinuria (trace to 1+) because of the secondary inflammation induced by the proximity of the tail of the pancreas to the left kidney.

 B. **Leukocyte count** The leukocyte count and the differential count have no specific diagnostic significance except in children; the finding of leukopenia with lower abdominal pain is suggestive of acute viral infection (e.g., measles) rather than acute appendicitis. Patients with mesenteric adenitis as the cause of abdominal pain usually exhibit a leukocyte count between 6,000 and 16,000, exactly the same range as in acute appendicitis. A shift to the left suggests an acute inflammatory disease or abscess but does little to differentiate surgical from nonsurgical inflammatory conditions. Serial leukocyte counts in a patient with obscure or variable findings may be helpful in that a rising leukocyte count may represent an indication for surgical exploration.

 C. **Serum, urine amylase** Obtaining amylase or lipase values (amylase is preferred because of the greater ease with which the test is performed) in patients with acute abdominal disease can provide evidence that the patient has acute pancreatitis. Levels over 400 Somogyi units/100 ml serum or over 700 Somogyi units in the urine are definitely suggestive of acute pancreatitis. Values over 700 Somogyi units in the serum and over 1,200 Somogyi units in the urine are diagnostic of acute pancreatitis. Amylase also may be elevated in a number of acute abdominal diseases, e.g., intestinal obstruction, perforated peptic ulcer, and mesenteric thrombosis, and following the administration of drugs such as morphine sulfate. However, the level does not approach the diagnostic values indicated above for pancreatitis. On the other hand, it must be remembered that acute pancreatitis may occur with normal or minimally elevated amylase levels (see Table 5-2).

IV. **OTHER DIAGNOSTIC APPROACHES** Following a careful history and physical examination, the diagnosis may still be obscure and further diagnostic tests may be indicated.

 A. **Routine x-ray studies** Four films of the abdomen and chest should be made routinely during the initial period of evaluation of patients with acute abdominal disease.

1. **Upright PA film of the chest** is utilized to exclude pulmonary parenchymal disease, to detect subphrenic free air suggesting perforation of the GI tract, and to demonstrate air-filled viscera in the chest (traumatic diaphragmatic hernia), mediastinal abscess, or spontaneous perforation of the esophagus.

2. **Flat film of the abdomen** can be used to delineate the pattern of gas in the intestinal tract, to differentiate gaseous from fluid distention, to detect fluid-filled loops of intestine, and to visualize abnormal soft tissue densities or calculi. Some 90% of urinary tract calculi contain sufficient calcium to be radiopaque and will be seen. Conversely, only 10% of biliary tract stones will be seen. Of great diagnostic value is the detection of air in the biliary tree, indicating biliary-intestinal fistula, and possible gallstone ileus as the cause of small-intestine obstruction. Further, the psoas shadows can frequently be seen, and bony abnormalities of the vertebra or pelvis may also be detected.

3. **Upright film of the abdomen** is used to detect the presence of air-fluid levels, especially at different heights, in mechanical intestinal obstruction. In addition, masses or soft tissue densities and their relationship to air-filled loops of intestine may be helpful in arriving at the diagnosis.

4. **Left lateral decubitus film** is taken after the patient has been lying on his left side for at least 10 min to allow any free air which may have escaped detection in the upright view of the chest to gravitate upward to the space between the right lobe of the liver and the parietal peritoneum. Furthermore, a long air-fluid level on the right side of the abdomen, representing the ascending colon air-fluid interface, will be seen in patients with colon obstruction.

B. Diagnostic abdominal paracentesis

1. Of great importance is the concept that a negative, or "dry," abdominal paracentesis has no diagnostic significance; in other words, if no fluid is obtained, the abdominal tap cannot be assumed to have yielded any information and should be ignored. It is common, though considerable fluid is present, for none to be aspirated even by several needle insertions into the peritoneal cavity.

2. Paracentesis should not be employed until after abdominal roentgenograms have been obtained, since small amounts of air inadvertently may be introduced during needle paracentesis and lead to an erroneous x-ray diagnosis of perforation.

3. The technique commonly employed for simple abdominal paracentesis involves turning the patient on his left side for 5 min, allowing the fluid to gravitate into the left paracolic area, and then inserting a needle into the abdomen, with the patient still in the left ducubitus position, halfway between the umbilicus and the pubis at the left lateral edge of the rectus sheath. This puncture site will obviate laceration of the deep inferior epigastric artery.

4. It is **important not to use local anesthesia of the peritoneum** so that penetration will be perceived by the patient as a sharp pain, thus serving to identify the level of the peritoneum. Gentle suction should be applied to the needle with a sterile 10-ml syringe after it has been determined that the needle has entered the peritoneal cavity. The hub of the needle should not be moved about in an arc in an attempt to obtain fluid, as this will markedly increase the chance of causing serious injury to subjacent viscera.

5. If the left lower quadrant paracentesis is negative (no fluid is obtained), the right side should be aspirated in the same fashion. It is not desirable to use the upper quadrants, as damage to the liver, spleen, or stomach may occur.

6. Another technique, which has proved somewhat more sensitive than bilateral needle aspiration, involves placing a plastic **catheter** into the peritoneal cavity in the lower abdominal midline, 1 in. below the umbilicus (see Chap. 25). The catheter used is one of the commercially available needle-plastic catheter combinations customarily used for IV fluid therapy. When the catheter has been placed and the needle withdrawn, 500 ml of sterile saline solution buffered with 50 ml of 7.5% sodium bicarbonate should be allowed to flow into the peritoneal cavity over a 10–15-min period. The fluid is then aspirated and examined as indicated below.

7. A logical plan is to utilize simple needle aspiration first and, if no fluid is obtained, to proceed to catheter irrigation.

8. **Study of paracentesis fluid** should consist of measurement of pH, test for bile with Smith's reagent or other appropriate material, laboratory evaluation of amylase content, and microscopic examination of the fluid for leukocytes or erythrocytes. The presence of blood, large numbers of polymorphonuclear cells, or bile or the detection of acid pH of the fluid usually represents a solid indication for exploratory laparotomy.

9. An alternative to abdominal paracentesis in the female is **colpocentesis.** To perform this procedure, the patient must be in stirrups on a gynecological examining table. A spinal needle with a short bevel, usually 17- or 18-gauge, customarily is employed. With a vaginal speculum in place, the needle is introduced posterior to the cervix and directed straight cephalad. The needle should never be introduced more than half of its length in order to avoid perforation of intestine in or above the cul-de-sac. The technique is useful in patients thought to have a pelvic abscess or other pelvic disease. In a seriously ill patient it is more troublesome and more difficult to perform than simple abdominal paracentesis.

C. **Diagnostic pneumoperitoneum**   The instillation of 500 ml of air into the peritoneal cavity gives an excellent outline of the liver and spleen on an upright chest roentgenogram made to include the upper half of the abdomen. In the patient with a ruptured liver, ruptured spleen, and subphrenic or subhepatic abscess, the air will not enter the subphrenic space on the affected side, thus indicating the site of disease. Pneumoperitoneum should never be used until the customary x-rays of the chest and abdomen have been obtained and examined.

D. Special x-ray studies   Under certain circumstances, the use of contrast material in the GI tract or the injection of dye into the arterial tree may yield significant information.

1. **Contrast material by mouth**   Two types of medium can be given by mouth: diatrizoate (Gastrografin) and barium. The former is a water-soluble dye which is very helpful in elucidating the size of the intestine and the presence of obstruction in the upper GI tract. It has little value in detecting mucosal lesions; for these, barium is the more satisfactory contrast medium. Barium should not be given by mouth to a patient with gaseous intestinal distention. Use of oral barium should be limited to those patients with acute abdominal disease in whom no perforation of the GI tract is judged to be present and in whom the abdomen is scaphoid.

2. **Barium enema**   This is usually indicated to differentiate small-intestinal from large-intestinal obstructions. Barium enema should not be utilized under any circumstances in patients with diffuse abdominal tenderness, frank peritonitis, or other signs of a perforated viscus. The examination should always be done with great care in patients with acute abdominal pain, under the direct supervision of the radiologist, and barium flow should be stopped immediately if there is either aggravation of the abdominal pain or fluoroscopic evidence of barium leak during the procedure.

3. **Injection of stab wounds**   There has been some enthusiasm for detecting peritoneal penetration by sewing a catheter into the subcutaneous area of the wound of the abdomen, injecting dye, and obtaining a lateral abdominal x-ray to determine whether the dye is within the peritoneal cavity. This has not proved to be particularly effective or desirable, since penetration of the peritoneum does not require operation in small stab wounds of the abdomen unless the wound results in findings of peritoneal irritation or other signs suggesting injury to the viscera. In gunshot wounds, operation ordinarily is indicated without the use of this diagnostic technique.

4. **Ultrasound, echography**   Sophisticated instruments utilizing the Doppler principle of ultrasound detection have been developed and are quite helpful in detecting masses in the abdomen and in determining whether those masses are solid or fluid-filled. When a mass is palpated, it is sometimes helpful to subject the abdomen to ultrasound study, so that the precise nature of the mass may be ascertained. Abscesses, twisted cysts, and encapsulated hematomas are identified as fluid-filled, whereas solid tumors or other solid lesions are identified as such.

5. **Angiography** has become increasingly valuable in determining the site of GI bleeding. A Seldinger catheter is inserted by the femoral or brachial

route, and cannulation of the celiac or superior mesenteric arteries may be done. The same technique is applied to patients who have experienced abdominal trauma, in whom rupture of the spleen or liver is suspected. The kidney which has been injured is precisely evaluated by this technique. Flush aortography, in which individual vessel cannulation is not attempted, is helpful in diagnosis of splenic or renal rupture, but is of no benefit in patients with rupture of the liver.

SUGGESTED READING

Cope, Z.   *The Acute Abdomen* (13th ed.). New York: Oxford University Press, 1968.

Gelin, L. E., Nyhus, L. M., and Condon, R. E.   *Abdominal Pain: A Guide to Rapid Diagnosis.* Philadelphia: Lippincott, 1969.

Requarth, W.   *Diagnosis of Acute Abdominal Pain.* Chicago: Year Book, 1958.

6. MASSIVE UPPER GASTROINTESTINAL HEMORRHAGE

I. GENERAL COMMENTS A diagnostic and therapeutic revolution has occurred in this field in recent years. **Endoscopy** of the esophagus, stomach, and duodenum, plus **angiography** of the arterial tree of the same organs as well as of the liver and pancreas, has altered completely our basic approach to these difficult problems. The causes of massive hemorrhage are legion; thus, the determination of an accurate diagnosis is imperative for appropriate therapy.

A. Definitions

1. **Massive GI hemorrhage** is the rapid loss of at least 1 liter of blood, or acute blood loss of any volume that is sufficient to cause hypovolemic shock.

2. **Upper GI hemorrhage** refers to bleeding from the esophagus, stomach, or duodenum. Lower GI hemorrhage refers to bleeding originating distal to the ligament of Treitz. Massive hemorrhage is more frequent with upper than with lower GI tract lesions.

3. **Hematemesis** means vomiting of bright red blood. **Melanemesis** (coffee-ground emesis) means vomiting of altered brown or black blood. Either indicates that the source of bleeding is above the ligament of Treitz, usually in the esophagus, stomach, or duodenum.

4. **Melena** refers to the passage of black blood per rectum. **Hematochezia** means passage of bright red blood per rectum. The color of blood passed in the stool does not imply anything regarding its source, the color of blood passed per rectum is a function of both the source of hemorrhage and the intestinal transit time. As blood passes through the GI tract, the action of bacteria and digestive juices changes the character of the blood from bright red to black and tarry; this process requires some hours. Blood in the GI tract also may act as a cathartic, producing rapid transit. If transit is sufficiently rapid, blood shed in the stomach or duodenum may be passed unaltered per rectum. While melena is more characteristic of upper GI bleeding, it can occur with bleeding from a distal lower GI lesion. Hematochezia, conversely, is more characteristic of mucosal lesions of the rectum and rectosigmoid but is seen not uncommonly with upper GI hemorrhage.

B. Other comments

1. **Causes of hematemesis,** with the exception of very rare lesions, are, in approximate order of frequency, as follows:

   Duodenal ulcer
   Gastritis (acute, chronic, corrosive, infectious, stress)
   Gastric ulcer
   Esophageal varices (portal hypertension)
   Esophagitis or esophageal ulcer
   Gastric carcinoma
   Swallowed blood (epistaxis, hemoptysis)
   Esophageal trauma (foreign body)
   Esophageal carcinoma
   Aortoduodenal fistula
   Carcinoma of ampulla of Vater
   Hematobilia
   Blood coagulation dyscrasia (congenital or acquired)
   Postemetic laceration (Mallory-Weiss syndrome)
   Benign gastric tumor (hemangioma, leiomyoma, etc.)
   Multiple telangiectasia
   Pseudoxanthoma elasticum

2. **A duodenal or gastric ulcer or gastritis is the cause of 85% of cases of upper GI hemorrhage.**

3. **Most patients with upper GI hemorrhage (85%) stop bleeding** either just before or just after admission to the hospital. Patients in whom bleeding continues or recurs following admission are unusual and probably will need intra-arterial infusion therapy or operative control of their bleeding.

II. IMMEDIATE MANAGEMENT

A. Every patient with massive GI hemorrhage must be **admitted to a hospital** for further care. Of course, many patients develop this complication during hospitalization following admission for burns or admission to intensive care units for such complications as shock, gastric distention, respiratory embarrassment, and sepsis. The diagnostic approach is similar; the therapeutic approach may be different.

B. Resuscitation and diagnostic maneuvers are used simultaneously. Hypovolemic shock must be corrected before this dual approach.

C. There are **two prime objectives of initial therapy:**

1. **Replace the volume of lost blood** to stabilize the patient's condition.

2. **Determine the source** and approximate volume of the hemorrhage and whether or not bleeding is continuing.

D. The volume of blood lost is best estimated by findings on physical examination. The history is apt to be exaggerated in this regard. Estimating the volume of blood loss from the response of the blood pressure and pulse to a change from supine to sitting position is outlined in Table 9-4.

E. A rapid **physical examination** should be conducted, paying particular attention to evidences of diseases that are associated with GI bleeding. Look for melanin spots, telangiectases, hemangiomas, and stigmas of cirrhosis. An enlarged liver, enlarged spleen, spider nevi, collateral circulation over the abdomen and chest, and loss of body hair all are indications of portal hypertension. Point tenderness in the epigastrium suggests duodenal or gastric ulcer.

F. Place a **large-bore CVP monitor catheter** in one arm, and a second IV catheter in the other arm. The flow-directed balloon-tipped catheter (Swan-Ganz) may greatly facilitate hemodynamic studies in these critically ill patients.

G. **Type and crossmatch whole blood**   The number of units ordered will depend on the estimate of the volume of blood lost. Have the blood bank crossmatch 2 pints more than the estimated volume of hemorrhage. As blood is used, have more units crossmatched. Keep at least 2 crossmatched units of blood always available for at least 48 hr and until the patient's condition is stable and there is no indication of continued bleeding.

H. Treat **hypovolemic shock** as the first priority. Give blood or plasma expanders as rapidly as possible, pumping them in if necessary. Once shock is reversed, transfusion should continue at a reasonably rapid rate to replace blood until (1) blood pressure and pulse are normal and stable, (2) an effective circulating blood volume has been restored, and (3) the hematocrit level is about 35%. Follow the precepts of shock therapy outlined in Chapter 1.

I. The following **laboratory examinations** should be carried out.

1. Hematocrit   During and immediately after a major hemorrhage, the hematocrit does not reflect the amount of blood lost. Time is required for fluid shifts to replenish the circulating blood volume and cause a dilutional decrease in the hematocrit. Nonetheless, serial determinations of the hematocrit are useful in following patients with GI hemorrhage. Allowing for mixing time, about a 3% change in hematocrit can be expected for each 500 ml of blood lost by bleeding or gained by transfusion.

2. Leukocytosis is to be expected; leukopenia suggests that esophageal varices are the source of bleeding (portal hypertension produces secondary hypersplenism).

3. If cirrhosis is suspected, measure the prothrombin time and serum albumin. Sodium sulfobromophthalein (Bromsulphalein) retention is not reliable if the patient is or recently has been hypotensive.

J. A careful **history** should be obtained after replacement of lost blood volume has begun. *The history usually will provide the best clues to the source of bleeding.* Because the patient may be frightened or even incoherent, an effort must be made to obtain information and to corroborate the history with relatives or friends. Inquire particularly regarding symptoms of duodenal or gastric ulcer, alcoholism, and hepatitis.

K. Physicians who have treated the patient previously should be contacted. Old x-rays and records should be obtained for review, although rarely will they arrive in time to be of much help in making the initial decisions regarding therapy.

L. The **"vigorous diagnostic approach"** should be followed in all patients with a major upper GI tract hemorrhage in order to provide or confirm a diagnosis.

  1. **Lavage the stomach** with iced saline solution via an Ewald tube; remove all old blood and clots. Lavage is continued until the returns are clear.

  2. As soon as the patient's condition is stable, perform **upper GI endoscopy:** esophagoscopy, gastroscopy, and duodenoscopy. A definitive diagnosis should follow.

  3. If after these studies the diagnosis is still in question and the patient continues to bleed, **selective angiography** of the visceral arteries (superior mesenteric, gastroduodenal, splenic, and left gastric) with injection of contrast material should be performed. Depending on the specific source of the hemorrhage, the catheters may be left in place for 2-6 days for injection of vasopressin.

  4. If these diagnostic techniques are not available, an **upper GI series** with barium is performed; the esophagus must be carefully surveyed for varices or ulceration.

III. THERAPEUTIC APPROACH

A. Bleeding stops

  1. Place a **nasogastric tube** on suction to provide a means of early warning of recurrent upper GI bleeding. **Antacids** should be instilled into the stomach. The pH of the gastric aspirate should be monitored frequently and kept above 3.0.

  2. After the volume of estimated blood loss has been rapidly replaced, transfusions should stop. Maintenance IV fluids are continued. The recording of blood pressure and pulse at frequent intervals is continued. These data, together with the character of the nasogastric suction output, the presence or absence of borborygmi or hyperactive bowel sounds by auscultation, and the direction of change in the hematocrit, will allow early recognition of recurrent bleeding.

  3. After assurance that bleeding has stopped, the nasogastric tube may be removed. Antacids should be given hourly. Milk and cream, despite their popularity, are not efficient antacids. The patient should be kept at bed rest or at restricted activity, and small doses of sedatives administered around the clock for the first few days. No anticholinergics should be given to patients soon after a major GI hemorrhage. A caffeine- and alcohol-free general diet can be ordered. Depending on the source of the hemorrhage, definitive operation on an elective basis may be indicated.

B. Bleeding continues

1. Assuming that the patient is hemodynamically stable and can be maintained on modest blood replacement (less than 1,500 ml/24 hr), an attempt should be made to control the hemorrhage by use of **intra-arterial vasopressin.** This technique particularly applies to hemorrhage from varices, gastritis, or stress ulceration. It is less effective for bleeding from chronic duodenal or chronic gastric ulcer, so this method of treatment for ulcer should be reserved for high-risk patients who would be poor operative risks.

   a. Preparation of vasopressin solutions. Mix 100 units of vasopressin (Pitressin, 20 units per vial) and 500 ml of either normal saline or 5% dextrose in water. Infuse using a continuous-infusion pump.

   b. Infusion into superior mesenteric artery **for varices:**

      (1) Pituitrin (posterior pituitary injection), 0.2 units/min for 24 hr.

      (2) Then Pituitrin, 0.1 unit/min for 48 hr.

      (3) Then Pituitrin, 0.05 unit/min for 12 hr.

      (4) Then 5% glucose in water or normal saline at 1 ml/min for 24 hr.

      (5) Catheter removed on fifth day.

   c. Infusion into left gastric or gastroduodenal artery **for gastric hemorrhage:**   Vasopressin, 0.2 units/min for 12 hr. Cessation of bleeding should be prompt. If not, operative intervention is mandatory. The concentration of vasopressin may be increased for several hours to 0.3 or 0.4 units/min, but higher doses have not proved more effective in controlling gastric bleeding.

   d. Cautions. Effect on liver of direct vasopressin infusion is unknown. Do not infuse hepatic artery. There is a measurable antidiuretic effect of intra-arterially infused vasopressin. Care must be taken to prevent fluid overload.

C. Special problems in therapy of GI hemorrhage

1. The single most difficult problem relates to the decision to discontinue

nonoperative therapy (e.g., ice-water lavage or vasopressin infusion). A few **guidelines to when to operate** on the patient are helpful.

a. Older patients tolerate continuing hemorrhage and prolonged resuscitation poorly. Although not a fixed rule, 24 hr should be sufficient time to control bleeding fully. *Older patients who have persistent or recurrent bleeding should be operated on sooner* than a younger patient with the same problem.

b. Operative therapy should be considered seriously for all chronic alcoholics.

c. Patients over 50 yr of age who have a history of chronic duodenal ulcer and who present with a first major bleeding episode should be considered seriously for operation.

d. Operative therapy also should be considered seriously in patients who have hematemesis, severe pain persisting during hemorrhage, or complete absence of pain but a proven duodenal ulcer.

e. Operative therapy frequently is necessary in any patient who bleeds massively from a gastric ulcer.

f. **Immediate operative therapy is mandatory** in the following conditions:

   (1) Perforation and hemorrhage coexist.

   (2) Blood pressure and pulse are not normal and stable after rapid transfusion of 2,500 ml of blood.

   (3) Following initial stabilization, more than 1,500 ml of blood needs to be transfused in less than 24 hr to maintain a normal pulse and blood pressure.

   (4) Bleeding, even of small amounts, continues for more than 24 hr from onset. In young, vigorous patients, persistence of bleeding for up to 48 hr may be tolerated in selected cases.

   (5) Having initially stopped, bleeding recurs while the patient is hospitalized and receiving nonoperative treatment.

   (6) There is a shortage of compatible blood.

2. **Esophageal varices and balloon tamponade**   If intra-arterial vasopressin techniques are not available, the triple-lumen (Sengstaken-Blakemore) tube is both a diagnostic and therapeutic tool. The stomach first must be lavaged free of old blood. With a triple-lumen tube, the gastric aspirate can be isolated effectively from the esophagus. Balloon tamponade is a temporary, not a definitive treatment; half of these patients will bleed again when the balloon is deflated. Great care in the use of tamponade technique is essential. Rupture of the gastric balloon with asphyxiation and rupture of the esophagus may occur. Constant bedside attention by intensive care unit personnel is mandatory during periods of balloon inflation.

SUGGESTED READING

Baum, S., Athanasoulis, C. A., Waltman, A. C., and Ring, E. J.   Gastrointestinal hemorrhage. Angiographic diagnosis and control. *Adv. Surg.* 7:149, 1973.

Welch, C. E., and Hedberg, S.   Gastrointestinal hemorrhage. General considerations of diagnosis and therapy. *Adv. Surg.* 7:95, 1973.

7. INTESTINAL OBSTRUCTION

I. GENERAL COMMENTS

A. Normal peristalsis

1. **Electrical activity** of bowel smooth muscle is characterized by slow waves and spike discharges.

2. **Slow waves** (pacesetter potentials, basic electrical rhythm) are omnipresent, regularly recurring depolarizations of smooth muscle membrane which have a relatively low amplitude and long duration. Slow waves are generated intrinsically, are propagated aborally, and are not easily stimulated or inhibited by external influences.

3. **Spike discharges** occur singly or in short bursts, are of high amplitude and very short duration, and are superimposed on the slow wave at or just after maximal slow-wave depolarization. The percentage of slow waves carrying spike discharges can vary from 0-100%. Spike discharges are easily stimulated or inhibited by external influences. Feeding and certain drugs and hormones (morphine, gastrin, cholecystokinin, histamine) increase the number of spike discharges. Fasting, sleeping, and some agents (secretin, glucagon, prostaglandins) decrease the percentage of slow waves carrying spikes.

4. **Muscular contraction** of bowel occurs only in conjunction with a spike discharge. Contraction most frequently is limited to a small region of bowel. These contractions are called segmental (pendular, churning) contractions.

5. **Peristalsis** is brought about by the conduction of contractile stimuli from one bowel segment to the next. There is a gradient of rhythmic intrinsic activity and excitability which steadily decreases from mouth to anus. Impulses, therefore, spread more readily downward (aborally), producing propulsion of bowel content. The extent of impulse transmission in an upward (adoral) direction (reverse peristalsis) is limited by the gradient of excitability.

6. Peristalsis does not depend on extrinsic neural activity. Extrinsic stimuli serve only to modify intrinsic peristaltic activity. In general, sympathetic stimuli inhibit and parasympathetic stimuli augment intrinsic bowel mo-

tility. Nonadrenergic inhibitory neural activity also has been identified recently.

7. Preganglionic sympathectomy usually is followed by some increase in peristaltic activity. Postganglionic (celiac, mesenteric) sympathectomy has been followed by profuse diarrhea in dogs and sometimes in man. Truncal vagotomy (parasympathectomy) usually has little effect on bowel motility, but in a few cases it is associated with episodic or persistent diarrhea; the mechanism is not clear.

B. Types of bowel obstruction

1. Obstruction means that **bowel content does not pass normally** to the rectum. The block may involve either the large or the small bowel and may be complete or incomplete, mechanical or paralytic in origin, and may or may not involve compromise of the vascular supply. A **closed-loop obstruction** implies obstruction at two levels so that content in the intervening loop of bowel cannot progress in either an aboral or an adoral direction, i.e., the loop is "closed" in both directions.

2. Obstruction is a disease of the very young and the very old. Of all deaths in infancy, 10% are due to bowel obstruction. The incidence of obstruction rises progressively with age throughout adulthood, but there is a sharp increase in incidence after age 50, and a second sharp rise after age 70.

3. **Simple mechanical obstruction** is a result of a physical block to passage of bowel content without compromise of bowel blood supply. The obstruction may be extrinsic (adhesions, hernia), intrinsic (tumor, hematoma), or luminal (gallstone, polyp, fecal impaction, foreign body). Mechanical obstruction occurs in distinct clinical patterns: pyloric obstruction, high (jejunal) small-bowel obstruction, low (ileal) small-bowel obstruction, and colonic obstruction. In patients with mechanical obstruction, the site of obstruction is in the small bowel in 80% and in the colon in 20%.

4. **Paralytic (adynamic, neurogenic) ileus** means that peristalsis is ineffective or nonpropulsive. Motor activity, though diminished, is never completely absent. The bowel is functionally blocked but there is no physical obstruction to passage of bowel content and no compromise of blood supply.

5. **Strangulation obstruction** means that compromise of the blood supply leading to gangrene of the bowel is superimposed on a mechanical obstruction.

6. **Vascular ileus** represents a primary problem of gangrene caused by interference with venous drainage or arterial supply to the bowel. The clinical picture begins as a paralytic ileus and therefore resembles a bowel obstruction.

II. SIMPLE MECHANICAL SMALL-BOWEL OBSTRUCTION

A. Causes

1. In adults who have previously had an abdominal operation, 90% of mechanical obstructions are a result of **adhesions.** The cause of adhesions remains unproved, but they are most likely related to ischemic injury to visceral or parietal peritoneum.

2. In infants, segmental intestinal **atresia** and **imperforate anus** are the most frequent causes of obstruction.

3. In patients who have previously not been operated on, an **external hernia** is the most common cause of obstruction.

4. Some of the myriad of other causes of mechanical obstruction are listed in Table 7-1.

B. Pathophysiology

1. The disturbed physiology engendered by mechanical small-bowel **intestinal obstruction results in increased peristalsis, distention by gas and fluid, contraction of extracellular fluid volume leading to shock, and increased bacterial growth.**

2. **Increased peristalsis** is a result of enhanced intrinsic motor activity of the bowel both proximal and distal to the point of obstruction. The patient complains of colic or cramps; on examination, hyperactive bowel sounds are heard. The distal bowel is evacuated, after which the patient passes no flatus or feces if the obstruction is complete. After 24–28 hr, edema and muscular exhaustion supervene; bowel sounds are diminished and colic relents but usually does not disappear.

3. **Gas** accumulates in the bowel proximal to the obstruction, producing distention. Intestinal gas is derived almost entirely from swallowed air; minor volume contributions are made by bacterial fermentation and diffusion from blood gases.

4. **Fluid** accumulates in the bowel proximal to the obstruction, also producing distention. The increased fluid in the bowel lumen is caused chiefly by diminished absorption, but increased secretion also occurs. The fluid within the bowel lumen forms a "third space" and functionally is lost to the body. The small bowel may partially decompress itself by regurgitation into the stomach, resulting in vomiting.

5. **Contraction of extracellular (interstitial and plasma) volume** follows vomiting or sequestration of fluid in the obstructed bowel. In normal bowel, fluid turnover is about 7 liters each day. In obstructed small bowel, up to 50% of the plasma and interstitial fluid volumes (i.e., about 10 liters) may effectively be lost into and from the gut within 24 hr after onset of

TABLE 7-1. Some Causes of Intestinal Obstruction

Classification	Causes
Mechanical—extramural	Adhesions[a]—postoperative, peritonitis, enteritis, abscess, carcinoma Hernia[a]—external or internal Carcinomatosis Volvulus[a]—spontaneous, resulting from adhesions, congenital defect Intra-abdominal mass—tumor, abscess, cyst duplication Malrotation Annular pancreas Meckel's diverticulum Congenital bands Arteriomesenteric compression (superior mesenteric artery syndrome)
Mechanical—intramural	Carcinoma Stricture or stenosis—congenital, trauma, regional enteritis, radiation, tuberculosis, lymphopathia, endometriosis, enteric-coated potassium ulcer Hematoma—trauma, anticoagulants, hemophilia Diverticulitis Intussusception (lymphoid tissue in children, cancer in adults) Stoma/ostomy—stricture, edema, ulcer Polyp Congenital atresia or diaphragm Imperforate anus Meconium Gallstone ileus Bezoars, foreign bodies Fecal impaction
Paralytic—intra-abdominal	Inflammation, infection—appendicitis, cholecystitis, pancreatitis, etc. Peritonitis—bacterial (perforated bowel), chemical (bile, pancreatic juice, acid gastric juice) Wound dehiscence Mesenteric embolus[a]—arterial Mesenteric thrombosis[a]—venous, arterial Mesenteric ischemia[a]—shock, heart failure, vasopressors Blunt trauma[a] Distended bladder Gastric dilatation Hirschsprung's (aganglionic) megacolon Postcoarctation syndrome—mesenteric arteritis
Paralytic—retroperitoneal	Infection—pyelonephritis, abscess Ureteral stone or obstruction Vertebral fracture—lumbar, thoracic Pelvic fracture Central nervous system—trauma, tumor Hematoma—trauma, anticoagulants, hemophilia Tumor—primary (sarcoma, lymphoma) or metastatic Strangulation of spermatic cord, testicular torsion

[a]Gangrene may be present with these lesions.

TABLE 7-1 (Continued)

Classification	Causes
Paralytic—systemic	Potassium depletion Sodium depletion Drugs—ganglionic blockers, anticholinergics Emphysema Uremia Diabetic ketosis, neuropathy Lead poisoning Porphyria Septicemia Pneumonia, especially lower lobes Pulmonary embolus Empyema Meningitis

obstruction. Shock may result unless the lost fluid is replaced. Shock compounds the problems of a patient with obstruction, since it results in decreased arterial perfusion of the bowel.

6. While pyloric obstruction tends to produce alkalosis, resulting from loss of acid gastric juice, obstruction of small bowel results in predominant losses of sodium and in a tendency toward acidosis. In addition, there are significant losses of water and potassium.

7. Normal resting intraluminal pressure in small bowel is about 2-4 mm Hg, reaching 20-30 mm Hg with vigorous peristalsis. The intestinal vascular supply is oriented so that most vessels travel transversely within the bowel wall; the effects of peristalsis are thereby minimized. Intraluminal pressures up to 30 mm Hg have no appreciable effect on bowel vascular dynamics; pressures above 30 mm Hg cause lymphatic and capillary stasis, above 50 mm Hg result in occlusion of venous drainage, and above 90 mm Hg produce occlusion or arterial inflow. The bursting pressure of small bowel in man is 120-230 mm Hg.

8. Accumulation of fluid and gas within the obstructed bowel results in **increased intraluminal pressure.** In simple small-bowel obstruction, pressure may increase to 8-20 mm Hg, resulting in compromise of lymphatic drainage and promoting further fluid accumulation, but the small bowel is not in danger of bursting. The rise in intraluminal pressure is limited because the obstructed bowel decompresses itself by regurgitation of its contents into the stomach. In a closed-loop obstruction of small bowel (e.g., incarcerated external hernia), intraluminal pressures of 40-70 mm Hg may develop. The bowel is still in little danger of bursting because of increased pressure per se, but these high intraluminal pressures seriously interfere with blood and lymph flow. Submucosal vessels are occluded first as intraluminal pressure rises so that ischemia and subsequent necrosis initially affect only the mucosa. Later, necrosis may involve the entire muscular bowel wall and lead to perforation if very high pressures are maintained for several hours.

9. Distention also **reduces effective pulmonary ventilation** by elevating the diaphragm and reducing the effectiveness of abdominal respiratory movements.

10. Interference with lymph drainage as a result of increased intraluminal pressure produces **edema** and a further decrease in absorptive capacity of the mucosa, setting up a vicious cycle of fluid sequestration in the bowel lumen. Edema also interferes with effective muscular contraction so that ileus will persist for a time even after relief of the obstruction. Finally, edema may alter the permeability of the mucosa so that bacterial diapedesis and absorption of bacterial toxins occur.

11. **Bacterial growth** in the small bowel is enhanced by stasis. In early simple obstruction this may be of little consequence, but after a few hours of obstruction the small bowel must be regarded as filled with fluid feces. The high bacterial concentration is associated with an increased incidence of peritonitis, abscesses and wound infections, should resection of bowel be necessary to treat the obstruction or if the bowel is opened to decompress it.

C. **Signs and symptoms**

1. Clinical signs and symptoms of obstruction in **adults** are summarized in Tables 7-2 and 7-3.

2. In **infants,** obstruction should be suspected when any of these cardinal signs are present: (1) failure to evacuate meconium within 12 hr of birth, (2) green or bilious vomitus, or (3) abdominal distention.

3. **Colic** (cramps) coinciding with rushing peristalsis and sometimes with audible borborygmi is the classic pattern of pain in small-bowel obstruction. **Visible peristalsis** is frequent in children and is seen in 10% of adults with obstruction. Later in the course of untreated obstruction, when the bowel has "decompensated" and is too distended or edematous to contract effectively, colic is diminished or absent and is replaced with mild, dull, nonlocalized, steady discomfort.

TABLE 7-2. X-ray Signs in Intestinal Obstruction

Sign	Paralytic Ileus	Mechanical Obstruction
Gas in stomach	+ + +	+
Gas in bowel	+ + +	+
	Scattered in both large and small bowel	Only proximal to obstruction
Fluid in bowel	+	+ + +
Ladder pattern supine	+ +	+
Ladder pattern upright	+	+ +
Air-fluid interfaces at opposite ends of a bowel loop (upright film)	All tend to be at about same level across midabdomen; U-loops seen	Tend to be at different levels; J-loops seen

TABLE 7-3. Clinical Features in Intestinal Obstruction

Type Obstruction	Pain	Distention	Vomiting	Bowel Sounds	Tenderness	Temperature°C (°F)
Simple mechanical						
High small bowel	++ Cramps, mid- to upper-abdominal	+	+++ Early, bilious, persistent	Increased	Minimal, diffuse	<37.7 (<100)
Low small bowel	+++ Cramps, midabdominal	Early +++	++ Later, feculent	Increased, rushes	Minimal, diffuse	<37.7 (<100)
Colon	++ Cramps, mid- to lower-abdominal	Later +++	+ Very late, feculent	Usually increased	Minimal, diffuse	<37.7 (<100)
Strangulation	++++ Continuous, may localize, severe	++	+++ Persistent	Variable, usually decreased	Marked, localized	Normal
Paralytic ileus	+ Diffuse, mild	Very early ++++	+	Decreased	Minimal, diffuse	None
Vascular ileus	++++ Continuous, midabdominal and midback, may be severe	Early +++	+++	Decreased or absent	Marked, diffuse or localized	Usually >37.7 (>100)

4. **If pain is localized, steady, and intense, suspect strangulation.**

5. **Obstipation** is present early in complete obstruction, as soon as the initial reaction of hyperperistalsis has evacuated the distal bowel. Continued passage of small amounts of feces (often diarrheal) or flatus means that the obstruction is intermittent or incomplete.

6. **Distention** usually is present and is most prominent with low small-bowel obstructions. Distention is absent early in the course of obstruction, may be minimal with closed-loop obstructions, and often is not prominent and limited to the upper abdomen in high small-bowel obstruction.

7. **Vomiting** begins early and is bilious and persistent in high small-bowel obstruction. Vomiting appears later with more distal obstructions; it is initially bilious but later feculent. The early appearance of vomiting in low small-bowel obstruction suggests strangulation.

8. **Fever** is never caused by fluid loss in obstruction. If the temperature is above 37.7°C (100°F), suspect strangulation or perforation.

9. **Leukocytosis** is not usually prominent in simple obstruction. A high or a low leukocyte count suggests perforation or strangulation.

10. **Serum amylase** levels may be elevated, particularly if there is vomiting, but more often than not the amylase is normal.

11. Clinical signs of **saline depletion** (furrowed tongue, increasing hematocrit, oliguria, hypotension) and **water depletion** (thirst, dry axillae, increasing serum sodium) are present to some degree in every case (see Chap. 9). Fluid losses may account for all the systemic effects in many cases of obstruction.

12. Supine AP x-rays of the abdomen show distended bowel proximal to the obstruction and absence of gas distally. Multiple air-fluid levels are noted on upright or lateral decubitus views (see Table 7-2). Gas in the small bowel may be a normal finding in children less than 3 yr of age.

D. Treatment

1. Treatment of a simple mechanical obstruction is aimed at (1) relief of distention, (2) correction of fluid imbalances, and (3) removal of the obstruction.

2. **Nasogastric tube suction,** using an 18 Fr or larger tube, effectively short-circuits swallowed air, prevents further gas accumulation, and removes fluid regurgitated into the stomach, reducing the risk of aspiration.

3. Decompression with a **long intestinal tube** should be initiated in nearly all cases of mechanical small-bowel obstruction since a nasogastric tube alone will not as effectively decompress already distended bowel. Use an

18 Fr or larger tube: smaller tubes are not effective. Have the patient lie on his side; the tube can then most easily leave the stomach. Fluoroscopy usually is not needed.

4. Bowel preferably should be decompressed before operation. Decompression can be accomplished by "aseptic" aspiration during operation, but this procedure is associated with a high risk of infection and should be avoided. Intraoperative decompression via the long tube is preferable. The tube can be left in place postoperatively and may act as an intraluminal splint.

5. **IV fluid therapy** should be vigorous (see Chap. 9) and aimed at rapid restoration of major deficits. All patients need sodium- and potassium-containing fluids. The plasma volume deficit should be replaced with plasma substitutes, the interstitial fluid deficit with Ringer's lactate, and the intracellular fluid deficit with dextrose in water and added potassium. *A history of heart disease never should deter administration of saline solution.* Administration of only electrolyte-free water easily may produce water intoxication. Major fluid deficits and imbalances should be repaired before any operation is undertaken for uncomplicated simple mechanical obstruction.

6. **Antibiotics** in experimental animals reduce mortality from obstruction associated with strangulation. In patients without strangulation, the evidence is less clear that antibiotics are of benefit, but they should be administered preoperatively since bowel ischemia cannot be positively excluded in any patient until the abdomen has been explored. Neomycin or kanamycin is instilled via the long intestinal tube. An aminoglycoside plus clindamycin should be given systemically preoperatively. Systemic antibiotics should be continued postoperatively if indicated by the operative findings; otherwise, antibiotics need not be continued.

7. **No enemas** of any kind should be used. Enemas only confuse the x-ray picture by introducing gas into bowel distal to the obstruction. They are of no help in complete small-bowel obstruction and may make a partial obstruction worse.

8. **Oxygen** by nasal tube or mask may be of slight benefit in promoting absorption of intestinal gas but probably is of more benefit in partially overcoming the hypoxia resulting from pulmonary ventilatory restriction induced by distention.

9. **Watch out for strangulation!**   Repeated observations must be made during the period of initial tube and fluid treatment to detect signs of strangulation. The patient should be steadily improving, and colic and abdominal girth decreasing. Pain is usually decreased following intubation and beginning decompression in simple obstruction. If, instead, pain increases in intensity, localizes, or becomes continuous, strangulation may be present and the patient should be explored. If signs of peritonitis (rigidity, tenderness) appear, if a palpable abdominal, pelvic,

or rectal mass appears, or if the temperature or the leukocyte count goes markedly up or down, bowel ischemia must be presumed and urgent exploration of the abdomen carried out.

10. **Nonoperative treatment with a long intestinal suction tube may be continued** beyond the period of initial decompression and fluid therapy in these situations:

   a. An incomplete obstruction which is progressively improving.

   b. Obstruction occurring in the immediate postoperative period.

   c. Decompression resulting in conversion of a complete to an incomplete obstruction.

   d. The "frozen abdomen"—patients with a history of many previous operations for relief of obstruction resulting from adhesions, or patients with proven abdominal carcinomatosis.

11. **Long-tube treatment should be abandoned** if progressive improvement does not continue in any 12-hr period of treatment. Complications of tube treatment are usually minor, but mucosal necrosis and other complications do occur with prolonged intubation.

12. **Operative treatment**   "Never let the sun rise or set on an intestinal obstruction" is a reasonable rule. An uncomplicated mechanical obstruction of small bowel, however, is not an emergency. Time must be taken to replace fluid and electrolyte deficits prior to the operation. Operative relief is needed in nearly every case of complete small-bowel obstruction and in many cases of incomplete obstruction. The objective of operative treatment is release, removal, or repair of the cause of the obstruction. Diseased or necrotic small bowel must be resected. A primary anastomosis is much preferable to exteriorization. Proximal decompression (enterostomy) is only palliative and often leads to difficult postoperative fluid management problems. Bypass of the obstruction is acceptable only when definitive treatment is neither safe nor feasible; a bypass may be followed by a blind-loop syndrome (chronic diarrhea, malabsorption, and weight loss). Mortality of operative treatment is between 0.5 and 3% and is influenced by both the patient's general condition and the cause of the obstruction. In patients presenting with obstruction caused by adhesions, recurrence of obstruction after operative release occurs in 10%. In cases of such recurrent obstruction, intestinal plication can be considered.

III. SIMPLE MECHANICAL OBSTRUCTION OF THE COLON

A. Causes

1. **Carcinoma** causes 90% of colon obstructions; of these, 90% are between the splenic flexure and the rectum.

2. **Volvulus** (sigmoid, cecum) is the other frequent cause of mechanical colon obstruction.

3. **Fecal impaction** is common among aged patients and may resemble a colon obstruction.

B. Pathophysiology

1. The consequences of colon obstruction are similar to those of small-bowel obstruction; distention though greater occurs later and vomiting much later than in small-bowel obstructions.

2. Increased peristalsis produces colic which progresses to eventual exhaustion.

3. Accumulation of gas is very marked. Swallowed air still contributes the major volume, but methane, hydrogen sulfide, and other products of bacterial fermentation provide about one fourth of the gas volume in colon obstruction.

4. Accumulation of fluid in the obstructed colon is also marked, resulting from failure of normal water absorptive mechanisms in the right colon.

5. Fluid losses into the luminal "third space" have the same consequences as in small-bowel obstruction: contraction of the extracellular fluid volume progressing to shock.

6. Accumulation of fluid and gas behind the obstruction leads to progressive distention of the small bowel if the ileocecal valve is incompetent (50-60% of patients) and eventually to feculent vomiting.

7. The intraluminal pressure in unobstructed colon is 2-4 mm Hg. In a complete mechanical colon obstruction, if the ileocecal valve is competent and does not yield, a closed-loop obstruction (i.e., obstructed at both ends) is present. A pressure of 50-70 mm Hg is needed to force open a competent ileocecal valve. The bursting pressure of normal colon is about 70-80 mm Hg, considerably lower than the bursting pressure of small bowel. The pressures necessary to decompress the obstructed colon rapidly approach the bursting pressure. Primary rupture of the colon, usually at the cecum, is a definite threat. The high intraluminal pressure also blocks the lymphatic and capillary circulation, as in small-bowel obstruction, and may lead to patches of ischemic gangrene and perforation.

C. Signs and symptoms

1. Clinical signs and symptoms are similar to those of low small-bowel obstruction but develop more slowly.

2. Distention is marked; vomiting occurs late. Alternating diarrhea and constipation may have preceded frank obstruction. With volvulus, a large loop of colon often is visible on x-ray.

3. If the diameter of the distended cecum exceeds 12 cm or the distended transverse colon exceeds 8 cm, rupture is an imminent threat.

D. Treatment

1. Treatment, as in small-bowel obstruction, has three objectives: relief of distention, correction of fluid imbalances, and removal of the obstruction.

2. Sigmoid volvulus usually can be reduced by careful entry of a sigmoidoscope or a rectal tube into the twisted loop. Be prepared for a sudden and copious passage of flatus and feces. If sigmoidoscopic reduction is successful, the patient may then be prepared for elective resection of the redundant loop. Failure of sigmoidoscopic reduction often means that strangulation of the twisted loop has occurred. If reduction is not successful, or if volvulus recurs, sigmoid resection should be carried out at once.

3. In other colon obstructions (carcinoma, cecal volvulus, etc.), **principles of preoperative treatment** are:

   a. A nasogastric tube should be passed in all patients and put on suction.

   b. Vigorous IV fluid therapy (see Chap. 9) should prepare the patient for the operation as quickly as possible.

   c. Enemas for the purpose of evacuating the bowel are not indicated; they only serve to confuse the x-ray picture. A diagnostic barium enema under careful supervision sometimes is useful in confirming that carcinoma is the cause of the obstruction. Barium should not be allowed to pass proximal to an incompletely obstructing carcinoma, since it may become inspissated and convert the partial obstruction to a complete one, requiring immediate operative relief.

   d. Antibiotic bowel preparation (see Chap. 14) should be started in every case and completed whenever possible. If diverticulitis is present, or if there is any suspicion of strangulation, systemic antibiotics should be started preoperatively and, if indicated, continued after the operation.

4. **Treatment of a colon obstruction** (other than a sigmoid volvulus) **always involves an early operation.** There is no place for prolonged nonoperative tube suction therapy.

5. Resection of the obstructing lesion and primary end-to-end anastomosis may be elected in cases of obstruction seen early with no evidence of peritonitis and only minimal bowel wall edema. A proximal colostomy always should be done in such cases to decompress the new anastomosis; a cecostomy is not adequate decompression.

6. Resection of necrotic bowel is mandatory. An adequate exploration must be made to ensure that all the obstructed bowel not resected is viable. If the bowel ends are judged unsuitable for primary anastomosis, they should be exteriorized through separate wounds as an end colostomy and a mucous fistula.

7. Resection of an obstructing descending or sigmoid carcinoma and exteriorization of the bowel ends is preferred to a loop colostomy if the patient can tolerate this more extensive procedure.

8. Proximal diverting loop colostomy is the minimum operative treatment in colon obstruction. The colostomy sometimes may be placed just proximal to the obstruction so that later the colostomy can be resected with the obstructing lesion.

IV. PARALYTIC (adynamic, neurogenic) ILEUS

A. Causes

1. The fundamental mechanism producing paralytic ileus is unclear, but it is probably related to extrinsic inhibition since intrinsic contractility is not altered.

2. The more common lesions associated with paralytic ileus are:

   a. Neurogenic—spinal cord tumors and trauma, lead poisoning.

   b. Retroperitoneal—vertebral fractures, infection, hematoma.

   c. Intraperitoneal—peritonitis (chemical, bacterial), enteritis, colitis.

   d. Systemic—pneumonia, uremia, diabetes, porphyria, ganglionic blocking drugs.

   e. Other causes of paralytic ileus are listed in Table 7-1.

B. Pathophysiology

1. Decreased peristaltic activity and failure of progressive peristalsis occur without loss of intrinsic ability of the bowel to contract.

2. Gas derived from swallowed air accumulates in the involved segments of bowel producing marked, early distention which may seriously impair pulmonary ventilation.

3. Fluid also accumulates in the involved bowel because of failure of normal absorptive mechanisms. While significant volumes of fluid may be sequestered in such a "third space," the potential loss of extracellular fluid volume is not as great as in mechanical obstruction. Shock resulting from fluid loss is unusual in uncomplicated paralytic ileus.

4. The accumulation of gas and fluid causes only a small rise in intraluminal pressure. Lymphatic drainage may be slightly compromised so that some edema may accumulate in bowel wall but, again, such changes are slight as compared with those seen in mechanical obstruction. The intraluminal pressure does not reach levels that interfere with capillary blood flow or threaten rupture.

C. Signs and symptoms

1. Gaseous distention is prominent and the abdomen may be very tense and tympanitic.

2. Pain is dull, diffuse, and related to the degree of distention. Colic sometimes is present early in paralytic ileus and reappears as the ileus clears and progressive peristalsis is resumed, but it is never as prominent a part of the clinical history as in mechanical obstruction.

3. Obstipation is rarely complete, and small amounts of flatus may be passed throughout the period of ileus.

4. Peristalsis is usually depressed and bowel sounds may be infrequent, but peristalsis does not completely disappear. High-pitched and tinkling sounds are characteristic of paralytic ileus; the quality of bowel sounds is not a reliable criterion in differentiating paralytic ileus from mechanical obstruction.

5. Vomiting occurs as a result of ingestion of food or fluid but frequently does not occur if the patient does not eat or drink. The volume of vomitus is less than in mechanical obstruction.

D. Treatment

1. Therapy first should be directed at the underlying cause of the ileus.

2. Treatment of the ileus itself involves:

    a. Provision of IV fluids.

    b. Prevention of further distention by passage of a nasogastric tube. A long intestinal tube usually will not leave the stomach, so that long-tube therapy is not effective in paralytic ileus.

3. A wide variety of other treatments have been proposed which seem to be more emotionally than objectively oriented: hot stupes, repeated enemas, Pituitrin, neostigmine (prostigmin), pilocarpine, choline, pantothenic acid, spinal anesthesia, and electrical intraluminal stimulators. None of these measures has proved to be of real value.

4. The best adjunctive therapy in paralytic ileus would appear to be observation and the passage of time.

V. STRANGULATION OBSTRUCTION

A. Causes

1. Strangulation involves the small bowel more often than the colon; a closed-loop type of obstruction is usually present.

2. The most common cause of strangulation obstruction is an incarcerated external hernia; internal hernia and volvulus are other frequent causes.

3. Vascular compromise may be caused by the same factors that produced the mechanical obstruction (e.g., restricting hernial ring). Alternatively, strangulation may occur after the onset of obstruction and be caused by increasing pressure within a closed loop or twisting of the vascular pedicle of a fluid-filled loop resulting in ischemia.

B. Pathophysiology

1. The disordered physiology seen in strangulation obstruction is superimposed on that of mechanical obstruction and is the result of:

   a. Entrance of bacteria and bacterial products both into the circulation and into the peritoneal cavity through the necrotic bowel wall.

   b. Marked losses of plasma and whole blood into the bowel lumen.

2. Bacteria multiply rapidly in the lumen of obstructed bowel but do not pass through normal mucosa. Ischemia removes the mucosal barrier, permitting absorption of bacterial products from the bowel lumen. Bacteria invade the bowel wall, producing:

   a. Thrombosis of small blood vessels and necrosis of tissue.

   b. Diapedesis of live bacteria across the bowel wall to contaminate the peritoneal cavity.

3. A vasodepressor substance (kinin) which can cause shock appears in portal vein blood promptly after the onset of bowel ischemia.

4. The primary cause of toxicity and shock in strangulation obstruction is related to the presence of coliform endotoxin in the strangulation fluid found both within the bowel loop and in the peritoneal cavity. Exotoxins, primarily clostridial alpha-toxin, also enter the bloodstream and can produce septic shock. In many cases of strangulation, absorption of toxic materials is minimal until the venous obstruction is released, but then it occurs very rapidly.

5. Protection against the lethal effects of strangulation is obtained in experimental animals by either of the following:

   a. Preventing access to the body of the contents of the strangulated loop by placing it in a plastic bag.

   b. Pretreating the intestinal lumen with antibiotics. Confirmation of the importance of bacteria in producing the lethal effects of strangulation is provided by the fact that strangulation in germ-free animals is not fatal.

6. Fluid and blood losses are also important elements in the consequences of strangulation. Arterial obstruction produces an ischemic necrosis. Venous obstruction produces hemorrhagic necrosis. Hemorrhagic necrosis leads to more marked losses of blood, leading to shock.

C. Signs and symptoms

1. Clinical signs and symptoms in strangulation obstruction are initially those of the underlying mechanical obstruction (colic, distention, vomiting), but there is rapid progression and an early deterioration in the clinical state.

2. It is often difficult to differentiate simple obstruction from strangulation obstruction. Cramps may be replaced by severe, constant abdominal pain. Distention may not be so prominent. Vomiting, in particular, tends to be severe and persistent early in strangulation obstruction and is probably caused in part by stimulation of reverse peristalsis by the ischemic bowel. Fever and leukocytosis are usually present, although with peritonitis the leukocyte count may be low. Serum amylase and lactic dehydrogenase levels are sometimes elevated but cannot be relied on to make a diagnosis of strangulation. Blood ammonia levels also may be increased.

3. Strangulated loops do not become filled with gas and so are not visualized on plain x-rays of the abdomen.

D. Treatment

1. Strangulation obstruction is a surgical emergency.

2. Treatment involves systemic administration of an aminoglycoside and clindamycin plus oral administration of nonabsorbable neomycin followed by nasogastric suction, whole-blood transfusion, and IV fluids in rapid preparation for operation.

3. Inadequate blood replacement is a prime cause of death in patients with strangulation, so that a short period spent in preparing the patient preoperatively with transfusions is rewarded with a lowered operative mortality.

4. All necrotic bowel must be resected. The vascular pedicle should be approached first and control obtained to minimize entry of bacteria and their toxins into the portal vein on release of the obstruction.

5. In general, the simplest possible operative procedure should be carried out. Resection and primary anastomosis may be possible in early cases of strangulation without gross peritonitis, but temporary exteriorization of bowel ends more usually will be the prudent course.

VI. VASCULAR ILEUS (mesenteric infarction)

A. Between 1900 and the present, mortality from simple bowel obstruction has been reduced from 60% to about 1%. The mortality with strangulation obstruction is still 30%, and in vascular ileus it is an appalling 60%! Necrosis of the bowel is a very lethal lesion.

B. Vascular ileus may be present with any of the following:

1. **No vascular obstruction**   A triad of congestive heart failure, digitalis intoxication, and hemoconcentration is associated with a low cardiac output and mesenteric ischemia.

2. **Thrombosis**   Either venous or arterial thrombosis may be traumatic, atherosclerotic, inflammatory, cancerous, or spontaneous.

3. **Embolism**   This is always arterial. The clot may originate in the heart (atrial fibrillation, ventricular infarction, or aneurysm), but more usually the embolus originates on an ulcerated atherosclerotic plaque located proximally in the arterial system.

C. The pathophysiological changes in vascular ileus are similar to those in strangulation obstruction, but they tend to be quantitatively more severe and life-threatening since a larger segment of bowel usually is affected.

D. Clinically, vascular ileus presents as paralytic ileus, but it is accompanied by more severe midabdominal pain than simple paralytic ileus. Tenderness often is absent or minimal. Midback pain often is present. X-rays usually show only scattered small amounts of gas; the rigid loop sign should be sought. There is a rapid deterioration, with persistent vomiting, sweating, bloody stools, and shock. Sometimes there is an asymptomatic interval between the onset of symptoms and later evidence of frank bowel necrosis and peritonitis. This period of apparent improvement should not delay urgent operative treatment.

E. **Mesenteric arteriography** is indicated in any older patient presenting with abdominal pain and an apparent paralytic ileus for which an explanation is not readily apparent on completion of the history, physical examination, and screening laboratory tests. Arteriography should be done at once in any patient with atrial fibrillation or a recent myocardial infarction who develops "obscure abdominal pain." Aggressive use of arteriography may result in an earlier diagnosis of arterial or venous obstruction of bowel.

F. Despite the best attempts, definitive treatment of vascular ileus often is not initiated early enough for embolectomy or thrombectomy to preserve bowel viability. Nonetheless, unless the bowel is completely gangrenous, attempts at restoration of circulation are worthwhile. Preoperative preparation is the same as that for strangulation obstruction. All necrotic bowel must be resected, but if some question of viability of a major portion of small bowel remains after a reasonable period of observation, the abdomen should be closed and reexplored 12–24 hr later, when viability or lack of it will be more obvious.

8. CARE OF THE PATIENT BEFORE AND AFTER OPERATION

I. ROUTINE ORDERS Orders are used to convey to other members of the surgical team—nurses, physical therapists, technicians—exactly what the surgeon wants done for his patient. Orders must be clear, concise, and inclusive.

A. Patient admitted for elective operation

1. **Diagnosis** A record of the admitting diagnosis is helpful to alert the hospital staff to the care the patient needs and complications that may arise.

2. **Diet** Selection of a diet should provide adequate caloric and vitamin intake for the patient's overall condition and the present surgical problem.

   a. **Dentition** Patients without teeth, with poorly fitting dentures, or with an oral tumor or other lesion cannot chew solid foods well. Order a soft or liquid diet.

   b. **Debilitation** Chronic illness may cause loss of weight and appetite. Such patients need frequent small feedings of high-caloric food with supplements such as milk shakes. If the appetite is so poor that the patient refuses food, a small tube should be passed through the nose into the stomach and liquified high-calorie foods dripped in continuously (see Chap. 10). In some cases, IV hyperalimentation may be necessary to supplement oral intake to insure that the patient is in positive nitrogen balance (see Chap. 10).

   c. **Heart disease** Patients may be on a low-salt diet, which usually should be continued. If they also take diuretics, the diet should contain foods high in potassium content.

   d. **Diabetes** Specify the carbohydrate content and the caloric intake desired. Diabetic patients may need supplemental snacks at bedtime.

   e. **Esophageal lesions** These usually are obstructive. The diet will depend on the degree of stricture, but baby food or a high-caloric liquid diet may be all that can be swallowed.

   f. **Ulcers** Patients with active stomach and duodenal ulcers require a bland diet. Coffee, tea, alcohol, and spicy or fried foods are prohibited.

g. Cholecystitis and **pancreatitis**   These patients should be given a low-fat diet.

h. Colon disease   Patients with diverticulitis may have the residue content of their diet altered. At the present time, controversy exists whether a high- or low-residue diet is the best choice. Certainly, foods known to cause irritability in a patient should be eliminated.

3. **Activity**   As a general rule, maximal activity commensurate with the patient's condition should be allowed. Inactivity leads to thromboembolism, muscle atrophy, and other complications.

4. **Vital signs**   These include temperature, pulse, blood pressure, and respirations. Vital signs do not need to be recorded more than once daily unless the patient is ill or his condition is changing. If temperature readings are desired more often than once daily, the frequency with which the temperature is to be recorded should be stated, and the method—oral or rectal—should be specified. Nothing is to be gained by recording the temperature more often than every 4 hr, even in a very ill patient.

5. **Sedation**   Most preoperative patients are anxious, and an appropriate sedative should be ordered. Short-acting barbiturates are preferred for most adults but may act as stimulants in elderly patients. Chloral hydrate or diphenhydramine HCl (Benadryl) are excellent sedatives if liver function is compromised. Do not use narcotics or tranquilizers for bedtime sedation.

6. **Headache**   An anxious patient frequently develops minor headaches and similar problems. An order for aspirin is worthwhile.

7. **Constipation**   Elderly patients frequently are bothered by this problem, and an order for a mild laxative is helpful.

8. **Medications currently used**   The patient may be taking medication for other diseases or for the surgical problem. These medications should be continued unless contraindicated by the surgical problem or its proposed treatment. The management of diabetic patients and of those on steroids is discussed in Chapter 13.

9. **Vitamins**   The water-soluble B and C vitamins are especially indicated in the debilitated patient prior to operation. B vitamins are essential in intermediary metabolism of carbohydrates. Vitamin C (ascorbic acid) aids in wound healing. There are no great body stores of B or C vitamins, and they need to be provided daily. Vitamin K is indicated preoperatively in jaundiced patients, as their prothrombin may be low; it should be given parenterally.

10. **Daily bath,** with special attention to the area of the planned incision.

11. **Lung function**   Many elderly patients, those at any age who smoke cigarettes, and patients with chronic bronchitis or emphysema are in-

creased risks for general anesthesia. Postural drainage, mucolytic agents, and, when indicated by positive sputum cultures, appropriate antibiotics should be ordered to help improve lung function prior to the operation (see Chap. 12).

B. Emergency admission for urgent operation   These patients are extremely ill with possibly life-threatening problems. The diagnosis may or may not be obvious.

1. **Diet**   Any patient who is a candidate for emergency operation should have nothing by mouth (NPO); this includes water and oral drugs.

2. **Medications**   The special problem in this group of patients is usually pain. Since pain may be the only clue to diagnosis and the only symptom which can be followed to determine whether the patient's condition is getting better or worse, it should not be masked by giving narcotics or other anodynes. As a general rule: **No medication should be given for relief of pain until a diagnosis has been established and a decision has been made whether or not to operate.** If the patient has sepsis, appropriate antibiotics should be started (see Chap. 14).

3. **Fluid therapy**   Almost all the patients in this group will require IV fluid therapy to correct dehydration and electrolyte imbalance (see Chap. 9).

C. Preoperative orders   These orders are written the day before a planned operation.

1. **Nothing by mouth** is indicated usually for at least 8 hr preoperatively to allow the patient's stomach to empty and to reduce the risk of vomiting and aspiration on induction of anesthesia. The most convenient regimen is to discontinue solids after the patient's evening meal and liquids after bedtime the night before he is to undergo the operation.

2. **Bath before bedtime** from head to toe, including a shampoo.

3. **Enema**   The evening before operation, order an emema to empty the distal colon. On induction of general anesthesia, patients may relax their sphincters and defecate on the operating table if the distal colon and rectum are not empty.

4. **Voiding**   The patient should void before leaving for the operating suite, for the same reason as above. If he is unable to void, consider placing an indwelling catheter to remain through the early postoperative period.

5. **Sedation**   An appropriate sedative should be ordered for bedtime, to be repeated as necessary.

6. All **oral medications** that must be taken by the patient during the few hours immediately prior to operation should be changed to parenteral (IM or IV) administration.

7. **Local anesthetic**   For patients who will have local anesthesia, premedication orders should be written by the surgeon. A combination of drugs usually is used, the particular combination and dose depending on the size and condition of the patient. A healthy young adult patient weighing 150 or more pounds may require IM administration of meperidine (Demerol), 100 mg; secobarbital (Seconal), 100 mg; promethazine (Phenergan), 25 mg or diazepam (Valium), 10 mg; and atropine, 0.4 mg, ½ hr before an operation under local anesthesia. Premedication should make the patient very drowsy. Reduce these doses to meperidine, 50 mg; secobarbital, 75 mg; promethazine, 25 mg or diazepam, 10 mg; and atropine, 0.4 mg for an adult patient weighing less than 150 lb; reduce doses of all drugs except atropine by half after age 50. Eliminate all narcotics and sedatives in any patient with chronic respiratory or liver disease. Eliminate barbiturates in patients over age 60 and narcotics in patients over age 65. A 70-year-old, 125-lb patient may need only 0.4 mg of atropine.

8. **Preoperative medication for general or regional anesthetics is usually ordered by the anesthetist.** If not, the regimen outlined above for local anesthetics will prove satisfactory.

9. **Consent** should be obtained by the surgeon the day prior to operation. A full explanation of what is to be done should be given at this time along with answers to any questions the patient may have. In some hospitals patients may visit postoperative areas, such as the recovery room and intensive care unit; an explanation of activities in each area is given by the nurse. Such steps are helpful in relieving anxiety.

D. **Postoperative orders**   Orders for the postoperative patient follow the same general outline as that for admission. All orders must be rewritten postoperatively. No order is carried over from preoperative orders. As the patient's condition changes and improves postoperatively, orders will have to be revised daily. Generally this involves increases in diet and activity and decreases in medication.

1. **Operation**   A statement of what was done should be included in the orders for the same reasons that the diagnosis was stated on admission: to inform the staff of the nature of the operation so that they can anticipate the kinds of care that may be needed and the complications that need to be sought.

2. **Vital signs** may be unstable for a few hours after an operation. For this reason, vital signs should be recorded half-hourly for the first few hours and then less often after they stabilize. If the patient's condition is so unstable that vital signs need to be recorded more often than half-hourly, a responsible physician should be in constant attendance and the patient should be in an intensive care unit.

3. **Diet** is dependent on the type of operation and the type and duration of anesthesia. In general, the patient initially is kept NPO. Oral intake is started when bowel sounds are present and the patient is passing flatus. Start with liquids and, if they are tolerated for one or two meals, pro-

gress to a general diet or other solid foods. Stepwise advancement of the diet (clear liquid, full liquid, bland-soft) is not necessary. As soon as the patient can eat, start the appropriate solid diet.

4. **Activity**   This, too, will depend on the operation performed, the type of anesthetic used, and the duration of anesthesia. Most patients having a general anesthetic and an operation in a major body cavity will be at bed rest during the afternoon after the operation. Beginning in the evening or certainly by the next morning they should be up walking around the bed with assistance; they should progressively increase activity each day. Remember, inactivity leads to complications. Connection of tubes for IV fluids, nasogastric suction, catheters, etc., may complicate but does not contraindicate ambulation.

5. **Narcotics**   The patient should receive sufficient narcotic medication to relieve pain. Remember that narcotics depress the respiratory center. Administration of large doses can be associated with hypoventilation, hypercapnia, atelectasis, and hypoxia. Small doses of morphine (5-8 mg) or meperidine (50-75 mg) given frequently (q2-3h) are more effective in relieving pain than larger doses given on the more traditional 4-hr schedule. Pentazocine (Talwin) is an effective nonnarcotic anodyne said to cause less respiratory depression than narcotics.

6. **Sedatives**   In the immediate postoperative period, narcotics given for pain relief provide more than adequate sedation. Beginning on the second or third postoperative day, when pain has subsided and the patient is taking liquids, narcotics may be reduced or stopped and sedatives for sleep may be given orally at night.

7. **Vomiting**   Nasogastric intubation and suction should be used in patients who vomit repetitively after an abdominal operation. Antiemetics, such as prochlorperazine (Compazine), are effective in controlling short-term postanesthetic nausea. Remember that the patient who has gastric distention secondary to a plugged nasogastric tube also will vomit; antiemetic drugs will not correct this problem. Be sure of the etiology before you treat.

8. **Turn, cough, and hyperventilate**   A "stir-up" regimen should be ordered every few hours in the early postoperative period. It prevents splinting of one side of the chest resulting from lying continually in one position, helps to prevent accumulation of secretions, and reduces the tendency to atelectasis. Mucolytic agents or bronchodilators should be given by nebulizer if the patient needs them. The management of patients with compromised respiratory function is discussed in Chapter 12.

9. A daily record of **intake and output** and of **body weight** should be kept to help decide the volume and type of fluid replacement required.

10. **IV fluids and parenteral nutrition** are discussed in Chapters 9 and 10.

11. Care of **drains and tubes** is discussed in Section V of this chapter.

12. **Specific medication required by the surgical problem** depends on the nature of the disease and its operative treatment.

13. **Medication for concurrent problems,** such as chronic heart failure, should be restarted as soon as possible. Usually these drugs will have to be given by injection at first. Diabetic patients and those on steroids have special problems which are discussed in Chapter 13.

14. **Notify the surgeon** of (a) unstable vital signs (set specific limits), (b) unusual drainage on dressings or via catheters or tubes, (c) inability to void (set time limit), and (d) any other specific problem, as appropriate.

II. EVALUATION OF RENAL, CARDIAC, AND PULMONARY FUNCTION

A. Renal function

1. **Preoperative evaluation** Routine **urinalysis** and measurement of **serum creatinine** provide sufficient screening evaluation for a healthy person with no history of renal disease. Patients with prior renal disease, advanced age, arteriosclerosis, hypertension, diabetes mellitus, cardiac disease, urinary infection, or urinary obstruction also should have preoperative testing of glomerular and tubular function by **creatinine clearance** and **urine concentration tests.**

   a. **Urinalysis**

      (1) **Specific gravity** Random urine samples usually have a specific gravity of 1.012-1.025. Higher specific gravity reflects dehydration or the abundance of unusual solutes such as radiographic dye (after IVP or angiography) or glucose (each gram of glucose per 100 ml of urine increases the specific gravity by 0.003). Dilute urine (specific gravity less than 1.007) reflects overhydration, diuretic therapy, water intoxication, or diabetes insipidus. A fixed specific gravity in the range of 1.010 to 1.014 (isosthenuria) signifies lack of renal tubular concentrating ability and occurs in renal parenchymal disease, congenital tubular defects, and acute tubular necrosis.

      (2) **Urine pH** ranges from 4.3 to 8, reflecting diet and acid-base balance. Persistent aciduria may result from metabolic or respiratory acidosis, potassium depletion (paradoxical aciduria), starvation, or fever. Alkaline urine may result from metabolic or respiratory alkalosis, certain urinary infections, and carbonic anhydrase inhibitor diuretics.

      (3) **Protein** Transitory proteinuria may result from acute stress (fever, exposure to cold, strenuous exercise, acute abdominal crisis). Persistent proteinuria signifies renal disease and, when present, should be quantitated in a 24-hr urine collection (normal is less than 250 mg/24 hr).

(4) Glucose   Glycosuria usually signifies diabetes mellitus but may result from benign renal glycosuria, renal tubular disorders, pregnancy, and IV glucose infusion. Ascorbic acid, cephalosporins, salicylates, paraldehyde, and chloral hydrate may produce positive reactions to urine tests for reducing agents.

(5) Ketone   Ketonuria, the hallmark of diabetic ketoacidosis, also occurs in conditions accompanied by excessive vomiting, starvation, or cachexia, and may occur after strenuous exercise or exposure to cold.

(6) Occult blood   The dipstick test for occult blood reacts positively if there are more than 10 red blood cells per high-power field in the spun urine sediment. The test is also positive with myoglobin or hemoglobin in the urine.

(7) Urine sediment   The spun sediment of normal urine contains few epithelial cells, occasional red and white blood cells, and occasional hyaline or granular casts. More than five cells or casts per high-power field indicate possible renal parenchymal or urinary tract disease.

b. Serum creatinine and BUN   The BUN concentration varies with dietary nitrogen consumed, hepatic production of urea, and endogenous catabolism of protein; it also may be elevated by excessive protein ingestion, GI bleeding, hemolysis, and tissue breakdown in trauma, shock, or sepsis. The serum creatinine concentration more reliably reflects renal function. Creatinine production is related to muscle mass and remains nearly constant from day to day.

c. Creatinine clearance   The excretion of endogenous creatinine reflects **glomerular function.** Urine volume and creatinine concentration are measured for a specific time interval; a 24-hr measurement is most accurate, but a 2-hr test is reasonably reliable. The patient empties the bladder and discards the urine at the start of the test. Then all urine up to and including the emptying of the bladder at the completion of the test is collected. Serum creatinine concentration is measured in the middle of the urine collection period.

   Creatinine clearance = UV/P, where U = urine creatinine concentration in mg/100 ml, V = urine volume in ml/min (there are 1440 min/24 hr or 120 min in 2 hr), and P = serum creatinine concentration in mg/100 ml. Creatinine clearance varies with lean body mass and is approximately 120 ml/min for adult males and 100 ml/min for adult females. A minimum creatinine clearance of 10 ml is necessary to maintain life without dialysis. Serum creatinine concentration may remain normal until creatinine clearance is less than half of normal.

d. Concentration test   Examination of the first-voided, morning urine specimen for osmotic concentration or specific gravity is a simple test of **tubular function.** Specific gravity of 1.025 or osmolality of 750 mOsm/liter implies normal tubular concentrating ability. Renal tubules are able to dilute or concentrate urine through a specific gravity range of 1.003 to 1.035 and an osmolality range of 50 to 1,500 mOsm/liter. Abnormal tubules are unable to dilute or concentrate glomerular filtrate appropriately; the urine resembles serum in its solute concentration (specific gravity 1.010, osmolality 320 mOsm/kg).

The concentration test can be performed over a 24-hr period. In the first 12 hr the patient takes a regular diet but restricts fluids to 500 ml/m^2 body surface (about 865 ml for a 70-kg patient). In the subsequent 12 hr (overnight) no fluids are allowed. In normal subjects, urine specific gravity will rise to 1.025 or greater and the urine osmolality to 750 mOsm/liter or greater when measured in the urine first voided the next morning.

2. Preoperative prophylaxis of renal failure

   a. An initial response to the stress of operation is redistribution of intrarenal blood flow, resulting in decreased glomerular filtration. This occurs with all major operations and may precipitate renal failure if other factors which compromise renal function are present.

   b. Urinary tract infection should be treated preoperatively by appropriate antibiotic therapy determined by urine culture and sensitivity tests.

   c. Obstructive lesions of the urinary tract should be removed or bypassed prior to other major operations.

   d. Dehydration hypovolemia and electrolyte imbalance should be corrected and adequate urine volume assured prior to operation.

   e. Nephrotoxic agents (e.g., kanamycin, gentamicin) should be used with caution.

3. Preoperative management of renal insufficiency   The management of postoperative acute renal failure is discussed in Chapter 11. The same principles apply in preparation of a patient with established renal insufficiency for an operation.

   a. Precise fluid and electrolyte balance   The diseased kidney, unable to concentrate urine, requires a greater urine volume to excrete metabolic end products, yet may be unable to excrete excess water and electrolytes. A slim margin exists between further renal insufficiency from underhydration and congestive heart failure from excess salt and water. Effective management requires monitoring body weight, intake, output, serum electrolytes and pH, and CVP. Urine output and specific gravity will not reliably reflect the state of hydration. Enough fluid should be given to provide a urine volume of 1,500-2,000 ml/day. Measuring electrolyte concentration in the urine and recording the volume of all measurable losses guide selection of appropriate IV solutions (see Chap. 9).

   b. Anemia should be partially corrected prior to operation. A hemoglobin of 9 gm/100 ml and hematocrit of 25% are satisfactory preoperative levels for patients with chronic renal insufficiency.

c. Patients with chronic renal disease frequently harbor **coagulation abnormalities** which should be identified and corrected prior to operation (see Chap. 16).

d. **Sodium bicarbonate** should be administered prior to operation to correct metabolic acidosis, even though compensated, because of the risk of sudden severe acidosis if hypoventilation occurs during anesthesia.

e. If **hemodialysis** is required, it should be planned for the day prior to operation. The next hemodialysis with its attendant anticoagulation can then be delayed until the second or third postoperative day.

f. **Hyperkalemia following operation should be anticipated**   Obtain frequent measurements of serum potassium in the postoperative period. Usually, increases in serum potassium can be managed by administration of intestinal potassium-exchange resin (Kayexalate), 40-80 gm mixed with 50 ml of sorbitol, by mouth, nasogastric tube, or retention enema (exchange rate is 1 mEq of potassium per gram of resin). Hemodialysis is necessary for hyperkalemia which cannot be controlled by potassium-exchange resin.

4. **Postoperative anuria and oliguria**   Postoperative urine output of less than 25 ml/hr requires immediate evaluation. Oliguria suggests either prerenal or renal (parenchymal) failure; total anuria suggests vascular obstruction, cortical necrosis, or urinary tract obstruction (postrenal failure). Acute renal parenchymal failure is discussed in Chapter 14.

B. Cardiac function

1. **Preoperative screening**

a. A careful **history** and **physical examination** are the most important measures of estimating cardiac function. Every patient should be specifically questioned for symptoms of dyspnea, chest pain, exercise intolerance, syncope, peripheral edema, nocturia, and orthopnea. Document any past history of rheumatic fever or heart disease. Record past or current use of diuretics, digitalis, coronary vasodilators, and antiarrhythmic agents. Examine the heart carefully for murmurs, gallop rhythm, and arrhythmias. Attempt to distinguish significant findings from innocent murmurs or rhythm irregularities which tend to disappear with brief exercise. Listen carefully for murmurs of aortic stenosis, pulmonary stenosis, and atrial septal defect which may be asymptomatic yet pose a significant risk to the patient undergoing a major operation.

b. Preoperative PA and lateral **chest x-rays** may disclose evidence of heart disease not suspected from the history and physical exam.

c. An **ECG** should be obtained in patients over age 40, and in any patient who has heart disease suspected from the history, physical examination, or chest radiograph.

d. The ability to walk up two flights of stairs without stopping and without development of dyspnea, angina, or significant tachycardia is a gross but generally reliable indicator of good cardiopulmonary function.

2. In patients with **evidence of heart disease,** further cardiac evaluation must be undertaken to determine the precise anatomical and functional impairment.

   a. Functional impairment is best determined by the severity of symptoms, the physical findings, and exercise intolerance.

   b. Cardiac catheterization and coronary arteriography may be necessary to define the anatomical abnormality.

   c. The **risk of a major operation** is generally proportional to the limitation of cardiac function, with the exception of aortic stenosis and coronary artery disease; in these the risk is increased regardless of the degree of functional limitation.

   d. Patients with heart disease for which surgical correction is indicated must be evaluated for priority of treatment of noncardiac conditions.

      (1) Elective procedures should be deferred until 6 mo after corrective cardiac surgery.

      (2) Urgent conditions (e.g., colon or breast carcinoma) take precedence over the cardiac condition if cardiac function can be controlled. However, valvular heart disease with intractable failure, aortic stenosis with angina, and coronary artery stenosis with serious risk of infarction should be corrected first and followed in 1–2 mo by the other urgent surgical procedure.

      (3) Emergency conditions (e.g., peritonitis, bowel obstruction) always take priority in management.

   e. **A recent myocardial infarction imposes additional risks** of arrhythmia, cardiac failure, and extension of infarction. After acute myocardial infarction, the excess mortality after a major operation is approximately 25% for operations within 3 wk of the infarction, 10% within 3 mo, and 5% within 6 mo. Only urgent operations necessary to save life or limb should be performed within 3 mo after a fresh infarction. Semiurgent operations should be delayed for 3–6 mo, and elective operations should be delayed for at least 6 mo.

3. **Preoperative preparation** of the patient with heart disease

   a. Assure proper fluid and electrolyte balance and adequate renal and pulmonary function. Potassium deficits are frequent in patients taking diuretics and in those receiving preoperative mechanical bowel preparation. Potassium administered preoperatively will reduce the risk of developing an intraoperative arrhythmia.

b. Arrhythmias are controlled pharmacologically, by electroconversion, or by pacemaker (see Chap. 3). Placement of a temporary transvenous pacemaker is indicated for conditions such as second degree AV block which predispose to complete heart block.

c. Congestive heart failure is treated with digitalis and diuretics. Rapid digitalization is necessary before urgent or semiurgent operations. Digitalis should not be employed prophylactically unless the patient has evidence of heart failure or has had congestive heart failure in the past.

4. Operative and postoperative management of the patient with heart disease. Every patient with significant heart disease undergoing a major operation needs **careful monitoring in an intensive care unit** for at least 48 hr postoperatively.

a. A central venous catheter is placed prior to induction of anesthesia for **serial measurement of CVP** during and after operation. In the presence of increased pulmonary vascular resistance, left atrial pressure will not be accurately reflected by CVP, but can be measured indirectly by a balloon-tipped (Swan-Ganz) pulmonary wedge catheter.

b. An **arterial catheter** provides continuous recording of blood pressure and the pulse curve as measures of cardiac output.

c. Arterial blood gases and pH are measured at frequent intervals after operation.

d. The **hematocrit** and **serum potassium** concentration should be determined at regular intervals. Blood is replaced when necessary to maintain a hematocrit of 35% or above. Serum potassium should be maintained in the range of 4.5–5.5 mEq/liter.

e. A **urethral catheter** should be placed so that hourly urine output can be monitored.

f. The **ECG is monitored continuously** to recognize arrhythmias promptly.

g. Nitroglycerin, 0.6 mg, is given sublingually to patients with coronary artery disease immediately prior to induction of anesthesia.

h. Drugs needed for cardiac resuscitation—atropine, calcium chloride, digoxin, epinephrine, glucagon, isoproterenol, lidocaine, oubain, potassium chloride, propranolol, and sodium bicarbonate—should be available in the operating room and postoperatively at the bedside (see Chaps. 3 and 4).

5. Postoperative cardiovascular deterioration

a. Postoperative **shock usually is caused by hypovolemia.**

b. Acute myocardial infarction always should be considered when postoperative hypotension cannot be attributed to a volume deficit. Angina may not be present or, if present, may be misinterpreted as operative pain. Diagnosis is made by noting ECG changes; serum enzyme changes are unreliable after operative trauma.

c. Other cardiac causes of postoperative hypotension include arrhythmia, tamponade, and acute congestive heart failure.

d. Postoperative hypotension also may be caused by hypoventilation, pulmonary embolus, sepsis, pulmonary atelectasis, acidosis, narcotic overdose, acute gastric dilation, adrenocortical insufficiency, antihypertensive drugs, and circulating vasoactive substances (such as bradykinin in bronchogenic carcinoma or cirrhosis).

C. Pulmonary function

1. Screening evaluation

a. History   Dyspnea with exertion signals respiratory impairment. Chronic smoking, occupational hazards, previous pulmonary infections, and chronic alcoholism indicate a probability of underlying pulmonary disease.

b. Physical examination   A barrel chest with poor diaphragmatic excursion, wheezes, a prolonged obstructive phase, and diminished breath sounds suggest chronic obstructive pulmonary disease. Ask the patient to cough; a paroxysm of coughing and rattling of sputum indicates chronic bronchitis.

c. Chest x-ray may show emphysema, pneumonitis, pulmonary fibrosis, or pulmonary hypertension. The x-ray may be normal in chronic obstructive pulmonary disease.

d. Exercise tolerance   A simple indication of respiratory function is the degree of dyspnea induced by climbing two flights of stairs, provided that dyspnea is not due to heart disease, anemia, or metabolic disturbance.

2. Patients with **evidence suggestive of respiratory impairment**

a. Spirometric testing and measurement of arterial blood gases and pH Spirometry will show reduced lung volumes with relatively normal flow curves in the presence of restrictive ventilatory impairment. The most sensitive indicator of obstructive ventilatory impairment is the timed forced expiratory volume (FEV). When obstructive pulmonary disease is present, the forced expiratory volume in 1 sec (FEV$_1$) is less than 80% of the total vital capacity. Arterial blood gases and pH reflect both the severity of ventilatory impairment and the degree of physiological compensation. Preoperative blood gases and pH also provide a baseline for future comparison.

b. Operative risk in patients with respiratory insufficiency is increased in proportion to the degree of functional pulmonary impairment. Postoperative pulmonary problems almost always occur in patients with preexisting pulmonary disease. Anesthetic gases and the mechanical ventilation required during general anesthesia adversely affect pulmonary function by inhibiting ciliary cleansing, increasing bronchial secretions, and reducing lung compliance.

c. Operative incisions, particularly in the upper abdomen, impair ventilation by imposing painful restriction of diaphragmatic and thoracic movement. In the presence of preexisting marginal pulmonary function, additional operative or postoperative impairment may produce respiratory failure.

d. In a patient unable to maintain adequate ventilation at rest, only urgent, life-saving operations are indicated. In a patient with compensated respiratory insufficiency, elective operations should be deferred until optimum respiratory function has been achieved.

3. Preoperative preparation

a. Training in **deep breathing** and **effective coughing** is the most important measure in prevention of pulmonary complications. A planned preoperative program of ventilatory therapy is necessary in preparation of patients with pulmonary disease for elective operation.

b. Smoking should be stopped for 2 wk prior to operation.

c. Acute respiratory tract **infections should be treated** with antibiotics as indicated by sputum culture and sensitivity tests. Operation should be delayed until 2-3 wk after convalescence from an acute respiratory infection.

d. Patients with chronic production of sputum should be given 5-7 days of preoperative antibiotic therapy based on culture and sensitivity studies of their sputum.

e. Intermittent positive pressure breathing (IPPB) improves ventilation and clearing of secretions in patients with obstructive or restrictive ventilatory impairments. Preoperative introduction of IPPB will familiarize the patient with it and allow more effective postoperative use.

f. Liquification of sputum is best accomplished through humidification (steam, vaporizer, or ultrasonic nebulizer).

g. Bronchodilators should be given to patients with chronic obstructive pulmonary disease.

h. Postural drainage is helpful in patients with bronchiectasis or chronic bronchitis.

i. Preoperative **corticosteroid** therapy may be necessary in patients with interstitial pulmonary fibrosis or severe bronchial asthma.

4. Postoperative management

a. Routine measures

(1) Encourage the patient to take deep breaths, carry out Valsalva's maneuver, and cough every 20-30 min after he awakens from anesthesia.

(2) IPPB has limited value for routine postoperative use in normal patients; its effectiveness depends on the patient's skill and cooperation in using the pressure apparatus. IPPB is more helpful in patients with chronic respiratory disease.

(3) Blow bottles and balloons are inexpensive measures which encourage lung expansion, particularly in children.

(4) Early ambulation contributes to reduction of postoperative pulmonary complications.

(5) Tracheal suctioning helps prevent atelectasis and pneumonia in the patient who cannot breathe deeply or cough effectively. A 12-18 Fr soft Silastic or rubber catheter is introduced through the nose; the patient takes a deep breath and the catheter is passed into the trachea. Vigorous coughing follows. Instillation into the trachea of 5 ml of sterile saline will enhance aspiration of thick secretions. *Remember that prolonged suctioning without periodic administration of oxygen leads to hypoxia and cardiac arrhythmias.* **Never maintain suction through the catheter for a period longer than you can hold your breath**—approximately 15 sec.

b. The **patient with respiratory insufficiency** demands energetic application of both routine measures (above) and the following additional maneuvers postoperatively:

(1) Determine arterial blood gases and pH frequently during operation and at intervals for at least 48 hr.

(2) Never remove the endotracheal tube nor stop assisted ventilation until adequate spontaneous ventilation is assured clinically and confirmed by blood gas analysis and spirometric testing. Measure tidal volume and vital capacity with a portable respirator attached to the endotracheal tube. A tidal volume of 500 ml and vital capacity of 800-1,000 ml indicate sufficient ventilation in the average-sized adult.

(3) Oxygen administration may cause respiratory depression by reducing the anoxic drive of patients with chronic hypercapnia due to pulmonary disease. Only low concentrations (28-40%) of oxygen should be administered, with blood gas monitoring to assure normal P_{CO_2}.

(4) IV fluid administration should be kept at the minimum required for maintenance and replacement of losses. Excess salt and water may lead to pulmonary edema with resultant decompensation.

(5) Bronchodilators should be employed postoperatively in patients with obstructive ventilatory impairment. Aminophylline is given by IV infusion (250 mg over a 30-min period every 6 hr), or isoproterenol may be given intermittently by nebulizer (0.5 ml of 1:200 solution mixed with 5 ml saline in the nebulizer every 6 hr).

(6) Narcotics or sedatives may produce decompensation of marginal pulmonary reserves. Low doses of narcotics at frequent intervals effectively control pain with less respiratory depression.

   c. Postoperative pulmonary decompensation is discussed in Chapter 12.

III. ANESTHESIA AND ANESTHETIC PREMEDICATION

A. Local versus general anesthesia

1. The pharmacodynamic action of all anesthetic agents depresses the CNS and other systems. In debilitated patients this poses a significant risk; local anesthesia often is preferable if careful attention is paid to the total dose of local anesthetic used and intravascular injection is avoided. Remember that local anesthetics also produce CNS and cardiovascular depression by intravascular injection, rapid absorption from highly vascular tissue, or rapid infiltration.

2. Inadequate local anesthesia, on the other hand, often has to be supplemented by depressant analgesics, producing respiratory and circulatory depression. If a general anesthetic then has to be used in order to maintain respiration and circulation, the patient (and surgeon) would have been better served by the use of a well-planned general anesthetic in the first place.

3. The multitude of anesthetic agents and methods available today permits the use of general anesthesia in the vast majority of patients.

B. Choice of anesthesia

1. The patient's age, previous anesthetic experience, complicating diseases, drugs being administered for these diseases, the operation to be performed, the habits of the surgeon, and the position required for the operation must be considered in choosing anesthetic agents and technique.

2. On the basis of past experience a patient may have formulated preferences that differ from those of the anesthesiologist. Frequently a clear explanation of the reasons for the proposed choice will lead the patient to

agree to a certain technique. However, the patient's preference has to be considered.

3. The patient's emotional status is important since psychological instability or apprehension may require heavy premedication and avoidance of local or regional anesthesia.

4. A prolonged operative procedure under regional anesthesia, even with perfect pain relief, may be quite trying because of the discomfort of lying in one position for a long time.

5. Spinal and epidural anesthesia, in the majority of instances, is used for operations on the lower extremities, inguinal area, or lower abdomen. Recent ingestion of food, airway abnormalities, and hepatic, renal, or metabolic disease support a choice for spinal or epidural anesthesia. Contraindications are previous technical difficulties with spinal anesthesia, neurological deficits, backache, skin infections of the back, and the preoperative use of anticoagulants. Hypovolemia, severe anemia, and cardiovascular instability are lesser contraindications.

6. Postspinal (puncture) headache is due to decreased intracranial pressure following escape of CSF through the dural opening after lumbar puncture. The headache is more severe in the head-up position and is more frequent in younger patients. Treatment consists of keeping the patient flat, administering analgesics, and carrying out IV hydration. The injection of 10 ml of fresh autologous blood into the peridural (extrathecal) space will seal the dural leak.

7. Epidural and caudal anesthesia are techniques which apply local anesthetics extrathecally. Indications and contraindications are essentially the same as those for spinal anesthesia.

8. **Special considerations**

   a. Respiratory insufficiency due to pulmonary abnormalities or neuromuscular or skeletal disorders, or central depression due to intracranial disease, drugs, or carbon dioxide retention, results in inadequate ventilation and impaired coughing and deep breathing. These patients are very susceptible to postoperative atelectasis. Narcotics are avoided in premedication because they depress alveolar minute volume, impair cough and sigh reflexes, and decrease sensitivity to carbon dioxide.

   b. Liver disease can influence the metabolism of anesthetic compounds. Acute hepatic disease is associated with a high mortality following anesthesia. Maximal improvement of liver function should be obtained prior to anesthesia. Serum albumin, prothrombin, Bromsulphalein retention, and alkaline phosphatase should have minimally acceptable values.

   c. Kidney failure affects excretion of anesthetic agents, acid-base balance, and water metabolism. Long-acting barbiturates, gallamine, and succinylcholine are avoided since they all are excreted primarily by the kidney. Dialysis may restore fairly normal homeostasis preoperatively.

C. Anesthetic premedication

1. The **purpose** is to facilitate induction of, maintenance of, and recovery from anesthesia by administration of agents to:

   a. Decrease fear and anxiety.

   b. Reduce secretions in the air passages.

   c. Prevent undesirable reflexes (e.g., cardiac arrhythmias) due to:

      (1) Afferent impulses from the trachea and the abdominal and thoracic cavities.

      (2) Volatile agents.

      (3) Succylcholine.

   d. Enhance analgesia during light anesthesia.

   e. Decrease nausea and vomiting.

   f. Aid in special techniques (e.g., chlorpromazine to facilitate hypothermia, diazepam for cardioversions).

2. **General considerations**

   a. After premedication, patients should be awake but drowsy, free of anxiety, and cooperative.

   b. Psychological rapport established during the preanesthetic visit will help to gain confidence and reduce the need for sedation. Frank discussion of the nature of the anesthetic, the operation, and immediate postoperative activities will help patient cooperation. Instruction, suggestion, and psychological support are important elements of preanesthetic preparation. The psychological preparation of a child and his parents is of utmost importance.

   c. Age, sex, weight, and physical and psychological status dictate the dose of premedicants. The severely ill, aged, and debilitated patient requires less sedatives and analgesics.

   d. In using a combination of drugs, keep each at a minimal dose in order to avoid depression of vital functions.

3. **Effects of concomitant drug therapy**

   a. Potentiation (additive or synergistic effects) can be produced (e.g., barbiturates potentiate ethanol).

TABLE 8-1. Premedication

Trade Name	Generic Name	Dose	Administration Time (min before induction of anesthesia)	Action Desired	Side Effects and Potential Hazards
Short-acting barbiturates					
Nembutal	Pentobarbital	0.5–1.0 mg/kg IM	90–120	Sedation	Possible "excitement" if pain present; omit in patients with porphyria
Seconal	Secobarbital	0.5–1.0 mg/kg IM	90–120	Sedation	
Nonbarbiturate sedatives					
Doriden	Glutethimide	125–500 mg orally	90–120	Sedation	Tolerance and dependence
Noludar	Methyprylon	50–200 mg orally	90–120	Sedation	Habituation
Tranquilizers					
Phenergan	Promethazine	0.5 mg/kg IM	90–120	Tranquilization	Marked potentiation of narcotics and sedatives; use with caution in patients with Parkinson's disease
Valium	Diazepam	0.01–0.02 mg/kg IM	90–120	Tranquilization	
Vistaril, Atarax	Hydroxyzine	0.5–1.0 mg/kg IM	90–120	Tranquilization	
Inapsine	Droperidol	2.5–10.0 mg IM	30–60	Tranquilization	
Narcotics					
	Morphine	0.01 mg/kg IM	45–60	Analgesia and sedation	Respiratory depression; omit in patients with respiratory disease
Demerol	Meperidine	0.5–1.0 mg/kg IM	45–60	Analgesia and sedation	
Sublimaze	Fentanyl	0.05–0.1 mg/70 kg IM	30–60	Analgesia	Muscular rigidity
Anticholinergics					
	Atropine	0.4–0.6 mg/60 kg IM	45–60	Drying effect on airway secretions	Tachycardia; prevents reflex bradycardia
	Scopolamine	0.4–0.6 mg/60 kg IM	45–60	Drying effect plus sedation and amnesia	
Robinul	Glycopyrrolate	0.1–0.2 mg IM	30–60	Drying effect	

TABLE 8-2. Pediatric Premedication

Body weight (kg)	Atropine (IM)	Meperidine (IM)	Morphine (IM)
0-10	0.1-0.2 mg	0	0
10-25	0.3-0.6 mg	20-50 mg	0
25-50	0.4-0.6 mg	0	6-10 mg

b. Enzyme inhibition produced by one drug can prevent metabolism of another (e.g., monoamine oxidase inhibitors prolong the action of meperidine).

c. Enzyme induction stimulation can lead to increased metabolism of another agent (e.g., phenobarbital stimulates metabolism of anticoagulants, requiring an increase in dosage of the latter).

d. Plasma or tissue protein binding can be altered (e.g., chloral hydrate displaces coumarin from carrier protein, leading to increased anticoagulant effect).

e. Diuretics may cause a loss of potassium, producing abnormal responses to muscle relaxants or digitalis.

f. Monoamine oxidase inhibitors can cause a release of a mixture of catecholamines from nerve terminals.

g. Cessation of chronic drug therapy existing prior to anesthesia is frequently undesirable (e.g., antihypertensive agents should be maintained in order to avoid a state of hypertension). Safety lies in the knowledge that these drugs are being used.

h. Aminoglycoside antibiotics (neomycin, streptomycin, kanamycin, gentamicin) and others enhance the neuromuscular block created by nondepolarizing muscle relaxants.

i. Phenothiazine drugs potentiate opiates, cause peripheral vasodilation, and may produce severe hypotension during anesthesia.

j. Disulfiram (Antabuse) used in the treatment of alcoholics may have a synergistic depressant effect with thiopental.

4. **Drugs used for premedication** in adults are listed in Table 8-1. Pediatric premedication is listed in Table 8-2.

SUGGESTED READING
Green, N. M.   Halothane anesthesia and hepatitis in a high-risk population. *N. Engl. J. Med.* 289:304, 1973.

IV. ACUTE PSYCHOSES

A. General considerations

1. **Preoperative psychological evaluation** includes any history of previous emotional difficulties, drug ingestion, or alcoholism, and a mental status examination. Since many postoperative psychoses are depressive in nature and interfere with convalescence, elective operations should be postponed in cases of frank psychotic depression.

2. In psychoses, the predominant behavior reflects lack of reality testing and one or more of the following: (a) defects in consciousness, orientation, or judgment, (b) inability to control behavior, (c) disordered thinking, (d) mood alteration, or (e) motor disturbance.

3. The **mental status examination** includes investigation of:

   a. Orientation (awareness of time, place, and person).

   b. Level of consciousness (fluctuating, stable).

   c. Judgment and intelligence (observed ability to manipulate numbers, words, arithmetic problems of addition and subtraction).

   d. Memory (recent and early).

   e. Communication (clear or distorted thinking).

   f. Affect (mood is even and stable, depressive and withdrawn, or euphoric).

   g. Motor changes (impulsive, aberrant discharges seemingly without provocation, or behavior that is withdrawn).

B. Description of acute psychoses

1. There are **two categories** of psychoses—organic and functional. **Acute organic psychosis** refers to potential reversibility, not duration. **Acute functional psychosis** refers to the suddenness and intensity of the disorder. The functional psychoses are either affective or schizophrenic.

2. **Depressive psychoses** are the most frequent postoperative functional psychoses and show the following behavior:

   a. Loss of esteem, self-depreciation, and suicidal thoughts.

   b. Psychomotor changes, either retardation or agitation.

   c. Affect changes, usually sadness or withdrawal.

3. Schizophrenic disorders include paranoid and catatonic reactions, and other forms marked by:

    a. Thinking disorders—delusions, loosened or incomprehensible associations, bizarre thoughts.

    b. Affect changes—fear or panic, inappropriate affect.

    c. Sensory and motor changes—visual or auditory hallucinations, bizarre and impulsive motor activity (including violence), states of autism and negativism.

4. Organic brain syndromes are recognized by marked or subtle deficits in cognition and awareness (delirium); deficits in orientation, memory, and intellectual functioning (acute and chronic brain syndromes); and those conditions in which confusion, instability, and visual hallucinations are prominent (toxic psychosis).

C. Management of acute psychoses

1. Once the physician is aware of mental status changes before or after operation, diagnosis must be directed to the possibility of mental reaction to drugs, brain damage and aging processes, blood-gas disorders, electrolyte disorders, nutritional and vitamin disorders, metabolic diseases (e.g., sepsis, uremia, or hypothyroidism), acidosis, hepatotoxicity, alcoholism, ingestion of hallucinogens or amphetamines, and isolation (as in the intensive care unit syndrome).

2. Management should be aimed at eliminating factors causing adverse mental reactions (e.g., hyponatremia, hypokalemia, uremia, hypoxia, hypercapnia, drugs such as barbiturates, and anticholinergics).

3. Postoperative psychoses are more common in the elderly than in the young. Elderly persons are more sensitive to drugs, relative malnutrition, shifts in electrolyte balance, and fluctuations in oxygenation of the cerebrum during and after an operation. Treatment should be directed to immediate search and elimination of the offending drug, electrolyte imbalance, or cardiac imbalance reducing cerebral blood flow.

4. Psychological treatment of all organic syndromes should include continuous supervision in a well-lighted room with adequate stimulation from staff and tranquilization with the lowest doses of diazepam (2-5 mg) or chlorpromazine (25-50 mg) which control agitation.

5. Withdrawal reactions to opiates, alcohol, amphetamines, or hallucinogens may include delirium tremens (alcohol), convulsions (barbiturates, opiates), or paranoid states (amphetamines). In the face of excitement or cerebral irritability, sedate with chlorpromazine, 75-100 mg IM, and continue to maintain adequate electrolyte, nutritional, and vitamin balance. Immediate psychiatric consultation is indicated.

6. Immediate therapy for excited, paranoid patients is physical restraint and isolation, including continuous supervision, in an isolated room and tranquilization with chlorpromazine, 75-100 mg IM q4h.

7. Immediate therapy for a psychotic depressive reaction also is continuous care in a safe room with suicidal precautions enforced. If the patient is very agitated, diazepam, 5 mg, can be given; an antidepressant such as imipramine, 25 mg q4h, also can be initiated under psychiatric supervision.

SUGGESTED READING
Altschule, M. D.   Postoperative psychosis. *Surg. Clin. North Am.* 49:647, 1969.

V. CARE OF DRAINS AND TUBES

A. Management of drains

1. Drains are placed **prophylactically,** to prevent the accumulation of fluids, or **therapeutically,** to promote escape of fluids which have already accumulated.

2. **Gauze** acts as a drain only as long as capillary action in the fabric can absorb fluid. As soon as gauze becomes saturated, it acts as a plug rather than a drain. Use gauze only under special circumstances—to pack a cavity to prevent its closure or to control diffuse oozing.

3. **Rubber** is used as corrugated or flat strips or as hollow rubber tubes (Penrose). A Penrose drain which has gauze within it forms a "cigarette drain." Remember that in a cigarette drain material takes exit along and not through the gauze; the rubber acts as the conduit.

4. **Sump suction** is used to accomplish drainage against the force of gravity. Sump drainage prevents skin damage from irritating secretions and permits accurate measurement of the volume of drainage removed. Sumps are commercially available, but they also can be improvised with two rubber or plastic tubes tied side by side or one inside the other. The larger lumen drains the fluid to be aspirated, while the smaller lumen provides access of air to prevent vacuum plugging of the drain. Properly placed sump drains can be used for irrigations: irrigating fluid flows through the air vent tube while intermittent suction continues. Sump drains are particularly advantageous in drainage of pancreatic, duodenal, jejunal, and ileal fistulas as well as in drainage of the pancreas following trauma. One disadvantage of some sump drains is lack of pliability; pain and erosion of surrounding tissues may result. Sump drains should be fixed away from vital structures if long-term use is contemplated.

5. Drains should not be placed into joint spaces, across tendon sheaths, or in similar areas where reaction is detrimental to function. In the neighborhood of tendons, nerves, large blood vessels, and solid organs, only soft drains should be used; otherwise, necrosis of vital structures may result.

6. Intraperitoneally, only localized drainage is possible. Protective mechanisms rapidly wall off drains from surrounding viscera. Drains should be inserted purposely to "extraperitonealize" and drain surface defects of such organs as the pancreas or liver. Drains leading to the surface of such organs will drain secretions from them until their capsule has been closed by reparative processes. Drains in the presence of generalized peritonitis are deleterious to peritoneal resistance.

7. Drains to suture lines of most intestinal anastomoses are unnecessary. While drains probably do no harm to anastomoses in small bowel, they have been shown to interfere with healing of colon anastomoses. There is a significantly higher morbidity from intraperitoneal leakage following colectomy in patients who have drainage as compared to those without any drainage. Extraperitoneal anastomoses of the rectum probably should be drained. Esophagogastric-esophagoenteric anastomoses should be drained because of their high incidence of disruption and leakage.

8. The splenic fossa should not routinely be drained except in cases suspected of pancreatic damage.

9. As soon as the drain is removed, intra-abdominal movement should be stimulated to aid in the disappearance of remaining adhesions; feeding the patient is the best method.

10. **Removal of drains**

  a. **Drains placed prophylactically** should be removed as soon as it is obvious that there is no significant drainage and the drains will not be required. Drains placed prophylactically do not have to be shortened progressively. Remove them as soon as it is clear they are not needed, usually on the first or second postoperative day.

  b. **Drains placed therapeutically** should be left in place as long as they produce more than 25-50 ml of drainage. When drainage ceases, adhesions should be broken up by twisting the drain. If no further drainage ensues, remove the drain gradually, a few centimeters each day. In this way the drainage tract will fill up from its depths. If such a drain is pulled out completely at one time, the skin seals promptly while pocketing and suppuration develop in the tract.

11. **Complications** Since drains are foreign bodies, they call forth an inflammatory tissue response and production of a small amount of drainage. This is rarely of serious consequence and subsides following removal of the drain. A drain is a "two-way street"; it permits ingress of bacteria that may develop into local or invasive infection. Careful dressing of the wound and removal of the drain as soon as possible will reduce the possibility of significant infection. Because it permits bacterial ingress and because it prevents closure of a wound, a drain should never be brought through the operative incision. Drains placed into the

peritoneal cavity may promote paralytic ileus or stimulate adhesions that secondarily result in mechanical bowel obstruction.

A portion of a drain may become separated and be retained as a foreign body, causing secondary breakdown of the wound or necessitating reoperation for its removal. Drains should be tagged, usually with safety pins, or sutured to the skin with nonabsorbable material. A drain that is too hard or stiff may cause pressure necrosis of surrounding tissues.

12. In **summary**   Use a drain whenever contaminated or infected material, blood, bile, lymph, or exudative or transudative accumulations are encountered or anticipated. The drain used should be (a) soft, so as not to erode the surrounding tissues, (b) smooth, so as not to permit fibrin to cling to it, (c) of a material, preferably radiopaque, that will not disintegrate and leave foreign bodies in the wound, and (d) brought through a wound separate from the incision. The stab wound which gives access to the drainage cavity should be large enough so that free drainage can occur. The drain must be placed dependently if gravity alone is to accomplish drainage. A sump tube must be used to remove drainage "uphill," against the force of gravity.

B. Nasogastric tubes

1. Nasogastric tubes are placed (a) to remove fluid and gas present in or regurgitated into the stomach and (b) to prevent accumulation of swallowed air in a paralytic bowel.

2. Nasogastric suction decompression is an important part of treatment of intestinal obstruction, paralytic ileus, and postoperative abdominal distention. However, routine use of nasogastric tubes in every abdominal procedure is unnecessary.

3. Successful and uncomplicated nasogastric intubation requires **preparation of both tube and patient.** Instruct the patient in what is going to be done. The distance from the xiphoid to either ear lobe is measured with the tube. After insertion, with this point at the external nares, the end of the tube will be in the midstomach. The tube should be well lubricated. A rubber tube should be refrigerated or placed in ice to stiffen it prior to insertion. It is inserted without force through the nares into the posterior pharynx. The patient is asked to swallow and, in synchrony with a swallow, the tube is advanced into the esophagus. It can then be passed to the stomach; continued swallowing aids in this passage and helps prevent kinking in the pharynx.

4. Entry into the stomach is confirmed by aspiration of gastric contents; alternatively, air injected through the tube produces characteristic borborygmi, which can be heard over the stomach.

5. Irrigation of the nasogastric tube with 30-50 ml of air should be performed at least hourly to prevent blockage of the tube. Air is preferable to saline in cleaning nasogastric tubes since it does not complicate fluid

balance record keeping. In some cases, where blood or thick secretions occlude the tube, saline should be used.

6. Complications of nasogastric intubation are many and frequent:

a. Mouth breathing   Normal respiration through the nostrils is impossible with a tube through the nares. Breathing through the mouth results in dry oral mucosa and dry cracked lips; the patient is uncomfortable and liable to develop parotitis. Mouthwashes should be used frequently; lubricating glycerin is applied to the lips, tongue, and mucosa.

b. Ulceration and necrosis of the nares is caused by taping the nasogastric tube to the forehead. Swallowing advances the free portion of the tube until it is under tension, producing pressure necrosis of the margin of the naris. The tube should be fixed in line with the long axis of the nose; a single piece of tape placed along the nose from bridge to tip is continued straight along the tube for an inch or two; no other fixation is needed.

c. Interference with ventilation   A nasogastric tube reduces the volume of pulmonary ventilation and interferes with effective coughing; voluntary inhibition of deep respirations and cough because of discomfort is the likeliest explanation.

d. Loss of fluids   Nasogastric suction may remove large amounts of fluids from the upper GI tract, resulting in depletion of chloride, potassium, and hydrogen ions. If the tube is inserted into the upper GI tract beyond the pylorus, or if there is transpyloric regurgitation of large amounts of biliary and pancreatic secretions, sodium depletion also may occur. If the patient is allowed to drink water or ingest ice chips, even in modest amounts, the resultant electrolyte loss may be increased significantly.

e. Esophagogastric reflux   The presence of a nasogastric tube induces reflux of gastric contents into the distal esophagus as a result of functional incompetence of the cardioesophageal junction. Esophagitis can be produced; the patient complains of substernal burning discomfort or a sensation of a lump behind the xiphoid.

f. Esophageal erosion and stricture   Minor erosion of the lower esophagus is common in patients who have a nasogastric tube in place for more than a few hours. Though common, these erosions are unrecognized because of rapid spontaneous healing when the tube is removed. Esophageal stricture occasionally follows nasogastric intubation, presumably as a result of a deep erosion or ulcer. No definite relationship has been found between the length of time a nasogastric tube is in place and the subsequent development of esophageal ulceration or stenosis.

g. Other complications   Otitis media, sinusitis, traumatic laryngitis and hoarseness, traumatic rupture of esophageal varices, knotting of the tube and inability to withdraw it, nasal bleeding from trauma to mucous membranes during passage, pressure necrosis of the pharynx or the upper part of the esophagus opposite the cricoid cartilage, and retropharyngeal or laryngeal abscesses are occasional complications of nasogastric intubation.

C. Long intestinal tubes

1. Long intestinal tubes should be placed preoperatively or intraoperatively for decompression of dilated small bowel, to facilitate abdominal closure, or to splint the small bowel postoperatively. Long tubes also can be used in patients with multiple recurrent episodes of obstruction or disseminated carcinomatosis.

2. These are **five types** of long intestinal tubes:

   a. **Miller-Abbott**   16 Fr or 18 Fr double-lumen tube with distal balloon; one lumen is for suction, the other to fill and deflate the balloon at the distal end of the tube; the balloon is usually filled with air, less often with water or saline. The small suction lumen is easily plugged.

   b. **Cantor**   16 Fr or 18 Fr single-lumen tube with distal balloon; 1-2 ml of mercury is injected into the balloon; this is the best tube for long-term use. Multiple holes placed into the balloon with a 25-30-gauge needle will prevent overdistention with gas.

   c. **Johnston**   Large 26 Fr single-lumen tube with a steel weight at the distal end; no balloon; this is the best tube for initial decompression and short-term use.

   d. **Baker**   16 Fr double-lumen tube with distal balloon (similar to Foley balloon concept) which can be inflated with fluid or air; the tube can be manipulated intraoperatively to decompress dilated small-bowel loops.

   e. A variety of tubes incorporating wires or other means of manipulating the tube from outside the patient; usually single-lumen with no balloon.

3. **Long intestinal tubes will not pass into the small bowel in paralytic ileus or in late or complicated mechanical obstructions in which propulsive peristalsis is no longer present.** Attempts to pass a long tube in such circumstances are futile; pass a nasogastric tube instead. If you are not sure about the effectiveness of peristalsis, a long tube may be tried. If it does not enter the small bowel in 12 hr or so, give it up.

4. **Successful passage of a long intestinal tube** requires skill and effort. Measure the distance from xiphoid to an ear lobe; add 4 in. and note this distance from the tip of the tube. A Miller-Abbott or Cantor tube (and balloon) should be well lubricated and then passed through the nose into the pharynx. If a Cantor tube is being used, the balloon should be grasped

with a clamp when it is in the pharynx and brought out through the mouth so that mercury can be added to the bag. The tube is then passed into the stomach, advancing it to the previously noted mark. If a Johnston tube is used, it is often too large to pass through the nose; if so, pass it through the mouth.

Progression of the tube from stomach to duodenum is helped by elevating the head of the patient's bed to 30 degrees and turning him right side down. Fluoroscopy is not necessary in the routine case, but should the tube fail to advance, its position should be checked before abandoning long-tube treatment. Sometimes, in this situation, it is possible to place the tube in the region of the pylorus at fluoroscopy. When the tube is properly placed, the balloon of a Miller-Abbott tube is partially filled with air, mercury, or water. The remaining length of the tube is not advanced into the stomach, but remains untethered outside the patient so that peristalsis can advance it. The patient should be checked frequently to make certain that the tube is moving and that it is not plugged. Abdominal roentgenograms help to check the position of the distal tip of the tube. Once the tube passes the duodenum, it will advance rapidly to the point of obstruction. Once the tube has reached the mid small bowel, a nasogastric tube should be inserted through the opposite nostril to aspirate gastric contents.

5. Long intestinal tubes require the same care, attention, and irrigation to keep them patent as do nasogastric tubes (see above).

6. Withdrawal of a long intestinal tube from the small bowel takes time. The tube simply cannot be pulled up all at once. Withdraw about 6 in. of the tube and fix the tube to the nose or cheek so that this length cannot be reswallowed. After an hour or so, withdraw another 6 in., as before, When the end of the tube has been withdrawn into the stomach, it can be removed completely.

Once the tube has been withdrawn so that the bag is in the pharynx, it is desirable to grasp the bag with a hemostat and withdraw it through the mouth. The tube may be cut above the bag. When the bag contains a large amount of mercury or gas, considerable discomfort will result from pulling it forcefully out through the nose.

If the tip of the tube has passed the ileocecal valve, or if there is undue difficulty in removing the tube, cut the tube at the nose and allow it to pass per rectum. Operative removal of a long tube rarely is necessary.

7. **Complications** of long-tube therapy include all of those listed above for nasogastric intubation. In addition, there are a few complications unique to long tubes.

   a. **Gaseous distention of the balloon**   This complication is seen in those long tubes, such as the Cantor, with a closed balloon. Intestinal gases diffuse into the balloon, increasing its size and leading to difficulty in its removal. Rarely, the distention may be so great that it causes bowel obstruction; laparotomy may be necessary for relief. Multiple punctures of the proximal portion of the balloon with a needle before passage will prevent this complication.

  b. **Rupture of the balloon** may result from overdistention by irrigation of the balloon rather than the suction lumen, or by use of worn-out, defective balloons. It is best to test Miller-Abbott tubes before inserting them to make sure that the labels on the metal tips have not been reversed. The balloon of a Cantor-type tube may burst, spilling mercury into the bowel lumen. The presence of metallic mercury in the bowel lumen is of no great consequence although it may get trapped in the mucosa and not be passed immediately.

  c. **Reverse intussusception** during withdrawal may occur if the distal balloon cannot be deflated and the tube is withdrawn quickly.

  d. Perforation or strangulation of obstructed bowel must be listed as a complication of ill-advised or neglectful therapy with a long tube. Long intestinal tubes are extremely useful in those situations in which they are indicated; however, they are no substitute for careful examination and application of good judgment in managing the patient with an intestinal obstruction (see Chap. 7).

D. Sengstaken-Blakemore tube

  1. This is a multiple-lumen tube with esophageal and gastric balloons used for control of bleeding esophageal varices.

  2. Prior to insertion of the tube, blow up the esophageal balloon to 40 mm Hg using an anaeroid manometer, and instill 300 cc of air into the gastric balloon. Test both balloons under water for leaks.

  3. Place the tip of the gastric balloon at the xiphoid and note the marking at the side of tube at the nose. Anesthetize the patient's nasopharynx, lubricate the tube, and pass through a nostril into the stomach 15 cm beyond the mark noted at the nose.

  4. Inflate the gastric balloon with 250-350 cc air and record the gastric balloon pressure (using another anaeroid manometer) for future reference. Then clamp the inflating tube. Attach the main tube to 1¼-lb traction.

  5. Lavage the stomach; then insert a Levin tube into the upper esophagus through the other nostril and place on intermittent suction.

  6. Check position of gastric balloon by x-ray. If bleeding continues, withdraw the Levin tube to the pharynx and inflate the esophageal balloon to 40 mm Hg pressure. Replace the Levin tube in the upper esophagus and replace on suction.

  7. Recheck pressures in both balloons frequently in order to ensure proper inflation.

  8. **If respiratory distress develops, cut across the Sengstaken tube with a large scissors kept within easy reach of the patient and attendants.**

9. If bleeding continues from the stomach, reevaluation is necessary. If bleeding is documented to be from varices and tamponade controls it, the esophageal balloon may be deflated at the end of 24 hr, but the gastric balloon should remain inflated on ¾-lb traction for another 24 hr. Following this, the gastric balloon is taken off traction and deflated, and the Levin tube is removed. The uninflated Sengstaken tube remains in place for another 24 hr.

10. If bleeding recurs, reinflate the balloons.

11. If no bleeding occurs 24 hr after deflation of the gastric balloon, the Sengstaken tube may be removed ½ hr after the patient has swallowed 2 oz of mineral oil to facilitate its removal.

E. Common bile duct T-tubes

1. A T-tube is placed for the following reasons:

a. For **decompression** and **drainage of bile** after exploration of the common bile duct, after choledocholithotomy, or in cholangitis.

b. As a **splint** for repair of a common duct stricture.

c. Occasionally, **to form an external biliary fistula** in common duct obstructions not amenable to an internal bypass.

2. Long-arm T-tubes have a limb which enters the duodenum through the ampulla of Vater. These tubes may obstruct the orifice of the pancreatic duct, producing pancreatitis. They permit reflux of duodenal content into the common duct which may result in cholangitis. They are not generally recommended.

3. Any drainage tube within the common duct encroaches on the lumen. Any deposit inside these tubes increases the degree of obstruction, first in the tube and later in the duct itself, but the common bile duct has a remarkable capacity of dilation, and complete obstruction seldom occurs.

4. In the early postoperative period, deposits of biliary mud or blood clots may be flushed out easily by gentle irrigation of the tube with saline or water. Later this becomes more and more difficult and, ultimately, blocked T-tubes have to be removed. Solvents such as ether or irrigating fluids other than saline should not be used. Recently heparin solutions and chenodeoxycholic acid (not commercially available) have been infused through T-tubes and reported to dissolve retained stones; we have not been able to convince ourselves that irrigation with these agents has any advantage over saline irrigation.

5. T-tubes occasionally may slip or be pulled out of the duct during removal of a dressing or movement of the patient. To avoid this, care should be taken during operation to leave some slack in the tube intra-abdominally and the tube should be sutured to the skin.

6. When a tube becomes partially dislocated shortly after operation, it is usually best not to remove it immediately, since it still may provide a track for escape of bile to the outside. If there is distal obstruction of the common duct, there usually is a large amount of bile drainage around the tube. If signs of bile peritonitis develop, the tube must be replaced operatively.

7. A **cholangiogram through the T-tube** should be obtained prior to removing it. T-tubes placed prophylactically or to drain a nonobstructed common duct can be removed after 10 days. Simply put traction on the tube and pull it out; the small biliary leakage will stop in 24-48 hr. T-tubes placed as splints are meant to remain in place for at least 6 mo.

8. When larger T-tubes are used, removal is facilitated if a V-shaped piece has been cut out of the tube opposite the external limb. Occasionally, difficulty is encountered in removing a T-tube from the common duct. Gentle, persistent traction is needed. In particularly difficult situations, applying traction to the tube, then setting a clamp across it at skin level and having the patient walk about results in release of the tube.

F. Chest tubes

1. Intrapleural drainage tubes are placed in cases of chest trauma and after any intrathoracic operation regardless of its magnitude. These tubes serve to remove (a) any accumulating fluid or blood, (b) any air leaking from lung, and (c) any air entering the pleural space through the wound.

2. A single tube is used after nonpulmonary thoracic operations in which there is no injury to lung and a major air leak is not expected. Usually a polyethylene tube is placed through an interspace below the thoracotomy wound in the midaxillary line. This permits the patient to lie either on his back or the opposite side without kinking the tube. The intrapleural portion of the tube is placed posterior to the lung.

3. When air leakage, together with fluid, can be anticipated, two chest tubes are used. One tube is placed as described above. A second tube is introduced through a separate interspace below the thoracotomy wound and placed anteriorly in the pleural space.

4. Chest tubes are not placed after pneumonectomy, since transudative fluid is allowed to fill the empty pleural space. Infrequently, a chest tube connected to a water seal is placed following a pneumonectomy if empyema is anticipated.

5. In trauma cases, or whenever a tube must be introduced into the chest by less experienced physicians, the safest method is the sixth intercostal space midaxillary line technique (see Chap. 25).

6. Chest tubes must never be left open to atmospheric pressure as this produces complete pneumothorax.

7. Chest tubes should be connected either to water seal drainage or to a chest suction apparatus. Water seal drainage is useful where only minimal fluid or air drainage is expected. Suction drainage should be used whenever significant drainage of fluid or air is expected.

8. Water seal drainage involves the placement of the external end of the drainage tube 1-2 cm below the surface of water in a container placed at least 15 cm below the patient's chest. During inspiration (increased negative intrapleural pressure), water is drawn up from the container into the chest and drainage tube, preventing entrance of air; during expiration or during coughing, as soon as intrapleural pressure exceeds the depth of the tube below the water surface, i.e., 1-2 cm, air is blown out of the tube and bubbles away. The water seal thus acts as a one-way valve, permitting escape of air from the chest.

9. Suction drainage, using either the classic three-bottle technique or one of the commercial devices incorporating this principle, is used whenever significant drainage of fluid or air is expected. Usually 15-20 cm of effective negative suction is applied to the chest tube to produce gentle bubbling of air through the negative-pressure-limiting tube.

   The effective pressure relationships within the pleural space in this situation cannot be determined a priori, except within certain limits. If the pleural space and all tubing contain only air, the effective intrapleural suction pressure is that set externally, usually -15 to -20 cm H_2O. But, if the pleural space and all tubing are filled with fluid, the effective intrapleural suction pressure is the sum of the negative pressure set externally plus the negative siphon pressure created in the tubes between the level of the chest and the level of the suction device; usually this is of the order of -50 to -90 cm H_2O. These two situations—air-filled tubing or fluid-filled tubing—determine the limits of effective suction. Typically, the tubes are filled with slugs of fluid separated by air, and the effective intrapleural suction pressure falls somewhere between the limits outlined.

10. Chest tubes should be kept patent by frequent stripping, particularly when they are filled with fluid. If the tube must be irrigated, it should be done under strict aseptic conditions. Constant attention to maintenance of patency in chest tubes ensures prompt expansion of a collapsed lung and minimizes late pleural complications.

11. There is no rigid schedule for removal of tubes. They are removed when it is apparent that the lung is well expanded, there is no air leak from wound or lung, and less than 150 ml of fluid is aspirated in a 24-hr period. In most nonpulmonary operations, the chest tube may be pulled the first postoperative day. In typical pulmonary resections without excessive air leakage, conditions permitting removal of the chest tube may be met between the second and fourth postoperative day. When the air leak initially is large, the tube may be needed for a longer period and should be clamped for 24 hr prior to actual withdrawal of the tube to ensure that no further accumulation of air occurs.

12. Chest tubes are removed with suction maintained in the patent tube. The patient should be told to inspire and hold his breath (Valsalva's maneuver) while the tube is being removed. A previously prepared petrolatum gauze dressing is immediately applied to the wound as the tube is removed. A firm dry gauze dressing is placed over the petrolatum gauze dressing for 12–24 hr and strapped to the chest wall with adhesive tape.

VI. POSTOPERATIVE FEVER

A. General comments

1. Postoperative fever is produced in response to both infectious and noninfectious processes.

2. Minor elevations in body temperature which occur transiently in the postoperative period usually are related to fluid losses and altered metabolism.

3. Any postoperative elevation of body temperature more than one degree above normal or lasting over 2 days should be considered significant, and diagnostic studies to determine the etiology should be undertaken.

4. Postoperative fever often signals an impending complication that, unless identified and appropriately treated, will lead to prolonged hospitalization, increased morbidity, and, in some cases, death.

5. Fever in the immediate postoperative period (first 6 hr) usually is produced by metabolic or endocrine abnormalities (thyroid crisis, adrenocortical insufficiency), prolonged hypotension with inadequate peripheral tissue perfusion, or a transfusion reaction.

6. Septicemia, with or without endotoxin shock, secondary to operative manipulation of a bacterially contaminated area is an occasional cause of fever in the immediate postoperative period.

7. After the first 6 hr, pulmonary abnormalities provide the most common sources of fever until about the fourth to fifth postoperative day, at which time wound infections begin to appear. Fever resulting from thrombophlebitis or urinary tract infection may appear at any time, but is unusual before the second or third postoperative day.

8. If the patient has not been catheterized and has no urinary tract symptoms, postoperative fever rarely is due to urinary infection.

B. Pulmonary problems

1. Atelectasis and pneumonitis are the most common causes of postoperative fever. A diagnosis of atelectasis should be suspected in any patient with fever during the first 3 postoperative days.

2. Patients who smoke or who have chronic bronchitis, emphysema, thoracic kyphoscoliosis, obesity, or asthma are predisposed to postoperative pulmonary complications.

3. Factors which tend to increase the incidence of postoperative atelectasis are narcotics (depress cough reflex), prolonged postoperative immobilization, splinting from pain or constricting bandages, pulmonary congestion and edema, aspiration of foreign material, and weakness of respiratory muscles.

4. Postoperative atelectasis is produced by inadequate ventilation or by obstruction of the tracheobronchial tree.

5. If atelectasis is allowed to persist, bacterial pneumonitis will supervene. The presence of leukocytosis usually indicates a complicating bacterial infection.

6. The physical findings are diagnostic of postoperative atelectasis and appear many hours before a characteristic picture is visible on a chest x-ray.

    a. The patient with postoperative atelectasis usually has tachypnea and tachycardia.

    b. Cyanosis and tracheal shift rarely are present unless massive atelectasis has occurred.

    c. Localized moist rales and diminished breath sounds with bronchial breathing are detected, especially posteriorly toward the lung bases.

7. Treatment of atelectasis is aimed at removing obstructing mucus and reexpanding the involved pulmonary parenchyma before bacterial infection intervenes. Preoperative instruction in deep-breathing and coughing and postoperative use of blow bottles are of value.

8. Antibiotics are indicated only in patients with superimposed pneumonitis.

C. Postoperative urinary tract infection

1. Factors which predispose to development of infection are urinary stasis and the use of a urethral catheter.

2. The organisms involved usually are gram-negative enteric bacteria.

3. The site of infection usually is the urinary bladder (cystitis). Not infrequently, the infection then ascends directly to the upper urinary tract (pyelitis, pyelonephritis).

4. Any patient with a postoperative fever who has undergone a genitourinary operation or who has had a urethral catheter in place should be suspected of having a urinary tract infection.

5. Symptoms include dysuria, chills, increased frequency of urination, and pain localizing over the area of infection (flank, suprapubic).

6. A carefully obtained midstream urine specimen examined microscopically will show the presence of many leukocytes and bacteria.

7. Following urological instrumentation, the patient may develop septicemia heralded by a shaking chill and a sudden temperature elevation. Blood and urine cultures usually will grow gram-negative bacilli. If hypotension or shock develops, elaboration of bacterial endotoxins should be assumed and treatment started immediately (see Chap. 14).

8. Unless infection is severe, adequate hydration should be the only treatment until culture and sensitivity studies of the urine are available.

9. If the patient is acutely ill or if septicemia is suspected, a broad-spectrum antibiotic should be started IV after adequate specimens of blood and urine have been taken for culture.

D. Wound infection

1. Clostridial myonecrosis (gas gangrene) usually occurs dramatically during the first 24 hr postoperatively. One of the earliest symptoms is shock with tachycardia, fever, and hypotension. Skin discoloration (yellowish brown), crepitation, and a thin brownish, malodorous discharge are characteristic of severe clostridial infections.

2. Fever appearing after the fourth postoperative day commonly is caused by wound infection due to enteric aerobic (*Escherichia coli*) and anaerobic (*Bacteroides fragilis*) organisms or to staphylococci.

3. The location of the operative wound is important because tissue resistance to infection varies. Surgical wounds of the head and neck rarely become infected because of their excellent blood supply and rapid healing. Elderly patients with arteriosclerosis and obese patients may have a decreased blood supply in the area of the operative wound, leading to an increased incidence of wound infection.

4. Postoperative wound infection usually is signaled by increasing local wound pain followed by daily temperature elevations (spike pattern) similar to those of an abscess. The patient also may have tachycardia, chills, malaise, and leukocytosis.

5. Careful inspection of the wound discloses **marked tenderness and slight redness with enteric infections.** With staphylococcal infections, there is more obvious redness, swelling, elevated skin temperature, and, often, areas of fluctuation.

6. If the patient is receiving antibiotic therapy for another reason, infection may exist within the wound without many of the usual stigmas of inflammation.

7. Gram-staining and culture of the material found within the wound will lead to identification of the specific infecting microorganisms.

8. Treatment of a wound infection requires adequate drainage which is best provided by widely opening the operative wound. A common mistake is to open only a small portion of the wound. With enteric infections, this leads to further spread of infection and necrosis of tissue.

9. After adequate drainage, silver nitrate solution (0.5%) or Dakin's solution (¼ strength) is used to control bacterial growth in the wound and promote formation of granulation tissue.

10. Systemic antibiotics are used only when there is evidence of systemic toxicity. Antibiotics should be started only after cultures and Gram's stains of the infected drainage have been done.

E. Thrombophlebitis

1. Thrombophlebitis may occur at any time during the postoperative course.

2. Symptoms include fever, tenderness, and swelling of the involved area. Localized thrombophlebitis secondary to an indwelling IV needle or catheter rarely produces fever.

3. Adequate treatment, including anticoagulation, should be begun at the time of diagnosis to prevent pulmonary complications (see Chaps. 17 and 22).

F. Intra-abdominal abscess

1. Formation of intra-abdominal abscess is often first signaled by spiking fever in the postoperative period.

2. Pelvic abscess formation may occur as early as the third postoperative day. Diagnosis is easy when frequent rectal examinations have been made in the postoperative period.

3. Fever, hiccups, and fluoroscopic evidence of loss of movement of a hemidiaphragm suggest the development of a subphrenic abscess; these signs may appear as late as the seventh to tenth postoperative days.

VII. ASPIRATION PNEUMONIA

A. General comments

1. Vomiting with aspiration occurs in chronically **debilitated patients,** those under the influence of **alcohol,** in patients undergoing general **anesthesia,** and in patients receiving periodic or continuous **tube feedings.**

2. No measures are completely successful in preventing vomiting or regurgitation during anesthesia. Studies using intragastric dye show that over

10% of all patients aspirate a small amount of gastric content during general anesthesia.

3. Aspiration pneumonia is a **response to chemical irritation and is not caused primarily by growth of microorganisms.**

4. The acidity of aspirated material is critical in development of aspiration pneumonia.

5. Aspiration of liquid vomitus with a pH below 2.5 or the aspiration of solid food produces pneumonia in proportion to the amount aspirated.

B. Prophylaxis

1. If the patient has been kept NPO for at least 12 hr prior to operation, gastric emptying can be assumed and no extraordinary preventive measures are necessary during induction of anesthesia.

2. If **general anesthesia** is necessary in the face of possible **incomplete gastric emptying** (emergency, obstruction), a combination of these preventive measures should be used:

   a. **Awake intubation**   With the patient awake, an endotracheal tube is passed using local anesthetic spray. After passage the cuff of the endotracheal tube is inflated, occluding the trachea, and general anesthesia is induced. This method is safe and is preferred in most situations.

   b. **Crash induction**   The patient is given succinylcholine to paralyze muscles; this effectively prevents vomiting but not regurgitation. Just prior to the onset of muscular paralysis the patient is rapidly anesthetized with IV sodium thiopental (Pentothal), an endotracheal tube is passed, and the cuff is immediately inflated to occlude the trachea. This method carries some risk of aspiration as compared with awake intubation, but when skillfully done is safe and is less traumatic for the patient.

   c. **Mechanical gastric emptying**   Prior to administration of the general anesthetic, an Ewald, Johnston, or similar nasogastric tube (24 Fr or larger) is passed and the stomach contents emptied.

   d. **Induction of vomiting**   This can be accomplished prior to administration of the anesthetic, either pharmacologically with an emetic agent (apomorphine, syrup of ipecac) or mechanically (stimulation of pharyngeal mucosa by fingers or tube). This latter approach has the advantage of directness and simplicity although it is aesthetically unpleasant.

C. Management following vomiting   If vomiting does occur, the following measures are taken:

1. **Posture**   The patient's head is turned to one side and tilted down to allow dependent drainage of vomitus from the pharynx.

2. **Pharyngeal suction**   Immediate suctioning of the pharynx with a soft rubber or plastic tube is accomplished after the patient's head is positioned for dependent drainage. Solid material, if present, is cleared from the mouth and pharynx with a finger wrapped in gauze strips.

3. **Nasotracheal aspiration**   Once the mouth and pharynx are clear, the next step is to pass a plastic catheter into the trachea and both main bronchi. If gastric material returns with suctioning, one must assume aspiration.

4. **Bronchoscopy**   If a suspicion of aspiration exists, even though identifiable gastric content is not obtained on nasotracheal suctioning, or if the patient has copious secretions which cannot be raised by coughing and nasotracheal suctioning, bronchoscopy should be done. If the situation is urgent, local anesthesia can be omitted. If aspiration has occurred, all visible aspirated material should be removed by suctioning. The addition of tracheal lavage with saline and bicarbonate solution has been found experimentally to be of no benefit and may result in spread of pulmonary involvement.

D. Management of aspiration

1. Once aspiration of gastric content is evident, appropriate therapy should be begun immediately.

2. Clearing of the tracheobronchial tree by **nasotracheal suction or bronchoscopy** should be followed by early ventilatory assistance. Positive pressure ventilation should be employed for at least 72 hr in all patients, even when hypoxia initially is not evident.

3. **Bronchodilators** are helpful. Administer aerosolized isoproterenol (1:100–1:400), 0.2–1.0 ml tid or qid, depending on the severity of symptoms.

4. Broad-spectrum parenteral antibiotics should be given to help protect against secondary bacterial infection.

5. **Steroids**   The value of systemically or topically administered corticosteroids in aspiration pneumonia remains an unproved though clinically and pragmatically useful form of therapy. Steroids are given in the hope that their antiinflammatory properties will decrease the pulmonary injury resulting from gastric acid insult.

   a. **Parenteral steroids**   Hydrocortisone, 400–800 mg/day in four divided doses should be given IV and continued for 2–4 days, depending on the severity of symptoms, and then tapered rapidly. Equivalent doses of more potent steroids such as methylprednisolone or dexamethasone can be substituted.

b. Intratracheal steroids   Hydrocortisone, 50 mg in 5 ml of saline solution, may be administered via the respirator nebulizer three times a day for 1-2 days.

SUGGESTED READING

Cameron, J. L., Mitchell, W. H., and Zuidema, G. D.   Aspiration pneumonia: Clinical outcome following documented aspiration. *Arch. Surg.* 106:49, 1973.

Tinstman, T. C., Dines, D. E., and Arms, R. A.   Postoperative aspiration pneumonia. *Surg. Clin. North Am.* 53:859, 1973.

9. FLUID AND ELECTROLYTE THERAPY

I. FUNDAMENTALS

A. Clinical approach to fluid therapy

1. Since it is not possible to decide in advance the exact requirements of any patient for fluids or electrolytes, and since it is clinically difficult to measure outputs of fluid volumes and electrolytes from some sources, practical fluid therapy, even in the most difficult situations, must involve a semiquantitative approach, not a series of exact balance studies.

2. Fluid and electrolyte therapy is simplified if approached systematically. To arrive at a plan of treatment in any situation, answers to these questions are needed:

   a. What **imbalances** are present now and what is their probable magnitude?

   b. What **additional losses** can be expected during treatment?

   c. What are **daily maintenance requirements** for fluid and electrolytes?

3. Within each of these categories—imbalances, expected losses, and maintenance—determine next the needs for the following:

   a. Electrolyte-free water.

   b. Sodium, together with the water needed for its isosmotic solution.

   c. Potassium.

   d. Other electrolytes.

   e. Acid-base adjustment.

4. In the scheme to be outlined below, **two assumptions** are made:

   a. **The patient is a "typical 70-kg man"**   If the patient weighs more than 70 kg, no adjustments in fluid orders are necessary. If the patient weighs less than 70 kg, downward adjustments should be made using Figure 9-1 as a guide.

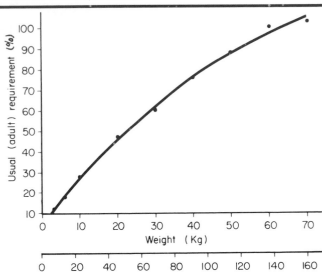

Figure 9-1. Relationship of body weight to percentage of full adult drug dosage. In addition to being useful in adapting fluid and electrolyte dosages for small adults and children, this curve also can be used to select a proper dose of *any* drug (sedatives and narcotics excepted). For patients weighing more than 70 kg, do not adjust dosage upward.

    b. Renal function is adequate   Children less than 2 yr of age have immature renal function, do not handle sodium well, and have higher proportional total body water than adults. Children less than 2 yr of age should have fluid and electrolyte therapy managed, in consultation with a knowledgeable pediatric surgeon or pediatrician, as outlined in Chapter 19. Patients having acute renal failure should be managed as outlined in Chapter 11.

B. Renal function

  1. Renal function is most easily assessed by measuring the **specific gravity and pH of the first urine voided in the morning.** If the patient is able to concentrate a protein- and glucose-free urine to a **specific gravity of 1.016 or higher** and is able to excrete urine with a **pH of 5.8 or lower,** renal function is adequate.

  2. Simultaneous determination of **serum and urine osmolality** is a more accurate way to measure the concentrating ability of the renal tubules. Normal serum osmolality is 280-300 mOsm/kg water. Typical normal urine contains 500-800 mOsm/kg water; the extreme range of urine osmolality is 40-1,600 mOsm. **After an overnight fast (12 hr), urine osmolality should be at least 850 mOsm/kg water and the ratio of urine to serum osmolality should be at least 3.0.**

  3. Adequate renal function simplifies fluid therapy enormously since as long as sufficient water and electrolytes are provided, the kidneys can make the

corrections necessary to keep the patient in electrolyte and acid-base balance.

4. Specific gravity persistently below 1.015, a persistently alkaline pH, or proteinuria greater than 100 mg/100 ml are signs of significant renal disease.

5. Patients with **chronic renal insufficiency** may have any of the following defects:

   a. **Metabolic acidosis** resulting from limited tubular capacity to excrete fixed acids. Such patients are as sensitive as young infants to chloride loads, so minimal amounts of saline solution should be used in supplying sodium. Sodium bicarbonate or lactate is tolerated better than saline solution.

   b. **Respiratory acidosis** develops easily during anesthesia or postoperatively. Patients with renal insufficiency should be given lactate or bicarbonate preoperatively, raising their serum bicarbonate concentration to about 30 mEq/liter, i.e., mild alkalosis. Frequent measurement of serum pH during and after operation is valuable.

   c. **Sodium retention** is a common feature of chronic renal failure and, when present, parenteral sodium intake should be limited.

   d. Conversely, some patients with chronic renal insufficiency are unable to retain sodium ion; they have **salt-losing nephritis**. Excretion of sodium in urine is increased and continues even in the face of a total body sodium deficit. The defect in renal tubular conservation of sodium must be made up by administration of additional parenteral sodium.

   e. **Water loss** is also common because of the inability of the renal tubules to concentrate, i.e., to excrete solute without additional water, resulting in urine of a fixed low specific gravity (hyposthenuria). These patients need additional electrolyte-free water.

C. **Facts and definitions**

   1. The limits of normal serum electrolyte concentrations are set out in Table 9-1.

TABLE 9-1. Electrolyte Concentrations in Serum

Electrolyte	Normal Range (mEq/liter)
Sodium	135–145
Potassium	3.5–5.5
Chloride	85–115
"Bicarbonate"	22–29
Calcium	4.0–5.5
Magnesium	1.5–2.5

2. Urine electrolyte concentrations are listed in Table 9-2.

3. Water comprises 55–70% of body mass. It moves freely throughout the body, crossing membranes to eliminate concentration gradients. **Total body water content is controlled by secretion of antidiuretic hormone (ADH) and regulates body osmolarity.**

4. Osmolarity, ignoring physicochemical nuances, is an expression of concentration of ions and proteins in solution in body water. If water is lost, either alone or in excess of solute, body osmolarity increases. If water is gained, alone or in excess of solute, body osmolarity decreases. Water moves freely in the body to prevent development of any compartmentalized osmolar concentration difference.

5. The **intracellular fluid (ICF)** compartment is that portion of body water from which **sodium is excluded.** The chief ion in ICF is potassium. Regulation of total body potassium is largely passive and secondary to changes in sodium and hydrogen ion excretion by the kidney.

6. The **extracellular fluid (ECF)** compartment is that part of body water in which **sodium is distributed** and is the chief electrolyte. The ECF compartment is subdivided into two portions: the plasma volume (about one third of the ECF, or 5% of body weight), located within blood vessels, and the interstitial volume, located outside both cells and blood vessels.

7. **Total body sodium content regulates ECF volume**   If sodium is lost, the ECF volume (and therefore the plasma volume) shrinks; if sodium is gained, the ECF volume expands. Sodium metabolism is controlled by aldosterone acting on the renal tubules.

8. A **third space** is a collection of ECF which, though present within the body, is functionally not available to normal physiological mechanisms maintaining fluid and electrolyte balance. Examples of third spaces are intestinal fluid content in paralytic ileus or mechanical obstruction, ascites in cirrhosis, and edema following burns or trauma. Such spaces collect at the expense of, and produce a deficit in, ECF volume. Later, they may be mobilized and (if the ECF volume has been replenished by parenteral therapy) excreted via the kidney, producing a diuresis.

9. **A tendency toward acidosis is a feature of normal physiology**   The daily load of acid metabolites is about 15,000 mEq, provided chiefly by oxidation of carbohydrate to carbonic acid and, to a lesser degree, by metabo-

TABLE 9-2. Urine Electrolyte Concentrations (random specimen, mEq/liter)

Tubular Activity	Sodium	Potassium
Normal	>40	>40
Conserving (early)	10–30	20–30
Maximal retention	<5	15–25

lism of fats (to carbonic and keto acids) and proteins (to carbonic acid and sulfate). The tendency to acidosis is accentuated in many disease states because of increased endogenous metabolism of body fat and protein.

10. **Alkalosis,** on the other hand, **is always secondary to altered homeostasis** (vomiting, hyperventilation). As a corollary of the normal physiological tendency toward acidosis, body defenses against acidosis are much better than those against alkalosis.

11. In acid-base imbalances, the presence of acidosis or alkalosis is defined on the basis of the arterial blood pH, which may or may not change in parallel with the intracellular pH. Defense of the normal extracellular pH of 7.4 is provided by buffer systems (bicarbonate, hemoglobin, phosphate, protein); later readjustments are made by the lungs and kidneys. The extreme limits of extracellular pH compatible with life are 6.8–8.0.

12. Pulmonary excretion of hydrogen ion is accompanied by conversion of carbonic acid to carbon dioxide and water; the carbon dioxide is then blown off. Disturbances of acid-base balance brought about by pulmonary insufficiency are called *respiratory acidosis* or *alkalosis.*

13. Renal excretion of hydrogen ion is accomplished by (1) direct excretion of hydrogen ion to a maximal urine concentration of 10^{-4} mEq/ml (pH 4.0), (2) exchange of hydrogen for potassium or sodium, and (3) synthesis of ammonia from glutamine. Acid-base imbalances brought about by renal insufficiency are called *metabolic acidosis* or *alkalosis.*

II. **DIAGNOSIS OF IMBALANCES**   The diagnosis of imbalances is the heart of any scheme of fluid and electrolyte balance. Diagnosis of the nature of imbalances present in the patient and an approximation of their magnitude are based on the history, clinical signs and symptoms, certain laboratory studies, and past clinical experience. Initial diagnoses always are more or less a guess. A more accurate diagnosis and an appreciation of the order of magnitude of any imbalance are obtained by assessment of the patient's response to initial therapy.

A. **Clues from the history**

1. **Gastric outlet obstruction** (duodenal ulcer, pyloric stenosis) results in vomiting and produces alkalosis (loss of chloride and potassium) and hypokalemia (loss of potassium), as well as losses of water and sodium.

2. **Vomiting** secondary to a cause other than gastric outlet obstruction produces loss of water, sodium, and potassium. If there is any shift in acid-base balance, it is toward metabolic acidosis. The electrolyte composition of various GI secretions is listed in Table 9-3.

3. **Diarrhea** (cholera, ulcerative colitis, ileostomy dysfunction) also results in loss of water, sodium, and potassium, and tends to result in acidosis.

4. **Burns** produce losses of plasma and ECF (water, protein, and sodium). The magnitude of fluid loss depends on the depth and extent of burn.

TABLE 9-3. Approximate Electrolyte Composition of GI Secretions (mEq/liter in adults)

Secretion	Usual Maximum Volume/Day	Sodium	Chloride	Potassium
Normal				
Saliva	1,000	100	75	5
Gastric juice (pH<4.0)	2,500[a]	60	100	10
Gastric juice (pH>4.0)	2,000[a]	100	100	10
Bile	1,500	140	100	10
Pancreatic juice	1,000	140	75	10
Succus entericus (mixed small-bowel fluid)	3,500	100	100	20
Abnormal				
New ileostomy	500–2,000	130	110	20
Adapted ileostomy	400	50	60	10
New cecostomy	400	80	50	20
Colostomy (transverse loop)	300	50	40	10
Diarrhea	1,000–4,000	60	45	30

[a] Nasogastric suction volume usually much less than this unless pyloric obstruction exists.

5. **Sweating,** if excessive, causes appreciable loss of both sodium and water, results in shrinkage of the ECF volume, and eventually results in vascular collapse.

6. A **low-sodium diet** coupled with **diuretic therapy** commonly induces a moderate state of salt depletion and consequent hypovolemia which normally is of no consequence. However, when such patients are given an anesthetic (which releases sympathetic vasoconstrictive tone), they may become hypotensive. Potassium is also lost as a result of diuretic treatment; unless replaced in the diet, hypokalemia ensues.

B. **Clinical signs and symptoms**

1. **Thirst is a very sensitive guide to need for water**

   a. Thirst needs to be differentiated from dry oral mucous membranes. Dry mouth is relieved by gargling a small amount of water; thirst is not.

   b. Thirst resulting from water depletion is such a compelling symptom that if the patient has access to water he will promptly correct any deficit.

   c. Clinical water depletion is found only in patients who are not able to drink water (feeble, comatose) or are prevented from drinking (restrained, NPO). Patients also may have increased water losses caused by high fever, diarrhea, or osmotic diuresis (glucose in diabetic acidosis, mannitol).

2. Moisture in the axilla and groin

 a. **A dry but otherwise normal axilla or groin should be interpreted as evidence of a major water deficit,** minimally at least 1,500 ml.

 b. Apocrine sweat glands in the axilla and groin normally are constantly active so that some moisture always is present.

 c. As a major water deficit develops, apocrine glands reduce their rate of secretion and finally stop; the axillae and groin become dry.

 d. The presence of dermatitis, chronic fungus infections, and similar lesions resulting in atrophy or malfunction of apocrine sweat glands may also produce a dry groin or axillae.

3. Body weight

 a. Short-term, i.e., minute-to-minute or hour-to-hour, changes in body weight reflect changes in both ECF volume and total body water. Repetitive measurements of body weight are so clumsy that body weight is not a useful measure over the short term.

 b. Longer-term trends in body weight over a period of days are a reasonably reliable guide to changes in total body water but should be interpreted with caution when a "third space" is developing.

 c. Measurements of body weight should be corrected for tissue losses in catabolic states (up to 500 gm/day) or for lean tissue gains in anabolic states (up to 150 gm/day). In most postoperative patients, a loss of at least 300 gm/day in body weight is expected.

 d. Weight gain is interpreted as indicating water retention. Weight loss in excess of 300–500 gm/day indicates water loss. Therapy should not be based only on correcting changes in body weight; other signs are used to determine if shifts in water balance are of ECF origin or are of electrolyte-free water.

4. Jugular veins

 a. With the patient supine, the external jugular veins normally fill to the anterior border of the sternocleidomastoid muscle. **These veins provide a built-in manometer for following changes in CVP.**

 b. CVP is:

  (1) Elevated by an increased plasma volume or by heart failure.

  (2) Depressed by a decreased plasma volume.

c. In the absence of heart failure, changes in neck-vein filling reflect changes in plasma volume. Since plasma volume is a part of the sodium-dependent ECF volume, alterations in filling of the neck veins are clues to changes in total body sodium content.

d. The presence of heart failure can be distinguished by the presence of **hepatojugular reflux.** The patient should be in a sitting-up or semireclining position for this test. Pressure on the abdomen over the liver causes a further increase in filling of the neck veins which persists as long as pressure is maintained. An expanded plasma volume in the absence of heart failure will not produce a positive hepatojugular reflux test.

e. In a supine patient, **flat neck veins reflect a contracted plasma volume and indicate a need for sodium-containing fluids.**

5. **Tissue turgor**

a. **Decreased turgor should be interpreted as indicating a contraction of the interstitial fluid volume and a need for sodium-containing fluids.**

b. **The tongue is the most reliable indicator of tissue turgor**   Normally, the tongue has a more or less single median furrow. Additional furrows which parallel the major median furrow appear with decreased interstitial volume.

c. Decreased skin turgor is another useful indicator of a diminished interstitial fluid volume. This is less reliable than tongue turgor since it is also influenced by loss of elasticity in older patients.

d. Eyeball tension is commonly mentioned as an indicator of turgor. The physician rarely has the opportunity to establish a baseline in a particular patient prior to the onset of fluid imbalance, so that this sign is often useless. If consistent with other findings, decreased eyeball turgor provides corroborative evidence of a decreased interstitial fluid volume.

6. **Blood pressure and pulse**

a. Changes in these measures are influenced chiefly by changes in the circulating blood volume (ECF compartment) (Table 9-4).

b. Tachycardia is the earliest sign of a decreased blood volume, followed by the appearance of postural hypotension and then hypotension when the patient is supine.

c. Bradycardia may accompany acute large losses in blood volume.

d. **Hypotension indicates a need for blood or sodium-containing fluids.**

TABLE 9-4. Response of Blood Pressure and Pulse to Hypovolemia

Blood Volume (ml)	Supine		Sitting	
	BP	P	BP	P
Normal	N	N	N	N
− 500	N	N	N	N or ↑
− 1,000	N	N or ↑	N or ↓	↑
− 1,500	N or ↓	↑	↓	↑ or ↓
− 2,000	↓	↑ or ↓	↓↓	↑ or ↓

7. **Edema and rales**

   a. **Edema reflects an increase in interstitial fluid volume and implies that total body sodium is increased.** Edema is not produced by retention of water alone.

   b. Edema is not a very sensitive indicator of sodium balance. A 20% increase in total body exchangeable sodium may accumulate before edema becomes very obvious.

   c. Barely perceptible pitting edema indicates that total body sodium has increased by at least 400 mEq (2.7 liters of saline).

   d. Rales in the absence of pulmonary disease indicate accumulation of alveolar fluid and imply heart failure or an acutely expanded plasma volume, or both.

   e. When rales are caused by expansion of plasma volume, the acute increase in volume is at least 1,500 ml.

C. **Interpreting laboratory values**

   1. **Serum sodium concentration** (mEq/liter)

      a. Serum sodium concentration reflects solute concentration in all body compartments. It is a **measure of the state of total body osmolarity.** Unless there is a disparity between the proportions of salt and water gained or lost, body osmolarity will not change and the serum sodium concentration will be unaltered.

      b. Acute changes in body osmolarity most often are caused by changes in total body water content.

      c. In **water depletion,** all body fluid compartments contract proportionately in volume, increasing the concentration of all solutes. This is reflected in an **increase in serum sodium concentration.**

      d. **In acute water depletion, the serum sodium concentration is a good guide to body need for water.**

e. **A decrease in serum sodium concentration** may be due either to water excess (common) or to sodium deficit (uncommon). Water excess due to stress-induced antidiuresis or to iatrogenic administration of only electrolyte-free IV solutions is seen frequently in surgical patients.

f. Differentiation between hyponatremia due to water excess and that due to sodium deficit is based on whether or not there are other signs of sodium depletion (ECF deficit) (see Table 9-6).

g. Water excess is treated by restricting water intake; administration of hypertonic sodium solutions is indicated only for convulsions (water intoxication).

h. Certain debilitated patients develop a low serum sodium concentration that is asymptomatic, the "hyponatremia of severe illness." The best treatment for this situation is no treatment at all. This syndrome is caused by a "resetting" of hypothalamic osmoreceptors; inappropriate secretion of ADH results in a chronic state of mild water excess. If one tries to raise the serum sodium concentration in such a situation by restricting water intake, signs of water depletion (thirst, oliguria) appear while hyponatremia persists. If one tries to raise the serum sodium concentration by administering salt, the salt is excreted via the kidneys; if not, the patient may become edematous, even while maintaining hyponatremia.

i. In neither acute nor chronic imbalances is the serum sodium concentration a reliable indicator of changes in total body sodium content or of sodium need.

j. **An increase in serum sodium concentration is interpreted as indicating a need for electrolyte-free water. A decrease in serum sodium concentration often indicates a need for restriction of electrolyte-free water intake;** sometimes there may be a need for administration of sodium-containing fluids to patients who are hypovolemic.

2. **Hematocrit**

a. Changes in hematocrit are interpretable in terms of fluid balance only when no changes are occurring in erythrocyte mass (i.e., no bleeding or hemolysis).

b. The whole-blood hematocrit provides a biopsy of both the intracellular compartment (erythrocytes) and the extracellular compartment (plasma).

c. The hematocrit changes little with disturbances of water balance, since when only total body water changes, the erythrocytes (intracellular compartment) swell or shrink proportionately and in parallel with the plasma volume (extracellular compartment). The percent volume of whole blood occupied by the erythrocytes (hematocrit) is not appreciably affected.

d. The plasma volume, as a part of the sodium-dependent ECF volume, changes in parallel with changes in total body sodium content. The erythrocytes (intracellular compartment) are little affected by changes in sodium balance. Therefore **changes in total body sodium are associated with changes in hematocrit.**

e. In sodium depletion, the plasma volume decreases and the hematocrit rises. An initial rough estimate of the magnitude of sodium deficit may be obtained by equating each 3% increase in hematocrit value from normal with a deficit of 150 mEq of sodium. Considerable clinical judgment enters into the assumption of "normal hematocrit," i.e., what the hematocrit in a given patient would be if no imbalance were present. The magnitude of any imbalances estimated in this way should not be rigidly interpreted but used simply as a guide to initial treatment.

f. In sodium excess, the expected decrease in hematocrit is not regularly seen.

g. Over the short term and as long as hemorrhage is not occurring, an **increase in hematocrit is interpreted as indicating need for sodium.**

3. Serum potassium concentration (mEq/liter)

a. The serum potassium concentration represents only a small fraction, about 1%, of the total body exchangeable potassium. Therefore, large changes in body potassium content can occur without producing a change in serum potassium concentration outside the normal range. Nonetheless, the serum potassium concentration, if properly interpreted, is a reliable but insensitive guide to potassium need.

b. Serum potassium concentration is increased in acidosis and decreased in alkalosis   This effect is caused by a shift of potassium out of (and hydrogen ion into) cells in acidosis or a shift of potassium into cells in alkalosis without any change in total body potassium content. The magnitude of the potassium-hydrogen ion shifts approximate a 1-mEq change in serum potassium concentration for each 0.2-unit change in serum pH. The approximate deficit or excess of potassium may be calculated from arterial pH and serum potassium concentration using the nomogram in Figure 9-3.

c. Some hormones (Pitressin, thyroxin) raise serum potassium concentration, while others (insulin, corticoids) lower it. Renal conservation or loss of potassium and potassium shifts into or out of cells are operative here.

4. Blood pH

a. This is the most **direct and accurate measure of the state of acid-base balance.** It should be used in preference to measurement of the serum bicarbonate.

b. Arterial samples should be used routinely. Venous samples have a lower normal value and their range varies considerably, depending on the state of tissues peripheral to the site of vein puncture, making interpretation less reliable in acutely changing situations.

5. Serum bicarbonate concentration

a. CO_2-combining power, usually reported as "CO_2," is the commonly available measure of bicarbonate concentration. Carbonic acid (H_2CO_3) concentration (dissolved CO_2 in blood) is measured as the P_{CO_2}, or CO_2 tension, usually by means of a modified pH electrode. CO_2 content is the sum of bicarbonate (HCO_3^-) and H_2CO_3, and is measured manometrically using a Van Slyke apparatus.

b. For most clinical situations, measurement of the bicarbonate concentration in serum is adequate, although an arterial pH is simpler and more direct.

c. Clinical disturbances of acid-base balance were classically described in terms of the Henderson-Hasselbalch equation for the bicarbonate buffer system because bicarbonate was the only buffer anion which could be measured easily in serum. Such a description is adequate so long as one remembers how the pulmonary and renal mechanisms for hydrogen ion excretion influence the bicarbonate buffer system:

$$pH = pK + \log \frac{HCO_3^-}{H_2CO_3} \begin{array}{l} \text{(controlled by kidney; measured as "bicarbonate")} \\ \text{(controlled by lung; equals } P_{CO_2} \times 0.03) \end{array}$$

d. Bicarbonate concentration is increased in respiratory acidosis and metabolic alkalosis; it is decreased in metabolic acidosis and respiratory alkalosis.

6. Urine

a. Volume output

(1) Record urine output at least every 8 hr in all patients on parenteral fluids. If there is a major imbalance, shock, or any suspicion of renal insufficiency, record urine output hourly.

(2) Expected volume output is $1,500 \pm 500$ ml/day (60 ± 20 ml/hr) in patients in a basal state.

(3) Following trauma or stress, output may decrease transiently to 750-1,200 ml/day (30-50 ml/hr).

(4) Output of 500 ml/day or less constitutes **oliguria.** In the absence of tubular failure or obstructive uropathy, oliguria is prerenal in origin and may be a result of either a deficit in ECF volume (total body sodium) or a deficit in total body water.

b. Urinalysis

(1) A random sample is sufficient. A 24-hr urine collection is not necessary to make any determination which is useful in managing fluid problems.

(2) Specific gravity reflects osmolar concentration of solutes in urine if performed on a protein- and glucose-free specimen. In oliguria resulting from water deficit, specific gravity is high (1.030) because of maximal tubular water resorption in the face of a continuing excretory solute load. Oliguria resulting from ECF (i.e., sodium) deficit tends to result in urine of low specific gravity (1.010) because of impairment of the sodium-dependent countercurrent mechanism of tubular water resorption, promoting relative diuresis as well as active sodium conservation which slightly reduces the excretory solute load.

(3) Urine osmolarity is measured directly by freezing point depression utilizing an osmometer. Normal urine osmolarity varies between 400 and 1,500 mOsm/liter. Simultaneous measurements of urine and serum osmolarity provide the most useful information regarding renal function. The urine-serum osmolarity ratio is calculated.

In **oliguria due to total body water deficit,** maximal tubular resorption of water in the face of a continuing excretion of solute produces concentrated urine with a high osmolarity; the urine osmolarity usually exceeds 1,200 mOsm/liter. The serum osmolarity is little affected and is usually normal, about 300 mOsm/liter. The **urine-serum ratio is 4 or higher.**

In **oliguria resulting from sodium (ECF) deficit,** as well as in acute tubular necrosis, there is failure of tubular concentrating and diluting mechanisms. The urine produced resembles glomerular filtrate which, in turn, resembles plasma in its osmolar concentration. **The urine-serum osmolar ratio approaches unity.**

(4) Urine pH reflects the pH in serum and helps confirm a diagnosis of acidosis or alkalosis. There are two exceptions: (a) paradoxical aciduria in hypokalemic alkalosis and (b) alkaline urine secondary to infection with urea-splitting bacteria.

(5) Urine electrolyte concentrations (mEq/liter) are set out in Table 9-2. Sodium retention begins promptly on renal tubular stimulation by aldosterone, but maximal conservation requires 3–5 days of constant stimulation. When maximally stimulated, renal sodium excretion can be brought to zero. In the absence of marked diuresis, **urine sodium concentration below 20 mEq/liter always indicates active conservation** which may be due to actual or functional plasma or ECF volume deficit or may be due to inappropriate secretion of aldosterone. Potassium retention is controlled by many factors (e.g., serum pH, tubular solute load, sodium balance) besides the state of total body potassium. Although some conservation of potassium occurs in hypokalemia, even with a large deficit in total body potassium there is still an **obligatory urinary loss of potassium of about 20 mEq/day.** Determination of urinary electrolyte concentrations is very helpful in confirming the presence or absence of deficits in total body sodium and potassium.

III. CLINICAL STATES OF FLUID AND ELECTROLYTE IMBALANCE   Imbalances rarely occur in pure form or in isolation: Clinical problems are always mixtures. Nonetheless, it is conceptually convenient to compartmentalize clinical diagnosis and treatment on the basis of theoretical pure states. It is far easier to determine first if the patient has an excess, is normal, or has a deficit in total body water and then to make a separate determination, using other criteria, regarding the presence of an excess, normality, or deficit in total body sodium or potassium, than to try to decide if the patient's problem is "hypotonic dehydration" or "acute desalting water loss." It must be reemphasized that the theoretical states to be discussed below rarely exist in pure form in patients. They are a conceptual and diagnostic convenience only.

A. Water depletion

1. Water depletion is caused either by unreplaced losses together with increased output (fever, osmotic diuresis, diarrhea) or by a lack of intake (NPO, coma).

2. A water deficit results in a decrease in volume of all body fluid compartments. Since solute content does not change, hyperosmolarity ensues. Osmoreceptors are stimulated and secretion of ADH is increased. More water is resorbed from the distal renal tubule.

3. The chief symptoms and signs of water deficit are **thirst, oliguria, and hypernatremia.**

4. A rough initial working **estimate of the magnitude of water deficit** can be made from clinical data (Table 9-5) or by assuming that each 3 mEq of serum sodium concentration above the normal range represents a deficit of at least 1 liter of total body water.

TABLE 9-5. Clinical Signs of Water Depletion

Magnitude of Deficit (adults)	Clinical Features
1.5 liters or less	Thirst
1.5–4.0 liters	Marked thirst Dry mouth, groin, axillae Serum sodium increased Urine specific gravity increased Hematocrit, skin turgor, and blood pressure normal
4.0 liters or more	Intolerable thirst Marked hypernatremia Oliguria Body weight decreased Slightly increased hematocrit Apathy, stupor If not corrected: hyperosmolar coma, death

5. In severe hyperglycemia, the serum sodium concentration will give a falsely low estimate of serum osmolarity. The estimate of water need based on the serum sodium concentration should be mentally corrected by adding 500 ml of water for each 100 mg/100 ml blood glucose elevation above normal.

6. **Treatment of a water deficit requires provision of additional sodium-free water**   If water depletion is severe, at least one half of the estimated deficit should be replaced in the initial 12 hr of treatment.

7. Combined saline and free water depletion (dehydration) often exists and clinically presents symptoms resulting from an ECF volume deficit (decreased total body sodium) and hyperosmolarity (decreased total body water). In such cases, the serum sodium is decreased. Initial treatment should be directed at correcting the sodium deficit (see paragraph **C**, below).

B. **Water excess, water intoxication**

1. Water excess is frequently **iatrogenic,** resulting from administration of electrolyte-free water to sodium-depleted patients or patients in whom ADH activity is increased, or by rapid administration of water in any situation in which oliguria exists. Water intoxication is occasionally caused by excessive intake (neurosis) or by injudicious administration of oxytocin (Pitocin) in an attempt to induce labor or stop bleeding from esophageal varices.

2. Water excess leads to an increase in volume of all fluid compartments. Since body solute content is not altered, a state of hyposmolarity ensues. Hypothalamic osmoreceptors are inhibited and pituitary secretion of ADH is decreased. The distal renal tubule resorbs less water, resulting in increased renal water excretion. These compensatory mechanisms are much less sensitive than those defending the body against a water deficit.

3. The symptoms and signs of water excess are related to both the degree of water overloading and the rate at which it develops. Moderate degrees of water excess often are well tolerated and clinically are asymptomatic. The only signs will be a **decreased serum sodium concentration, an increased urine volume, and an increase in body weight.** Pitting edema does not develop.

4. More marked water overloading causes swelling of brain cells and leads to nausea, vomiting, and ultimately convulsions (water intoxication). These symptoms rarely appear unless the osmolar shift has been rapid and the serum sodium concentration is below 120 mEq/liter.

5. **Treatment of water excess not complicated by convulsions requires only restricting water intake;** it is not usually necessary to do anything more. IV ethyl alcohol will inhibit ADH secretion and may be useful in the treatment of some cases of water excess. In severe cases, induction of enforced solute diuresis with mannitol may be needed. If the patient is in

renal failure and diuresis cannot be induced, dialysis is required. Convulsions should be treated by IV administration of small amounts (100–250 ml) of 5% sodium chloride solution. Convulsions or other CNS symptoms from water intoxication are the only good indication for use of IV hypertonic salt. Hypertonic salt is not the best treatment for a sodium deficit.

C. Sodium depletion

1. Severe sodium depletion may result from the following:

    a. Abnormal GI losses (suction, vomiting, diarrhea).

    b. Losses of ECF either externally (burns, marked sweating) or internally as a "third space" (peritonitis, ascites, ileus).

    c. Excessive urine sodium wastage (diuretics, chronic nephritis, adrenal failure, cerebrorenal shunt in hydrocephalus, vasopressin).

    d. Restricted dietary intake.

2. The **symptoms and signs** of sodium depletion are caused by decreased ECF volume (Table 9-6).

3. Acute changes in total body sodium content usually do not lead to any change in serum sodium concentration since equivalent amounts of water for isotonic solution of sodium are gained or lost in most acute situations (e.g., hemorrhage, burns, ileus). Therefore **serum sodium concentration is not a reliable guide to sodium need.**

4. **A low serum sodium concentration more often indicates water excess than sodium deficit.**

5. In extremely severe states of sodium depletion, the body abandons its defense of isotonicity and retains electrolyte-free water in an attempt to

TABLE 9-6. Clinical Signs in Acute Sodium Depletion

Magnitude of Deficit	Symptoms and Signs
Up to 450 mEq sodium (3 liters of ECF)	Furrowed tongue Neck veins collapsed Increased hematocrit Urine sodium <40 mEq/liter Tachycardia Anorexia Little or no thirst; craving for salt rare; serum sodium normal
More than 600 mEq sodium (more than 4 liters of ECF)	Marked increase in hematocrit Oliguria (prerenal) Hypotension (especially orthostatic) Apathy, nausea Some decrease in serum sodium If uncorrected and progressive: death in hypovolemic shock

preserve ECF volume. The resulting hyposmolarity is reflected in a lowered serum sodium concentration. This situation is also marked by signs of hypovolemia (flat neck veins, tongue furrowing, tachycardia, low blood pressure, oliguria) in contrast to the minimal signs and symptoms accompanying equivalent hyponatremia secondary to moderate water excess.

6. **Treatment of sodium deficit** consists of restoration of ECF volume by **administration of appropriate amounts of sodium-containing fluids.** Lost blood should be replaced with blood. Lost plasma should be replaced with plasma or, preferably, plasma substitutes (Plasmanate, albumin). Lost interstitial fluid (e.g., post-traumatic edema) should be replaced with electrolyte solutions. Exclusive replacement of plasma or blood loss with only electrolyte solutions requires about four times the volume of lost blood or plasma and results in overexpansion of the total ECF volume, since the distribution of sodium is not confined only to the plasma volume.

D. **Sodium excess**

1. Sodium excess usually is caused by abnormal renal retention of sodium related to inability to excrete a sodium load (starvation, severe illness) or to increased sodium resorption (increased activity of aldosterone or other hormones with salt-retaining action [cortisone, estrogens, testosterone]). Acute hypernatremia occasionally follows absorption of intrauterine hypertonic saline administered to induce abortion.

2. The only important clinical sign of total body sodium excess is **edema.** Even this is relatively late evidence, since 400 mEq of excess sodium (i.e., about 3 liters of fluid) may accumulate before minimal dependent pitting edema is evident. **Weight gain** will parallel accumulation of ECF. While disability resulting from edema is minimal, it is an undesirable situation since wound healing is impaired; plasma proteins are diluted, tending to bring about further sodium retention; and the patient is predisposed to develop heart failure and pulmonary edema.

3. Edema, of course, may be related primarily to other factors (increased hydrostatic pressure in congestive heart failure or in venous or lymphatic obstruction; increased capillary permeability in inflammation or allergic states; decreased plasma proteins in nephrosis and cirrhosis). These other abnormalities all bring about secondary renal sodium retention.

4. The hematocrit in sodium excess may be low, but often is normal; the serum sodium concentration usually is normal.

5. **Treatment of sodium excess** consists of sodium restriction and judicious use of diuretics and spironolactone. In edema accompanied by marked hypoproteinemia, the protein deficit also must be corrected; otherwise, sodium restriction alone will lead to a decrease in plasma volume.

6. Edema (sodium excess) accompanied by a low serum sodium concentration (water excess) is found in some severely debilitated patients. This situation is generally iatrogenic, resulting from efforts to treat a patient

with "hyponatremia of severe illness" by administration of large amounts of salt or to treat an edematous patient with poor renal function by salt restriction. In such patients, the kidneys have failed to respond to the osmotic stimulus to water excretion. This situation carries an extremely grave prognosis, since it means that the body has lost the ability to regulate its osmolarity. Treatment is aimed at maintaining a normal circulating plasma volume by judicious administration of plasma and sodium-containing fluids. The accumulating edema often will have to be ignored.

E. Potassium depletion

1. Hypokalemia may result from diuretic therapy, loss of GI fluids (suction, fistula, diarrhea), osmotic diuresis (mannitol, urea, diabetic glucosuria), adrenal hyperactivity (stress, Cushing's syndrome), or nephritis. Iatrogenic hypokalemia is not rare and results from prolonged parenteral administration of potassium-free fluids.

2. Hypokalemia may inhibit aldosterone secretion if the serum sodium concentration is normal. In combined sodium and potassium depletion, the stimulus to aldosterone secretion from the sodium deficit is overriding and potassium continues to be lost via the kidneys.

3. Renal mechanisms for hydrogen ion excretion are shared by potassium since both are excreted in exchange for sodium. If potassium depletion exists, hydrogen ion is excreted predominantly in exchange for sodium, since potassium is not readily available. This produces a relative depletion of plasma hydrogen ion (alkalosis) while at the same time an acid urine is being excreted (paradoxical aciduria).

4. Early **signs of potassium depletion are vague:** malaise and weakness. Paralytic ileus and distention are seen in some hypokalemic patients. Muscular paresis appears only with extreme depletion. Potassium-depleted patients are prone to develop ectopic atrial impulses or other signs of digitalis intoxication; hepatic coma may appear if the patient has liver disease; pseudodiabetic glucosuria may appear because of inability to transfer glucose across muscle cell membranes. ECG alterations are illustrated in Figure 9-2.

5. An approximation of the **magnitude of potassium deficit** can be obtained from an estimate of body potassium capacity and the measured blood pH and serum potassium concentration (Fig. 9-3).

6. **Potassium depletion is treated by parenteral administration of potassium salts**   Although large total amounts may be given in a single day when needed, the rate of infusion must be limited, so that transiently high venous blood concentrations do not affect the heart. In general, no more than 20 mEq of potassium should be administered per hour even in very severe hypokalemia.

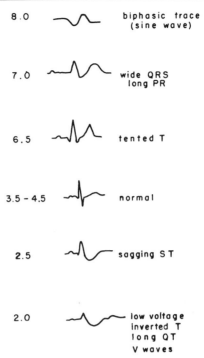

8.0		biphasic trace (sine wave)
7.0		wide QRS long PR
6.5		tented T
3.5 - 4.5		normal
2.5		sagging ST
2.0		low voltage inverted T long QT V waves

Figure 9-2. Changes in the ECG in hyperkalemia and hypokalemia. Serum potassium concentration is listed at the left and typical ECG tracings are depicted in the middle of the figure. The abnormal features of those tracings are listed at the right.

F. Potassium excess

1. Life-threatening potassium excess is usually associated with renal failure and is potentiated by concomitant tissue destruction or by depletion of sodium or calcium. Less threatening increases in total body potassium are seen in adrenal insufficiency.

2. Elevation of serum potassium above 6 mEq/liter may stimulate secretion of aldosterone, which enhances excretion of potassium by the normal kidney. This corrective mechanism is probably not available in renal insufficiency.

3. If the serum potassium exceeds 7 mEq/liter, intracardiac impulse conduction is slowed; arrhythmia, bradycardia, and hypotension may be followed by diastolic cardiac arrest (Fig. 9-2).

4. Treatment of hyperkalemia associated with renal failure is discussed in Chapter 11. Any patient showing a wide QRS complex or other evidence of hyperkalemic cardiac toxicity should be treated immediately with IV calcium (antagonizes potassium), bicarbonate (alkalization encourages

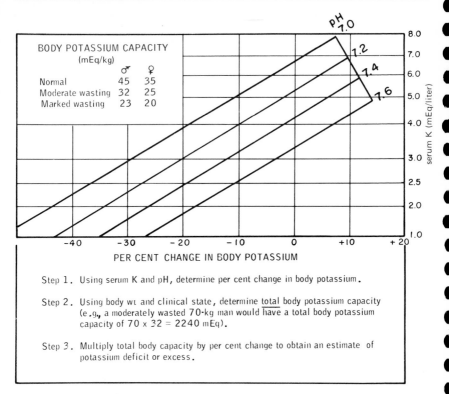

Step 1. Using serum K and pH, determine per cent change in body potassium.

Step 2. Using body wt and clinical state, determine total body potassium capacity (e.g., a moderately wasted 70-kg man would have a total body potassium capacity of 70 x 32 = 2240 mEq).

Step 3. Multiply total body capacity by per cent change to obtain an estimate of potassium deficit or excess.

Figure 9-3. Method of approximate calculation of depletion or excess of total body potassium.

potassium to shift into cells), and glucose plus insulin (potassium deposits with glycogen). These immediate treatment measures should be followed by administration of ion-exchange resins (Kayexalate) or by dialysis.

G. Calcium and magnesium

1. Body reserves of calcium are readily mobilized from bone and are so great that symptomatic hypocalcemia develops only in acute alkalosis (hysterical hyperventilation) or in hypoparathyroidism (see Chap. 13).

2. Chronic hypercalcemia is seen in hyperparathyroidism, sarcoidosis, vitamin D intoxication, and similar states, and results in formation of renal stones. Acute hypercalcemia producing coma is seen occasionally in hyperparathyroidism, but more often is a result of widespread skeletal metastases (usually responds to steroids).

3. Magnesium is the second most prevalent intracellular cation, but understanding of its metabolism in humans is incomplete. In experimental animals, magnesium deficiency causes vasodilation and convulsions and

is accompanied by myocardial necrosis. In humans, increased levels of serum magnesium are seen inconstantly in hypertension and chronic infections and more regularly in renal failure.

4. Hypermagnesemia produces sedation deepening to coma. Hypomagnesemia produces neuromuscular hyperexcitability similar to that seen in hypocalcemia.

5. Magnesium apparently behaves much like its intracellular partner, potassium, except that there is no obligatory renal loss of magnesium. Deficient diets can be tolerated for as long as a month, so that clinical magnesium deficiency in humans is rare. Cases of magnesium deficiency have been reported with prolonged GI suction or in delirium tremens. Administration of 2-4 gm of magnesium sulfate IM is probably indicated once weekly in patients on prolonged parenteral therapy (see Chap. 10).

H. Metabolic acidosis

1. Metabolic acidosis occurs whenever renal tubules fail to excrete sufficient hydrogen ion to maintain a normal serum pH. This may be a result of:

   a. Immaturity of renal function (premature infants).

   b. Chronic tubular failure (nephritis).

   c. Acute tubular failure (shock, toxins).

   d. Ketosis (diabetes, fever, starvation).

   e. Ingestion of excessive amounts of acidifying salts.

   f. Abnormal GI losses (diarrhea).

   g. Failure of oxidative metabolism (shock).

2. In acidosis caused by renal failure, GI loss, or ketosis, there is an increase in so-called fixed acids (SO_4, PO_4, etc.). In failure of oxidative metabolism, lactate is not converted to carbon dioxide and water for elimination via the lungs; "lactic acidosis" results. Respiratory attempts at partial compensation result in an increased rate and depth of breathing (Kussmaul's respirations); if respiratory compensation is interfered with (emphysema, pneumonia, anesthesia), a combined metabolic and respiratory acidosis develops in which the serum HCO_3^- is nearly normal but serum pH is very low.

3. **Mild to moderate acidosis usually requires no specific therapy** aimed at correcting pH. Therapy should be directed at the underlying cause of the acidosis. More severe acidosis (pH <7.30, serum bicarbonate <15 mEq/liter) requires treatment, per se.

4. In **severe acute metabolic acidosis,** IV bicarbonate is preferred to lactate, since its effectiveness is not dependent on intermediary hepatic metabolism. The amount of **bicarbonate needed can be estimated from the formula:** body weight (kg) $\times$ 0.3 $\times$ (25 – measured serum bicarbonate) = mEq bicarbonate needed. Lactate may be useful in states of chronic acidosis, but should not be given if hypoxia or shock is present, unless a volume deficit is the cause of shock, and should never be given to patients with liver failure. Amine buffers (tromethamine, or THAM) cannot be used in renal shutdown. In most cases of moderate acidosis, they probably have no advantage over bicarbonate.

I. Metabolic alkalosis

1. Metabolic alkalosis almost always is caused by loss of acid gastric juice and usually is accompanied by hypokalemia. Less frequently, metabolic alkalosis is caused by hypokalemia resulting from diuretic therapy, hyperaldosteronism, or a similar cause of renal potassium wastage.

2. Partial pH compensation is rapidly achieved by a clinically inapparent decrease in ventilation resulting in carbon dioxide retention, an increase in serum carbonic acid concentration, and partial restoration of the blood pH toward normal.

3. In all cases of metabolic alkalosis caused by loss of gastric juice, replacement of chloride is essential to successful therapy. Administration of saline solution is sufficient therapy in mild cases of metabolic alkalosis without hypokalemia, since the kidney will complete the job of correcting acid-base balance by retaining chloride and excreting sodium along with excess bicarbonate.

4. In moderately severe alkalosis, another problem arises. In addition to losses of potassium in gastric juice, renal potassium excretion is increased in order to permit the tubules to retain hydrogen ion. In this situation, administration of IV potassium chloride is the preferred treatment, since it will correct both the potassium and the chloride deficits.

5. In severe metabolic alkalosis which does not respond to saline or potassium chloride alone, it may be necessary to use ammonium chloride. Ammonium chloride is given slowly IV in doses up to 140 mEq (1 liter of the isotonic 0.75% solution). The blood pH should be checked frequently during ammonium chloride treatment. Severe metabolic alkalosis is the only good indication for administration of ammonium chloride.

6. Severe or rapidly developing alkalosis may lead to tetany because of a pH-dependent decrease in available ionized calcium. If this is symptomatic, 10 ml of calcium gluconate should be given IV slowly.

J. Respiratory acidosis

1. Respiratory acidosis is caused by pulmonary insufficiency, i.e., failure to excrete carbon dioxide via the lungs with normal efficiency (pneumonia, emphysema, fibrosis). It is usually accompanied by cyanosis.

2. Retention of carbon dioxide leads to an increase in serum carbonic acid concentration and a fall in pH. In acute respiratory acidosis, the serum bicarbonate may not be elevated, since renal compensatory mechanisms have not had time to act. The diagnosis can best be made by measuring serum pH and P_{CO_2}. In chronic respiratory acidosis, bicarbonate ion has been retained by the renal tubules, restoring the pH toward normal and, of course, resulting in an elevated serum bicarbonate concentration.

3. Treatment in respiratory acidosis must be directed to improving ventilation and aiding renal compensation.

K. **Respiratory alkalosis**

1. Respiratory alkalosis results from hyperventilation and is seen in hysteria, early in salicylate poisoning, in some brain stem lesions, in patients hyperventilated by a respirator, and occasionally during general anesthesia.

2. Hyperventilation leads to a fall in alveolar carbon dioxide concentration and a decrease in serum carbonic acid concentration. Tetany is seen if alkalosis is severe.

3. Most clinical situations are short-lived and well tolerated. When hyperventilation ceases, the carbonic acid concentration is rapidly restored and pH returns to normal.

4. If hysteria is the basis for hyperventilation, have the patient rebreathe into a paper bag. Other situations may call for the addition of small amounts of carbon dioxide to the inspired gas mixture.

IV. **ADDITIONAL LOSSES DURING TREATMENT**

A. **Sources of additional losses** during treatment may be:

1. GI secretion (Table 9-3).

2. Increased insensible losses resulting from fever, high environmental temperatures, and hyperventilation (Table 9-7).

TABLE 9-7. Allowances for Losses Resulting from Fever, Environmental Temperature, and Hyperventilation

Additional Allowance (per 24 hr)	Fever	Environmental Temperature (°F)	Respiratory Rate/Min
None	38.3°C (101°F) or less	85 or less	35 or less
500 ml water	38.4–39.4°C (101–103°F)	85–95	Over 35
1,000 ml water	39.5°C (103°F) or more	95 or more	...

Corrections are additive; thus, a patient with fever of 38.8°C (102°F) (+500 ml) in an ambient environmental temperature of 30°C (86°F) (+500 ml) would have a total correction of +1,000 ml water.

3. Increased water and salt loss from sweating (Table 9-8).

4. Increased renal loss of water and salt from an enforced osmotic diuresis (mannitol, urea, low molecular weight dextran).

5. Formation of a "third space" of sequestered ECF in traumatized and postoperative patients.

6. Plasma loss from burns, granulating wounds, chest tubes, and other drains.

B. GI suction is the most common and most important source of additional fluid losses occurring during treatment of surgical patients. GI losses should be measured. Postoperative nasogastric suction usually produces 500–1,000 ml/day. In most situations, the volume of GI fluid losses can be estimated in advance, the composition determined from Table 9-3, and the anticipated losses replaced as they occur.

C. Administration of each 12.5 gm mannitol will enforce additional excretion of about 125 ml water, 10 mEq sodium, and 2 mEq potassium. Prolonged use of mannitol leads to a predominant water deficit (hypernatremia) with accompanying mild sodium deficit.

V. MAINTENANCE REQUIREMENTS

A. Basal state   The requirements of fluid or electrolyte to provide for daily turnover needs and to maintain a patient in a basal state are as follows (Table 9-9).

1. Water

a. The largest source of **sensible water loss** (i.e., visible, measurable) is the urine. The excretion of urine with a solute concentration about the

TABLE 9-8. Allowances for Losses Resulting from Sweating

Degree of Sweating	Additional Allowance (per 24 hr)	
	Water (ml)	Sodium (mEq)
Moderate; intermittent	500	25
Moderate; continuous	1,000	50
Profuse; continuous	2,000 or more	75 or more

TABLE 9-9. Fluid and Electrolytes Required for Maintenance

Requirement	Per Day	Per Hr
Volume (ml)	2,000–2,500	100
Sodium (mEq)	40–100	3
Potassium (mEq)	40–80	2

same as that of serum involves minimum renal work and permits the most latitude in handling changes in solute load. The daily solute load which an adult surgical patient needs to excrete is of the order of 450 mOsm/liter. To excrete a load of 450 mOsm at a urine concentration of 300 mOsm/liter requires a volume of 1,500 ml/day.

b. Sensible water loss via the feces is small (50-200 ml/day) and can be ignored in the absence of diarrhea.

c. Insensible water losses (not visible or readily measurable) occur through the lungs (humidification of inspired air) and the skin (evaporation as a means of heat loss). These insensible losses amount to about 500 ml/m^2 body surface/day in a basal state. For an 80-kg man, body surface area is 1.75 m^2 and insensible water losses amount to 875 ml. Rigid calculations are unnecessary; for convenience, the insensible water loss in adults is assumed to be 500-1,000 ml/day.

d. Maintenance requirement for water, allowing for both sensible and insensible losses, is 2,000-2,500 ml of total fluid volume/day. The smaller figure is used when stress-induced antidiuresis may be present; the larger figure is used in routine situations.

2. Sodium

a. Sodium excretion in urine is usually of the order of 40-200 mEq/day in adults; basal losses via other routes are not important.

b. Maintenance requirements for sodium are met if 50-100 mEq/day is provided.

3. Potassium

a. Potassium excretion in urine is usually of the order of 40-100 mEq/day.

b. There is an obligatory daily urinary excretion of potassium that continues even in the presence of potassium depletion.

c. A daily maintenance allowance of 40-80 mEq potassium will cover minimal needs.

4. Calcium and magnesium

a. Daily excretion of calcium and magnesium in stool and urine balances amounts absorbed from the diet. When dietary intake stops, renal conservation mechanisms are very efficient and the daily loss of calcium and magnesium from the body is reduced to a few milliequivalents. Such losses are very small in relation to body stores. Deficiency of magnesium takes several weeks to develop; deficiency of calcium does not occur.

b. Daily losses of calcium and magnesium are so small that they do not usually require replacement.

5. Acid-base   In a basal state there are no abnormalities in acid-base balance and no replacements are needed.

B. The effects of trauma

1. Anesthesia and surgery, as well as external violence, constitute forms of traumatic stress to which the body responds by secreting additional aldosterone and antidiuretic hormone (ADH). There is a reduction in renal capacity to excrete both water and sodium loads, and renal loss of potassium is increased.

2. Trauma also results in formation of edema in and about injured tissues. The edema fluid is protein-rich and derived primarily from the plasma volume of the ECF compartment. Unlike normal ECF, traumatic edema is functionally sequestered as a "third space" and cannot readily be mobilized to meet body needs.

3. In the past, there has been a great deal of emphasis on the general response to stress: the demonstration in postoperative patients of a decreased capacity to excrete sodium and water loads. This led to recommendations that water and sodium intake be restricted in postoperative and post-traumatic patients.

4. Conversely, until recently, there has been little or no emphasis placed on the body's local response to trauma: functional loss of plasma volume. This loss must be replaced in postoperative patients by providing sodium- and protein-containing fluids.

5. Much of the activation of ADH and aldosterone secretion in association with an operation is related not only to stress but also to restriction of fluid intake preoperatively and to inadequate replacement of fluid losses during and after operation.

6. In general, daily maintenance fluid and electrolyte requirements are not altered by the fact of operation. The decreased capacity to handle sodium and water loads (the general response to stress) is balanced, in a sense, by the increased need for sodium and water to replace functionally lost traumatic edema (the local response to stress). Fluid requirements can be calculated just as for patients who have not been operated on, unless special circumstances exist, such as administration of exogenous steroids or a continuing state of inappropriate secretion of aldosterone (cirrhosis).

7. For most patients it is not necessary (and it is possibly harmful) to restrict fluid and electrolyte intake markedly in the early postoperative period.

VI. FORMULATION OF FLUID ORDERS

A. The approach

1. Fluid and electrolyte problems are greatly simplified if approached systematically. It is best to proceed as follows:

a. **Evaluate** the patient's present imbalances and their probable magnitude regarding water, sodium, potassium, and acid-base balance.

b. **Decide on the length in hours of the next treatment period.** For patients with no complications this is usually 24 hr, but for very ill patients it may be as short as 2 hr.

c. **Calculate requirements** for water, sodium, potassium, and acid-base balance for that treatment period by adding:

(1) **One half of the estimated magnitude of present imbalances** *plus*

(2) **The patient's maintenance requirements** for the number of hours in the treatment period *plus*

(3) **Losses anticipated during the treatment period.**

d. **Write fluid orders** to administer the total calculated requirements within the treatment period.

e. Make a mental **prediction of the outcome** of treatment.

f. **Check during the treatment period** to make sure that fluids are being given at the rates desired and that anticipated losses are occurring at expected rates. **Make adjustments** whenever necessary.

g. At the end of the treatment period, **reevaluate** the patient. Compare actual with predicted results of treatment.

h. At the beginning of each new treatment period, make a completely new evaluation just as if you were seeing the patient for the first time. Previous therapy is now history. When the new evaluation is complete, proceed again, beginning with paragraph **b,** above.

B. Writing orders and administering fluids

1. Convert the fluid and electrolyte requirements into bottles of standard IV solutions (Table 9-10) or use electrolyte additives in dextrose in water. A balanced electrolyte solution, such as Ringer's lactate, ordinarily is preferable as the medium for supplying sodium needs. If the patient is acidotic, use sixth-molar sodium lactate; if alkalotic, saline solution is indicated.

2. Write out the fluid orders: number bottles or bags consecutively and specify both the maximum rate of administration (Table 9-11) and the time for completion of each bottle.

3. Require the nursing staff to write on the label the time and date the bottle or bag is hung and infusion started, and the time and date infusion of that bottle or bag was stopped. Save all fluid containers: under the

TABLE 9-10. Composition of Commercially Available IV Fluids

Solution	Na	K	Cl	HCO$_3$	Ca	Mg	Calories
Ringer's lactate	130	4	109	(28)	3	...	...
Normal saline	154	...	154	...	...	...	...
5% dextrose in water	...	...	...	...	...	...	200
5% dextrose in normal saline	154	...	154	...	...	...	200
5% dextrose and 0.2% sodium chloride	34	...	30	...	...	...	200
5% dextrose and 0.45% sodium chloride	77	...	74	...	...	...	200
10% dextrose in water	...	...	...	...	...	...	400
Ringer's solution	147	4	155	...	4	...	...
0.6M sodium lactate	167	...	...	(167)	...	...	...
0.75% ammonium chloride	...	...	141	...	...	...	...
5% sodium chloride	864	...	864	...	...	...	...
Whole blood[a]	75	2	50	14	3	2	...

[a] Values listed are for 600 ml ACD unit.
Composition of parenteral nutrient solutions is listed in Chapter 10.

TABLE 9-11. Infusion Rates of Fluids

Drops/Min[a]	Approximate Ml/Hr	Approximate Liters/Day
5	20	0.5
15	60	1.4
30	120	2.9
50[b]	200[b]	4.8[b]
75	300	7.2
100	400	9.6
120	480	11.5
150[c]	600[c]	14.4[c]
200	800	19.2

[a] Standard commercial IV drip set.
[b] Maximum rate for hypertonic solutions via peripheral vein.
[c] Maximum rate for isotonic solutions without constant monitoring of CVP.

bed is a good place. Every container should be saved, whether empty or partially filled. This will allow you to check the actual amounts of fluids received by the patient. Nursing records in most instances are not sufficiently accurate for this purpose.

4. For children, subsidiary reservoirs limited to a volume of 50 ml are mandatory to obviate the danger of fluid overloading from a "runaway IV."

5. Except where profound sodium depletion or a similar problem requires rapid replenishment, limit infusion rates to 500 ml/hr. If large imbal-

ances are present or if the patient urgently needs an operation, faster rates of infusion may be used.

6. Limit potassium infusion rates to 20 mEq/hr; cardiac arrest may follow more rapid administration. Withhold potassium if serum creatinine or BUN is elevated or urine volume is low. The possibility of potassium excess must be eliminated by measuring the serum potassium or at least obtaining an ECG.

7. Use indwelling IV catheters for administration of hypertonic and irritating solutions.

8. Lower leg veins should be used only as a last resort or for very short periods, and only isotonic fluids should be infused through them.

9. In all patients with a history of heart failure or in whom rates of administration will exceed 500 ml/hr, insert a CVP monitor. Plastic venous catheters preferably are inserted via the subclavian vein (infraclavicular route) or via the jugular vein (posterior route). Use an antibacterial ointment and sterile dressings around indwelling IV catheters to reduce infection.

10. Add ascorbic acid and multiple B vitamins to at least one bottle daily. Surgical patients may require up to 300 mg of ascorbic acid daily. Needs for B vitamins are less well established, but since there are no significant body stores of these vitamins, empirical administration is warranted.

11. If IV antibiotics are administered, their electrolyte content must be taken into account when treating patients with renal failure.

12. Accurate records of all intake and output must be kept. Serum electrolytes and hematocrit should be measured after each 5 liters of IV fluids in routine situations and more often in complicated cases.

13. Urine output does not represent a loss, as such, but is a guide to the effectiveness of treatment. Do not attempt to replace urine losses; provide the standard daily volume allowance of 1,500 ml.

VII. EXAMPLES OF FLUID MANAGEMENT

A. Pyloric (gastric outlet) obstruction

1. **History**   A 55-year-old, 70-kg man with a long history of symptomatic duodenal ulcer enters the hospital with severe epigastric pain and vomiting present for five days. He has taken calcium carbonate to relieve pain. During the past two days, he has been thirsty and has drunk water copiously, most of which has been vomited. He complains now of severe thirst.

2. **Physical**   Fever 101.4°F, P 100, occ. irregular, BP 110/70, no postural hypotension; oral mucous membranes, axillae, and groin are dry; tongue is furrowed, skin turgor only fair; able to void only 30 ml of urine on

admission. Urine sp. gr. 1.032, pH 6.0, Na 22, K 30. Hct 38%. Serum Na 154, K 2.8. Arterial pH 7.52. Gastric aspirate pH 2.6.

3. Diagnoses

a. Severe water deficit—3,000+ ml (history, hypernatremia, thirst, dry membranes, concentrated urine; the +9 mEq serum Na indicates at least a 3-liter water deficit).

b. Moderate sodium deficit—150-300 mEq (history, poor turgor, tachycardia, low urine Na).

c. Severe hypokalemia (history, serum K, irregular pulse, paradoxical aciduria; using the nomogram in Fig. 9-3, the change in body potassium is −11% [pH 7.52, serum K 2.8] and with a normal capacity of 3,150 mEq [70 kg × 45] this indicates a total body potassium deficit of approximately 350 mEq).

d. Metabolic alkalosis (history, alkali ingestion, hypokalemia, arterial pH).

4. Fluid requirements for initial treatment period of 12 hr

	Water	Sodium	Potassium
Half of deficits	1,500	100	175
Maintenance	1,250	25-50	20-40
Losses			
Temperature	250	. . .	. . .
GI suction	1,000	60	10
	4,000	185-210	205-225

5. Fluid orders (one of many possibilities; the large estimate for potassium needed in this treatment period cannot be met safely).

a. Bottle #1, 1,000 5% dextrose in 0.45% saline; run at 200 gtt/min; complete at 0130. If urine output more than 50 ml, continue with IVs as ordered; if urine output less than 50 ml, notify me.

b. Bottle #2, 1,000 5% dextrose in 0.45% saline; add 40 mEq KCl; run at 120 gtt/min; complete at 0400.

c. Bottle #3, 1,000 5% dextrose in 0.45% saline; add 60 mEq KCl; run at 60 gtt/min; complete at 0800.

d. Bottle #4, 1,000 5% dextrose in water; add 60 mEq KCl plus 150 mg ascorbic acid; run at 60 gtt/min; complete at 1,200.

e. Measure and record CVP q 15 min during bottle #1; if CVP rises over 12 cm saline, slow infusion to 50 gtt/min and notify me.

f. Label all bottles: additives, time started, and time stopped.

g. Save all bottles; place in box under patient's bed.

6. **Follow-up**   At the end of 12 hr of therapy the patient is much improved although thirst persists. Temperature is 99°F, tongue is no longer furrowed, axillae are questionably moist. Urine output has been 920 ml, sp. gr. 1.028, pH 5.6, Na 40, K 36. Arterial pH is now 7.46. Nasogastric suction volume is 1,000 ml with pH 3.0. Serum Na 148, K 2.9.

7. **Reassessing** the situation, these diagnoses are made:

a. Moderate water deficit—more than 1,500 ml (persisting thirst).

b. Severe hypokalemia—about 230 mEq deficit (history, paradoxical aciduria).

c. Mild metabolic alkalosis (arterial pH).

No change in the allowance for GI suction need be made since the present rate of loss equals the estimate of 2,000 ml/day; no allowance now need be made for fever. Requirements for the next 12 hr of therapy will be:

	Water	Sodium	Potassium
Half of deficits	750	. . .	115
Maintenance	1,250	25-50	20-40
Losses—GI	1,000	60	10
	3,000	85-110	145-165

B. Peritonitis in a cardiac patient

1. **History**   A 72-year-old woman enters the hospital with a three-day history of abdominal pain culminating in prostration a few hours before admission. She had had severe congestive heart failure 2 yr previously, and since then had been on digitalis, a low-sodium diet, and a thiazide diuretic with potassium supplements.

2. **Physical**   She appears listless, has poor skin turgor, a furrowed tongue, and flat neck veins. BP 99/50, P 116 and thready, temperature 102°F. Abdominal signs are those of peritonitis, and exploration is required urgently. She is unable to void; an indwelling catheter is placed and 50 ml of urine obtained. Urine sp. gr. 1.014, pH 5.5, Na 28, K 53, Hct 46%. Serum Na 135, K 3.9, CO_2 20.

3. **Diagnoses**

a. **Sodium depletion**—600 mEq (physical findings, hypotension, tachycardia, low urine Na)

c. **Early metabolic acidosis** (low CO_2)

c. **Mild water excess** (hyponatremia, history)

4. Initial estimate of fluid requirements for 2 hr of therapy

	Water	Sodium	Potassium
Half of deficits	2,000	300	. . .
Maintenance	200	6	4
Losses			
Temperature	20	. . .	. . .
GI suction	100	6	1
Third space	500	75	5
	2,820	387	10

5. Treatment　A CVP catheter is inserted via the brachial vein; initial pressure is 5 cm saline. Since this patient requires very rapid correction, fluids, which also include appropriate antibiotics, are given by a physician in constant attendance who monitors the CVP. Two liters of Ringer's lactate are given in the first 90 min, after which the patient's BP is 130/80, P 100, CVP 9 cm. A third liter of Ringer's lactate is begun at a slower rate and the patient taken to the operating room. A perforated appendix with generalized peritonitis is found and appropriately treated.

6. Follow-up　Postoperatively, the patient is sweating, temperature 102°F, BP 110/70, P 110; Hct 42%. She has excreted 200 ml urine since admission. Reassessing the situation, the following diagnoses are made:

a. Sodium depletion—450 mEq (history, tachycardia).

b. Mild metabolic acidosis (probable).

c. Peritonitis; continuing development of a "third space" is to be anticipated.

Fluid requirements for the next 24 hr are estimated as:

	Water	Sodium	Potassium
Half of deficits	1,500	225	. . .
Maintenance	2,000	50	50
Losses			
Temperature	500		
Sweat	500	25	. . .
GI suction	600	60	6
Third space	1,000	150	10
	6,100	510	66

These requirements are too great to manage as a 24-hr treatment period in this ill patient. The next treatment period should be 6-8 hr, using an appropriate fraction of the above estimates. At the end of this first postoperative treatment period, a reassessment, including measurement of urine and serum electrolytes, is carried out and new estimates of deficits are made to guide subsequent treatment.

10. SURGICAL NUTRITION

I. TUBE FEEDING

A. General comments

1. Patients who are able to digest and absorb a diet providing sufficient calories for maintenance of nutrition and anabolism of new protein should be supported by tube feeding if they cannot eat. The complications associated with IV hyperalimentation dictate that the safer supply of calories via the GI tract should be chosen whenever possible.

2. Patients who may benefit from tube feeding are those with:

   a. An anatomically and functionally intact intestinal tract (burns, sepsis, cachexia, neurological disorders). Blenderized diets or a commercially prepared nutrient solution can be effectively utilized for caloric support.

   b. An anatomically altered but functionally intact intestinal tract (short bowel syndrome, internal and external fistulas). Low-bulk, or "elemental," diets have significantly expanded the clinical applicability of tube feeding regimens to include many patients in this category.

   c. An anatomically intact but functionally altered intestinal tract (ulcerative colitis, regional enteritis, pancreatitis, biliary fistulas). Low-bulk, elemental diets also are helpful in these patients.

3. Route of administration:

   a. **Nasogastric intubation** is easy and applicable in most clinical situations. Patient discomfort and gastroesophageal reflux can be minimized by use of a soft 5 Fr pediatric feeding tube.

   b. **Gastrostomy** is preferred over jejunostomy because of lower incidence of cramping and diarrhea. An 18 Fr Foley catheter or nephrostomy tube may be inserted under local anesthesia.

   c. **Jejunostomy** is preferred over gastrostomy in patients likely to aspirate gastric contents (patients with weak gag or cough reflexes) or with gastric or duodenal suture lines or fistulas. A 12 Fr red rubber (Robinson) catheter is suitable.

4. Sufficient calories, minerals, vitamins, and water must be provided for:

   a. Basal requirements   The required 30 Cal/kg/day usually is supplied 50% as carbohydrate (4 Cal/gm), 35% as fat (9/ Cal/gm) and 15% as protein (4 Cal/gm). Diluted with approximately 2,400 ml water, the average concentration is about 500 mOsm/liter. Minerals (Na, K, Cl, Mg, Ca) and vitamins are supplied in quantities outlined in Section II, below; the daily requirements of trace elements are less well defined.

   b. Replacement of abnormal losses (e.g., electrolyte loss with small-bowel fistula).

   c. Attaining positive nitrogen balance and anabolism of protein   For effective utilization of extra nitrogen for protein anabolism rather than as an energy source, each gram of nitrogen must be accompanied by 125 calories from a nonprotein source.

   d. Electrolytes (especially K^+, Mg^{++}) and **vitamins** (especially C) also are needed in increased quantitites for cell growth and wound healing.

B. Tube feeding formulas   There are three categories from which to select a specific tube feeding formula.

   1. Commercially prepared nutrient solutions (Sustagen, Meritine, Nutri-1000, Ensure). These are supplied premixed or in powdered form. After reconstitution with water, these formulas contain 1 Cal/ml. The protein is milk-derived. Their major appeal is ease of preparation. Sufficient minerals and vitamins are supplied in the formula for maintenance requirements, but supplements may have to be added when excess losses so dictate. The major disadvantages are:

      a. Diarrhea when concentrations of more than 1 Cal/ml are required.

      b. Cost.

   2. Blenderized feedings can be concocted from baby foods or any table food soft enough to be liquified, or a commercial preparation may be chosen (Compleat B, Cutter Formula II). Blenderized tube feedings supply calories in a balanced manner and are better tolerated. Two whole food complete diets which can be prepared easily and inexpensively are listed in Table 10-1.

   3. Low-bulk diets

      a. The protein is supplied as one of the following:

         (1) Crystalline amino acids (Vivonex, WT, Jejunal).

         (2) Casein hydrolysate (Flexical).

         (3) Egg albumin (Precision LR).

TABLE 10-1. Tube Feeding Prepared from Food

	1 Cal/ml	1.5 Cal/ml
Baby meat	210 ml	210 ml
Egg	50 ml (frozen)	60 ml (dried)
Applesauce	120 ml	. . .
Orange juice	240 ml (reconstituted)	100 ml (concentrated)
Whipped potatoes	200 ml	. . .
Refined cereal	100 ml	. . .
Oil	45 ml	45 ml
Milk	960 ml	480 ml
Strained carrots	100 ml	60 ml
Dextrose	60 gm	12 gm
Skim milk powder	. . .	60 gm
	2,000 ml	1,000 ml
% of calories		
Protein	16	23
Fat	40	46
Carbohydrate	44	31
Osmolarity (mOsm/liter)	567	1,000

   b. All contain the eight essential amino acids plus a number of nonessential amino acids and are quite similar to solutions used for IV hyperalimentation. The **advantages** of these diets are:

   (1) The composition is known precisely.

   (2) There is almost complete absorption.

   (3) Minimal digestion is required (important in short bowel syndrome).

   (4) Pancreatic, biliary, and gut secretions are diminished (important in inflammatory bowel diseases, fistulas, pancreatitis).

   (5) Stool bulk is lessened (important in ulcerative and granulomatous colitis).

   (6) Losses through fistulas are minimized.

   (7) The intestinal microflora is reduced.

   c. While these diets may be given orally, poor patient acceptance during long-term maintenance, in spite of a choice of flavors, eventually prompts introduction via a feeding tube. In full-strength dilution there is 1 Cal/ml and osmolarity varies from 500 to 1,200 mOsm/liter, depending on the flavor. Table 10-2 compares properties of several low-bulk diets currently in use.

TABLE 10-2. Properties of Some Commercial Low-Bulk Formulas

Product	Digestion Required	Osmolality (mOsm/l) of 1 Cal/ml Solution	% Total Calories CHO	% Total Calories Fat	% Total Calories Protein	Nitrogen (gm/100 Cal)
Vivonex	Minimal	500 (unflavored)	90	1	9	3.27
Vivonex HN	Minimal	844	81	1	18	6.67
WT	Minimal	646 (tomato)	91	1	9	3.00
Jejunal	Minimal	990 (unflavored)	90	1	9	3.37
Flexical	Yes	805	61	30	9	3.50
Precision LR	Yes	595 (cherry)	90	1	9	3.52

    d. Each preparation generally contains electrolytes in excess of the recommended daily requirements although certain trace elements may be missing (e.g., cobalt and molybdenum in Vivonex). Maintenance vitamins are included but an inadequate amount of vitamin K is common and must be administered separately (10 mg AquaMephyton IM twice a week). If therapeutic vitamin levels are necessary, a multivitamin preparation should be added. Since many multivitamins do not contain vitamins K or B_{12} or folic acid, these may have to be supplied separately.

    e. Medium-chain triglycerides (C8-10) (MCT oil) are absorbed without hydrolysis and pass directly into portal blood as free fatty acids rather than into lymph as chylomicrons. Used as a dietary supplement in doses up to 15 ml four times a day, MCT may produce more efficient absorption of fats in patients with short bowel syndrome, malabsorption states, and fistulas.

C. Methodology of tube feeding

    1. Start with a dilute (¼-strength) solution in maintenance volumes and then gradually increase the concentration every 2 or 3 days. Excess water must be provided with the more concentrated solutions to prevent hypernatremic dehydration. Thirst is a sensitive indicator of serum hyperosmolarity and of need for additional water, but may be lacking in obtunded and comatose patients.

    2. A constant infusion of diet over a 24-hr period is preferred and can be accomplished by either gravity drip or a mechanical (Barron) pump. Bolus feedings of 200-400 ml every 2-4 hr are less desirable.

    3. Gastrostomy and nasogastric tubes should be aspirated twice a day to check for gastric retention and then lavaged with saline to mechanically cleanse the tube of inspissated food material. Gastrostomy and jejunostomy tubes need time to seal and generally are not safe for infusion until 3 days after insertion. Every 3 days the skin around the tube should be washed and the tube sterilely dressed and securely taped to the skin to prevent accidental dislodgment.

4. Carefully monitor intake and output, body weight, serum electrolytes, osmolality, blood sugar, BUN, prothrombin time, and number and volume of stools. Serum levels of Mg, Ca, and P should be determined weekly.

D. Complications of tube feeding

1. Aspiration of gastric contents may occur in patients with weak gag and cough reflexes being fed intragastrically. Place the patient in the sitting position and avoid nighttime infusions.

2. Cramps, nausea, and vomiting often are related to jejunostomy feedings of too great volume and concentration.

3. Diarrhea, dehydration, and azotemia are due to hypertonicity of the nutrient solutions, especially when low-bulk diets are infused into the jejunum. Start with a dilute solution ($\frac{1}{4}$ Cal/ml) with additional supplies of water. The presence of small amounts of fat (less than 8%) may lessen diarrhea by increasing gastric emptying time.

4. Electrolyte imbalance. Increased quantities of electrolytes will be needed to replace abnormal losses and for anabolism of new protein.

5. Hyperglycemia, osmotic dehydration, and nonketotic, hyperosmolar, hyperglycemic coma. Elevated blood sugar is the response to an increased carbohydrate load in stressed or debilitated patients. By slowly increasing the carbohydrate in the diet, endogenous insulin output will compensate. Individuals with 3+ or 4+ urine sugar may require small subcutaneous doses of regular insulin (10-15 units) every 4-6 hr.

6. Bleeding most often is due to hypoprothrombinemia because of inadequate vitamin K intake.

7. Fluid retention is seen when the source of body energy is converted from oxidation of fat (starvation) to carbohydrates (feeding). Intermittent use of diuretics will control water retention. Water retention is more refractory if there is concomitant hypoalbuminemia.

8. Tube dislodgment, intraperitoneal leakage, skin infection and erosion, intestinal obstruction (jejunostomy), and mucosal erosions with bleeding also occur as complications.

SUGGESTED READING

Randall, H. T. Surgical Nutrition: Parenteral and Oral. In J. M. Kinney, R. H. Egdahl, and G. D. Zuidema (Eds.), *Manual of Preoperative and Postoperative Care*. Philadelphia: Saunders, 1971.

Stephens, R. V., and Randall, H. T. Use of a concentrated balanced, liquid elemental diet for nutritional management of catabolic states. *Ann. Surg.* 170:642, 1969.

Voitk, A. J., Brown, R. A., McArdle, A. H., Hinchey, E. J., and Gurd, F. N. Clinical uses of an elemental diet—Preliminary studies. *Can. Med. Assoc. J.* 107:123, 1972.

II. PARENTERAL NUTRITION (hyperalimentation)

A. Indications

1. Patients unable to maintain a normal state of nutrition who cannot utilize GI alimentation.

2. Patients in whom the caloric demands of illness are greater than can be met orally.

3. Nutritional therapy should be considered only in patients whose disease will last longer than 14 days. Patients who are in a terminal state should not receive parenteral nutritional therapy.

B. Principles governing parenteral nutrition

1. The parenteral requirement for a normal, average, resting adult is 24 Cal/kg/day.

2. Healthy young males will lose lean body mass more rapidly than females, or elderly and debilitated individuals.

3. If parenteral nutrition is provided in order to put the GI tract to rest, normal maintenance or 5-10% more, depending on the nutritional state at the time the therapy is being instituted, is sufficient.

4. In sepsis, needs increase by 5-8% with each degree rise in fever.

5. Peritonitis, even though associated with sepsis, imposes an additional caloric consumption of 20-40%.

6. Major fractures of long bones increase caloric demands by 10-25%.

7. The greatest demands are those of severe burn injuries (second and third degree). The need for extra calories may be 40-100% of normal intake.

8. The major factor limiting provision of calories is utilization of glucose, which maximally is 0.9 gm/kg/hr even with insulin administration.

9. Protein requirements for an average young adult will be 0.45 gm/kg/day. A ratio of 200 nonprotein Cal/gm of nitrogen must be reached before protein can be synthesized.

10. Young adults will require infusion of 2.4 mEq sodium and 2.0 to 2.3 mEq potassium/100 Cal/day. The cardiovascular and renal status of the patient often are limiting factors in calculating the total requirements for hyperalimentation fluid.

11. Calcium and phosphorous.   Give adults 200-400 mg Ca and 300 to 350 mg P/2500 Cal/day. When using casein hydrolysates, remember that they contain considerable amounts of both Ca and P. Casein, a phospho-

protein, has up to 200 mg of unbound P and 100-125 mg of Ca/liter. The fibrin hydrolysates have considerably less Ca and P; supplementary administration of these ions will be required, depending on serum levels.

12. **Magnesium.** Exact Mg requirements are not known with certainty. There appears to be no direct hormonal control of Mg metabolism; serum levels depend on intake and renal output. Deprivation lasting more than 3-4 wk can lead to hypomagnesemia. The fall in serum Mg is associated initially with neurological symptoms, and later with GI dysfunction (anorexia, nausea, and vomiting). The National Research Council recommends a daily dietary allowance of Mg for adults of 25 mEq; approximately one third of this is absorbed, so that 8 mEq enters the circulation. In infants, the recommended allowance range of Mg is 4-25 mEq/2500 Cal, so that 1-8 mEq enters the circulation.

13. Iron supplements are given parenterally as iron dextran once or twice a month. The estimated daily loss of iron in adults is 0.5-1 mg/day. For menstruating women, another 1 mg is added.

14. Trace elements (Table 10-3) can be replaced by giving a unit of plasma protein fraction (Plasmanate) every 1-2 wk.

15. **Vitamins**

   a. To utilize efficiently the carbohydrates and amino acids in hyperalimentation fluid, adequate amounts of water-soluble (B and C) vitamins are necessary (Table 10-4). Water-soluble vitamins have no serious toxic manifestations, even in renal insufficiency. To one bottle per day of hyperalimentation fluid, addition of 5 ml of the commercial parenteral vitamin preparation MVI plus 1-2 mg of folic acid will more than meet requirements for water-soluble vitamins.

   b. Care should be exercised in administration of the fat-soluble vitamins (A, D, E, K), since they do produce toxicity with overdosage. Only one bottle of hyperalimentation fluid each day should contain the fat-soluble vitamins. Vitamin K, 10 mg, should be administered twice weekly; additional vitamin K can be given if indicated by serum

TABLE 10-3. Suggested Intravenous Requirements of Trace Elements

Element	Infants and Young Children	Adults
Iodine	10 μg/kg	2 μg/kg
Copper	18 μg/kg	1 mg
Fluoride	1 μg/kg	? 1-2 mg
Zinc	50-60 μg/kg	5 mg
Manganese	? 10-40 μg/kg	? 1-2 mg
Chromium	? 0.5 μg/kg	? 15 μg

TABLE 10-4. Daily Requirements of Vitamins

Vitamin	Recommended Daily Allowance (1973)	Commercial Parenteral Vitamin Preparation (MVI, 5 ml)
Ascorbic acid	60 mg	500 mg
Thiamine	1.5 mg	50 mg
Riboflavin	1.7 mg	10 mg
Niacin	17.0 mg	100 mg
B_6	2.0 mg	15 mg
Pantothenate	10.0 mg	25 mg
Folate	0.4 mg	. . .
B_{12}	6.0 μg	. . .
Vitamin A	5,000 IU	10,000 IU
Vitamin D	400 IU	1,000 IU
Vitamin E	30 IU	5 IU
Vitamin K_1	5 mg	. . .

prothrombin studies. Administration of fat-soluble vitamins to patients on parenteral nutrition for more than 4-6 wk should be limited to once or twice a week.

c. For patients on long-term parenteral nutrition, 1,000 μg of vitamin B_{12} is given monthly.

C. **Administration of hyperalimentation**

1. **Insertion of central venous catheter**   Proper insertion and maintenance of the central parenteral nutrition catheter under strict aseptic technique is extremely important. This is the patient's "lifeline." Attention to details in its placement (see Chap. 25) and care will prevent serious, possibly life-threatening complications.

2. **Preparation of nutrient fluid**

a. **Protein hydrolysate basic fluid**

(1) Add 350 ml 50% glucose to 750 ml 5% glucose in 5% fibrin or casein hydrolysate under aseptic conditions of filtered air in a laminar flow hood. This results in:

Volume 1,100 cc
Calories 1000
Glucose 212 gm
Hydrolysate 37 gm
Nitrogen 7.4 gm/liter (fibrin)
    6.8 gm/liter (casein)
Phosphorous (free) 10 mg (fibrin)
    220 mg (casein)

Sodium 7 mEq
Potassium 13 mEq
Calcium 20 mg (fibrin)
     115 mg (casein)
Magnesium 2.2 mEq

(2) Add to each unit sodium chloride or bicarbonate 40-50 mEq, potassium chloride or phosphate 40-60 mEq, and magnesium sulphate 4-8 mEq.

(3) Add to only one unit once each day 5 ml of a multivitamin preparation and 1-2 mg folic acid.

(4) Additional additives as required by the patient: vitamin K 5-10 mg, calcium gluconate 4.5-9 mEq, and phosphate (potassium acid salt) 4-10 mEq.

(5) All of the above additives are injected into the basic fluid unit under aseptic conditions in a filtered air laminar flow hood. Parenteral nutrition solutions must be prepared in the pharmacy, and never more than 24 hr in advance of use. Those units that are not administered immediately are refrigerated until used.

b. **Crystalline amino acid solution**

(1) Add 500 ml 50% glucose to 500 ml 8.5% crystalline amino acids under aseptic conditions as described above. This gives a solution of 4.25% amino acids and 25% glucose containing the following:

Volume 1,000 cc
Calories 1170
Protein equivalent 39.0 gm
Nitrogen equivalent 6.25 gm
Sodium 10 mEq
Chloride 45 mEq
pH 6.5 (adjusted with acetic acid)

(2) Add to each unit sodium phosphate or bicarbonate 30-40 mEq, potassium phosphate 40-50 mEq, magnesium sulphate 4-8 mEq, and calcium gluconate 4-9 mEq (must be added last and slowly or insoluble precipitates form because of the acidic pH of the solution).

(3) Other additives can be added as with hydrolysate solutions, i.e., water-soluble vitamins and folic acid, and vitamin K as required.

3. **Infusion**

a. Each unit should hang at room temperature for no longer than 8 hr. All others are kept in a refrigerator, none longer than 24 hr.

b. A final filter should be used on each infusion unit: 0.45-μ pore size for drip; 0.22-μ pore size will require pump.

c. Starting infusion rate should be 75–100 ml/hr (1800–2400 Calories per day) for 2–3 days. Increases should be in steps of 25 ml/hr every 2–3 days to permit the pancreas to become tolerant of the added glucose load. Continue increasing the infusion volume until the desired caloric intake is reached.

d. Change all tubing and filter at least once a day.

e. Change the catheter dressing under aseptic conditions every 3 days. Change the catheter every 3–4 wk.

f. Change the catheter to a new site whenever sepsis is present. Culture the catheter tip as well as the blood.

4. Indicated laboratory investigations

a. Electrolytes (sodium, potassium, magnesium, carbon dioxide), glucose, and BUN daily for the first 7 days, then every other day.

b. SMA-12 every 3 days for the first week, then twice weekly.

c. Complete blood count weekly.

d. Serum osmolarity every day for the first week, then at least twice weekly.

e. Ammonia twice the first week, then once weekly.

f. Urine sugar and acetone qid the first week, and bid thereafter. Urine osmolarity qid the first week, then qd thereafter.

5. General measurements

a. Weigh qd in the morning.

b. Strict intake and output.

c. Measure body length and head circumference in infants qd.

6. Diabetic patients   When the patient is a latent or frank diabetic, or the pancreas has not adjusted to produce enough insulin to handle the glucose load, exogenous insulin may be necessary. Use only the subcutaneous route and only regular insulin, giving 5–10 units for 3+ and 4+ urine sugar. Do not add insulin to bottles of hyperalimentation fluid. Remember that insulin is adsorbed by IV bottles and tubing, reducing its effectiveness.

7. Do not use the parenteral nutrition catheter other than for infusion of hyperalimentation fluid. There should be no drawing of blood or "piggy-backing" of other fluids. If other IVs are needed, a secondary, peripheral IV should be started.

8. IV fat   Parenteral fat shows the best promise of providing large numbers of calories in a minimal volume of fluid. Soybean oil emulsified with phospholipid has been used successfully in Europe for a number of years but its use in the United States still is limited to a few research centers. The cottonseed preparation formerly used in this country was withdrawn from the market in 1963 because of its side effects.

D. Complications can be grouped into three areas:

1. Catheter

   a. Numerous complications related to the catheter and its placement have been reported, including pneumothorax, hydrothorax and hemothorax, brachial plexus injury, subclavian and carotid artery injury, catheter embolus, tracheal perforation, subclavian and internal jugular vein thrombosis, AV fistula, air embolus, thoracic duct injury, and cardiac perforation with tamponade.

   b. All of these complications can be prevented by meticulous attention to detail when placing the catheter.

2. Sepsis

   a. Contamination of the catheter puncture site due to improper technique during insertion.

   b. Long-term placement may be associated with superficial infection around the catheter site which could migrate internally. Pericatheter problems can be minimized by cleaning the puncture site and changing the dressing every third day.

   c. Catheter seeding from distant foci during bacteremia.

   d. Yeast and fungal septicemia secondary to long-term antibiotic therapy.

   e. Solution contamination due to a break in aseptic technique either on the ward or in the pharmacy.

3. Metabolic disorder

   a. Hyperosmolar nonketotic hyperglycemia and acidosis are most often associated with improper administration, i.e., too rapid an infusion rate, or not allowing time for the pancreas to adjust to a glucose load before making another increase.

b. Hypoglycemia may be due to exogenous insulin overdose or endogenous insulin overproduction by the stimulated pancreas.

c. Latent, unrecognized diabetes appears particularly in geriatric patients and in those with chronic pancreatic insufficiency.

d. Hyperammonemia appears in patients with chronic liver disease and in pediatric patients because of their inadequate liver function.

e. Renal failure may be potentiated in patients with chronic renal disease. This complication can be lessened by decreasing the amino acid load and utilizing a small volume of fluid while still giving calories needed to prevent tissue breakdown.

f. Calcium phosphate and magnesium overload or deficiency appears especially in chronic renal disease and can be minimized by monitoring serum values.

g. Anemia during long-term therapy can be avoided by administering parenteral iron, vitamin B_{12}, and folic acid.

h. Cardiac arrhythmias are rare and usually are associated with electrolyte abnormality, especially hypokalemia.

i. Acidosis can be associated with decreased peripheral perfusion, renal failure, or diabetic ketoacidosis. It also can be a complication when using crystalline amino acid solutions which usually are acidic chloride salts.

j. Coma can result from the rapid administration of hyperosmolar fluid which produces dehydration and hypernatremia.

k. Hypervitaminosis is most likely to occur with fat-soluble vitamins.

SUGGESTED READING

Cowen, G., Jr., and Schettz, W. (Eds.) *Intravenous Hyperalimentation.* Philadelphia: Lea & Febiger, 1972.
Dudrick, S., and Copeland, M. C.   Parenteral hyperalimentation. *Surg. Annu.* 5:69, 1973.
Vanamee, P., and Shils, M. E. (Eds.) *Symposium on Total Parenteral Nutrition.* Chicago: American Medical Association, 1972.

11. ACUTE RENAL INSUFFICIENCY

I. TYPES OF RENAL FAILURE Acute renal insufficiency is the rapid loss of glomerular filtration, commonly though not invariably associated with a diminution in urinary flow rate. It may be divided into three types, which require different forms of treatment: prerenal azotemia (renal underperfusion), acute parenchymal renal failure (acute tubular necrosis, vasomotor nephropathy), and obstructive (postrenal) uropathy.

   A. Prerenal azotemia results from persistent underperfusion of the renal vascular bed.

      1. The kidney behaves appropriately in response to underperfusion by retaining sodium in order to reexpand effective circulating blood volume.

      2. Total extracellular volume actually may be markedly expanded (congestive heart failure) or markedly contracted (persistent diarrhea). The common denominator is a deficit of effective arterial blood volume.

      3. Knowledge of the clinical setting preceding development of azotemia is essential for accurate diagnosis. Physical examination usually is of little value.

      4. Since the kidney retains salt in an effort to reexpand effective arterial blood volume, the urinary concentration of sodium and chloride will be low (<20 mEq/liter) and may even approach zero. The urinary potassium concentration will be high, reflecting the secondary aldosteronism that accompanies contraction of the effective arterial blood volume.

      5. Both sodium and chloride should be measured in the urine of patients with prerenal azotemia to detect those with superimposed metabolic alkalosis (vomiting, diuretic therapy), a common clinical occurrence. Such patients may have a high urinary sodium concentration, even though volume is contracted, as a consequence of loss of sodium bicarbonate in the urine, but will have a low urine chloride concentration. The combination of high sodium and low chloride has the same clinical connotation as the combination of a low sodium and low chloride in patients with volume contraction not suffering from metabolic alkalosis.

      6. Urinary osmolality in prerenal azotemia almost invariably is greater than that of plasma.

7. Resorption is stimulated in patients with prerenal azotemia. Since the kidney can resorb urea, the BUN rises out of proportion to the increase in serum creatinine concentration, though serum creatinine may become quite elevated in severe renal underperfusion.

8. **Treatment**   This disorder always is secondary to some other problem and must be attacked by treating the primary cause of renal underperfusion. If the kidney is underperfused because of fluid loss from the GI tract, skin, or secondary to hemorrhage, the fluid loss must be replaced. Doing so will bring about restoration of renal function to the level existing prior to the insult. On the other hand, if the renal underperfusion is secondary to a decrease in effective rather than absolute blood volume, as is seen in congestive heart failure, administration of large amounts of solute and fluid is contraindicated. Renal perfusion can be restored only if cardiac function is improved. This requires digitalis, bed rest, and therapeutic measures aimed at improving cardiac performance.

9. Patients with severe liver disease commonly have marked impairment of renal function; the so-called hepatorenal syndrome is best looked on as a severe example of prerenal azotemia. This type of renal failure may prove refractory because successful treatment depends on restoration of liver function, a therapeutic goal that may be unobtainable.

10. A mild form of prerenal azotemia seen in patients with the nephrotic syndrome is secondary to volume contraction as a consequence of a decreased plasma oncotic pressure.

11. The use of diuretic agents generally is not recommended in the treatment of prerenal azotemia, an exception being the treatment of congestive heart failure. Diuretic therapy may be a cause of the prerenal azotemia, in which case diuretics should be withdrawn and salt and water administered in amounts sufficient to restore volume.

B. **Acute parenchymal renal failure (acute tubular necrosis, vasomotor nephropathy)**

1. Causes of acute parenchymal renal failure are many and include acute glomerulonephritis, cortical necrosis, and bilateral renal artery thrombosis or embolization. The following discussion is limited to that form commonly referred to as acute tubular necrosis.

2. The term *acute tubular necrosis* is a misnomer since this syndrome may be seen in the absence of any identifiable histological abnormality. On the other hand, tubular necrosis can be present with few, if any, functional abnormalities.

3. The pathophysiology of this disorder is controversial, but involves the invariable presence of volume contraction secondary to shock, cardiovascular embarrassment, hemorrhage, toxins, and so forth, combined with hemolysis or rhabdomyolysis. The sequence of pathophysiological events involved in this syndrome is outlined in Figure 11-1.

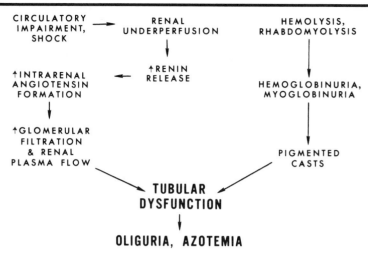

Figure 11-1. Pathophysiological events in acute renal failure.

4. Since volume contraction precedes the development of almost all cases of acute renal failure, prevention can best be accomplished by the prevention of volume contraction. Once the insult has taken place, the disease will run its course; attempts at attenuating the severity of acute renal failure with mannitol, furosemide, and saline yield disappointing results.

5. A good history combined with examination of the urine usually results in prompt diagnosis of this syndrome.

6. Since the tubules are diseased, there is impaired urinary concentration and tubular resorption of sodium. The resultant urine tends to have an osmolality equal to that of plasma and an elevated sodium concentration (>40 mEq/liter). The urine may contain pigmented casts. The presence of renal tubular epithelial cells is a helpful diagnostic sign.

7. The disorder in a typical patient with acute renal failure can be divided into an oliguric phase and a diuretic phase. Some patients have acute renal failure without ever going through an oliguric phase. Such an occurrence (high output renal failure) is typical of patients with methoxyflurane (Penthrane) nephropathy. It may also be seen following the administration of nephrotoxic antibiotics such as gentamicin.

8. The **oliguric phase** lasts from days to weeks during which the 24-hr urinary volume varies between 50-400 ml/day. The persistence of oliguria for longer than a month should suggest another diagnosis. The presence of anuria is atypical for this disease and should suggest another disorder (cortical necrosis, urinary tract obstruction).

9. The **diuretic phase** begins with a gradual increase in urinary volume. The increase in urine volume in excess of intake usually results from diuresis

of accumulated edema fluid, rather than from inability of the kidney to conserve fluid and electrolytes. Occasionally diuresis may be massive and result in circulatory collapse if adequate amounts of fluids are not administered.

10. Since the recovery of functional glomerular filtration usually lags behind in the diuretic phase, the increase in urine volume initially may not be accompanied by a fall in BUN or serum creatinine. After a period of several days, however, the BUN and creatinine will fall.

11. To estimate the need for fluid replacement, the patient should be weighed daily and the blood pressure and CVP monitored. Development of postural hypotension or a very low CVP suggest that diuresis has been excessive and that fluid and electrolytes should be promptly administered.

12. The main cause of mortality from acute renal failure is associated infection. The patient should be watched closely for development of signs of infection. Instrumentation that predisposes to infection, such as urinary catheterization, should be avoided.

C. **Obstructive uropathy** (postrenal azotemia) must be considered in any patient who develops acute renal failure. Since permanent impairment of renal function may develop if the obstruction persists more than seven days, early diagnosis is desirable but can be pursued during the normal working hours of the hospital, not as an emergency.

1. IVP, using a constant infusion of radiopaque medium, may aid in ruling in or out a diagnosis of obstructive uropathy. Satisfactory results may be obtained even when the serum creatinine is as high as 7 mg/100 ml.

2. If the clinical situation is suggestive of obstructive uropathy, retrograde catheterization of one ureter should be carried out to demonstrate its patency. Since infection, in the presence of acute renal failure, is a major cause of morbidity and mortality, this procedure should be carried out with the utmost attention to aseptic technique.

3. Following relief of a urinary tract obstruction, there may be a massive diuresis of water and solutes. This may result either because of the delivery of large amounts of edema fluid, in which case replacement of the fluid and electrolytes will only perpetuate the diuresis, or as a consequence of impaired resorption of salt and water. The latter event may result in circulatory collapse if fluid and electrolytes are not replaced.

II. TREATMENT OF ACUTE RENAL FAILURE

A. **Dialysis should be performed early in acute renal failure**   Management will be much more difficult if the patient is allowed to become uremic before dialysis is instituted. The use of arbitrary values of BUN, serum potassium concentration, acid-base status, and similar determinations as an indication for dialysis is best avoided. There is nothing to be gained by heroic attempts to manage acute renal failure "conservatively." **Most patients with acute renal failure, especially postoperatively or following trauma, need frequent dialysis.** Hemodialysis is preferred to peritoneal dialysis in patients who have suffered extensive tissue destruction, resulting in liberation of large amounts of potassium into extracellular fluid, and in patients who have recently undergone abdominal surgery. Hemodialysis can be performed with regional heparinization if systemic anticoagulation must be avoided. Other patients may be treated satisfactorily with peritoneal dialysis, which should be performed for periods of 36–48 hr, at 2- to 3-day intervals, for as long as is required.

B. Diet   It has been traditional to restrict protein in patients with acute renal failure. With use of early, daily hemodialysis this practice is not necessary. Almost all patients with acute tubular necrosis are markedly catabolic and in negative nitrogen balance. Hyperalimentation may be required. Protein should be administered in needed amounts. Likewise, zero potassium diets are unnecessary, since daily hemodialysis will maintain homeostasis.

C. Fluids

1. Most patients with acute renal failure receive more fluid than is prudent. Overhydration is the cause of the hypertension so commonly seen in renal failure patients. Proper management of fluid and electrolyte replacement will control the patient's blood pressure as well as avoid edema accumulation.

2. Daily weight is an essential measurement in management. Combined with CVP and arterial blood pressure, the weight provides an index of the state of hydration. In general, the patient should receive 5–7 ml fluid/kg/day plus a volume equal to urinary and GI losses. Patients with fever may require additional amounts of fluid.

D. Electrolytes

1. Frequent determinations of blood electrolytes are necessary for proper management of patients with acute renal failure. This is especially true in the postoperative patient who may have significant extrarenal electrolyte losses.

2. Sodium intake should equal that lost in urine and other sites of exit. It should be emphasized that the serum sodium concentration defines the relative osmolar state of total body water and gives no information whatsoever concerning the state of extracellular volume (see Chap. 9). Patients who develop hyponatremia during acute renal failure almost invariably are overhydrated and may have to have water intake restricted. Hemodialysis will correct electrolyte disturbances.

3. Hyperkalemia is a common cause of death in patients with acute renal failure and is particularly likely to be a major problem in patients who have extensive soft tissue destruction. Early and frequent hemodialysis is essential. Potassium should not be administered, save to replace identified

losses. Large amounts of potassium may be given inadvertently by administering penicillin as the potassium salt (1.7 mEq K/million units). If the serum potassium rises above 5.5 mEq/liter, sodium polystyrene sulphonate (Kayexalate) exchange resin, 15-30 gm, should be given up to four times daily. The resin may be given orally or as an enema. It also may be administered with 20% sorbitol.

   4. The physician should be familiar with the ECG changes of hyperkalemia, which may not always correlate with the serum potassium concentration. Peaked elevation of the T-wave, prolongation of the Q-T interval, widening of the QRS interval, prolongation of the P-R interval progressing to atrial arrest, and, ultimately, development of a sine wave and cardiac arrest occur in hyperkalemia (see Fig. 9-2).

   5. **Elevation of the serum potassium concentration to 6.5 mEq/liter or more should be considered a bona fide emergency** and be treated, even in the absence of ECG findings of hyperkalemia. Rapid infusion of 25 gm glucose (50% solution) combined with administration of 10-15 units of regular insulin will lower the serum potassium concentration in 30-60 min; the effect will last up to 6 hr. The effect is due to shift of potassium from the extracellular to the intracellular compartment. Alkalinization with sodium bicarbonate (45 mEq) will have a similar effect on the serum potassium and may be combined with glucose-insulin therapy. If the serum potassium concentration is above 7.5 mEq/liter, or if significant changes of hyperkalemia are present on the ECG, calcium salts should be administered (5-10 ml 10% calcium chloride IV over 2-5 min) while observing the ECG. Calcium ion antagonizes the effect of potassium on the myocardium. The result of administration of calcium salts is almost instantaneous and usually lasts 30-120 min. Hemodialysis should be started or restarted as soon as practicable.

   6. Magnesium intake must be restricted in patients with acute renal failure. Many common antacid preparations contain large amounts of magnesium which may be absorbed from the GI tract. An increase in the serum magnesium concentration may result in neuromuscular weakness, loss of deep tendon reflexes, complete heart block, hypertension, and respiratory depression. Only antacid preparations containing pure aluminum hydroxide should be administered to patients with renal failure. Intravenously administered calcium antagonizes the action of magnesium on the myocardium in the same way that it antagonizes that of potassium.

   7. Hypocalcemia occurs commonly in patients with acute renal failure although symptoms are extremely rare. An occasional patient may develop hypercalcemia during the diuretic phase of acute renal failure.

E. **Acid-base balance**   Most patients with acute renal failure develop metabolic acidosis secondary to reduced renal acid excretion. Therapy for acidosis is not necessary unless the serum bicarbonate falls below 15 mEq/liter. Frequent dialysis will control the bicarbonate concentration, but if it fails to do so, sodium bicarbonate should be administered orally or IV.

F. **Infections** Patients with acute renal failure are extraordinarily susceptible to severe infections. Indeed, infection is the major cause of death in such patients. IV catheters should be changed frequently. Catheterization of the bladder should be avoided; there usually is little need to know hourly urinary output and the risk far outweighs any benefit.

G. **Convulsions**

1. Uremia per se does not cause convulsions; it does, however, lower the seizure threshold and make the patient more likely to convulse. The common causes of convulsions in patients with acute renal failure are water intoxication and hypertension, both of which are preventable.

2. Treatment of convulsions requires elimination of the underlying cause. For short-term management, short-acting barbiturates which are excreted primarily by the liver may be administered IV. Diphenylhydantoin (Dilantin) should be administered in the same dose as in a patient without renal failure. Recent evidence suggests that uremic patients may metabolize Dilantin at an accelerated rate, so that it may be necessary to increase the dose in renal failure. Diazepam (Valium) also is a very effective anticonvulsant and may be administered in the usual dose.

3. Phenothiazine drugs, such as chlorpromazine (Thorazine), may produce cortical irritability and precipitate seizures in patients with renal failure.

H. **Congestion (overhydration)**

1. Congestion is very common in acute renal failure and results from the administration of both salt and water in amounts exceeding the capacity of the diseased kidneys to excrete them.

2. Congestion is not the same as congestive heart failure. Congestion may produce elevation of the CVP, pulmonary edema, and an increase in heart size, and still not be associated with heart failure. Heart failure exists only when the heart is unable to pump blood in sufficient amounts to meet the oxygen requirements of the tissues. The cardiac output usually is decreased (high output failure is an exception). In heart failure there is an increase in the AV oxygen difference and pH difference. Measurement of the circulation time often will provide a clue to distinguish congestion (normal or shortened circulation time) from heart failure (prolonged circulation time).

3. The distinction between congestion and congestive heart failure is important in that congestion does not respond to the administration of digitalis. Since digitalis administration is hazardous in patients with renal failure, the drug should be used only when it clearly will be of therapeutic benefit, and then only in reduced doses. Digitalis should be administered with decreased doses of the preparation to be used (see Table 11-1). If at all possible, plasma levels should be monitored.

4. Congestion, when it occurs, is rapidly correctable by dialysis.

TABLE 11-1. Drug Therapy in Renal Failure (% of usual dose/day)

Creatinine Clearance (ml/min)	Digoxin	Digitoxin	Kanamycin, Streptomycin	Gentamicin	Clindamycin	Carbenicillin
0	42	63	6	8	10	. . .
10	50	66	10	17	25	10
25	63	72	20	33	75	30
50	75	79	40	67	100	75
75	90	86	60	100	100	100

I. Anemia   Most patients with acute renal failure develop some anemia attributable to the renal disease. It is rare for such patients to require transfusion. A rapidly falling hematocrit in a patient with acute renal failure should alert the physician to seek some other cause.

J. Drug therapy   Drugs excreted primarily by the kidneys must be given in reduced doses. Table 11-1 provides doses of some commonly administered drugs. Antibiotics should not be administered prophylactically to patients with acute renal failure, but should be reserved to treat specific infections as they are identified.

K. Hypertension in acute renal failure almost invariably is a consequence of injudicious administration of salt and fluid. The best treatment is to remove the excess salt and fluid by dialysis. If the hypertension is of life-threatening proportions, it can be controlled by diazoxide, 300 mg IV push, while the patient is being prepared for dialysis. An occasional patient will be refractory to diazoxide; in such patients, hypertension may be controlled by constant infusion of sodium nitroprusside, 100 mg/liter 5% dextrose in water.

SUGGESTED READING
Flamenbaum, W.   The pathophysiology of acute renal failure. *Arch. Intern. Med.* 131:911, 1974.
Gessler, U., Schroder, K., and Weidinger, H. (Eds.)   *Pathogenesis and Clinical Findings with Renal Failure.* Stuttgart: Thieme, 1971.
Reidenberg, M. M.   *Renal Function and Drug Action.* Philadelphia: Saunders, 1971.

12. ACUTE RESPIRATORY INSUFFICIENCY

I. DEFINITIONS

A. **Acute respiratory insufficiency may exist whenever the Pa_{O_2} is less than 60 mm Hg or the Pa_{CO_2} is greater than 50 mm Hg.** The syndrome appears in association with serious illness, major surgery, or massive trauma, and afflicted patients experience a high mortality.

B. **Tidal volume** is the amount of gas (air) inspired or expired during a single respiratory cycle. **Minute volume** is the amount of air moving in or out of the respiratory system per unit time; minute volume is determined by multiplying tidal volume by respiratory rate.

C. **Physiological dead space** is the volume of inspired gas that never exchanges with pulmonary blood. It is composed of three parts.

   1. Anatomical dead space is the volume of the pulmonary conducting system (nasopharynx, oropharynx, larynx, trachea, bronchi), which approximately equals 1 ml/kg in a normal adult.

   2. Alveolar dead space refers to alveoli that are ventilated but not perfused.

   3. Alveolar excess ventilation is related to perfusion. The excess ventilation is wasted and must be placed in the dead space. The two alveolar parts of physiological dead space are highly variable and unpredictable in volume.

D. **Dead space to tidal volume ratio (VD/VT) represents the percentage of tidal volume that is wasted.**

   1. In normal individuals, the VD/VT ratio is about 30% (range 20-40%).

   2. **The VD/VT ratio is calculated** using Pa_{CO_2} (see below) and the measured mean carbon dioxide content of expired air (PE_{CO_2}) as follows:

$$\text{VD/VT} = (\ |Pa_{CO_2} - PE_{CO_2}|\ \div\ Pa_{CO_2}\ ) \times 100$$

   Example: Pa_{CO_2} = 55 mm Hg (measured in arterial blood) and PE_{CO_2} = 25 mm Hg (measured in gas from endotracheal tube at end of expiration). Thus, VD/VT = (55 − 25) ÷ 55 × 100 = 55%.

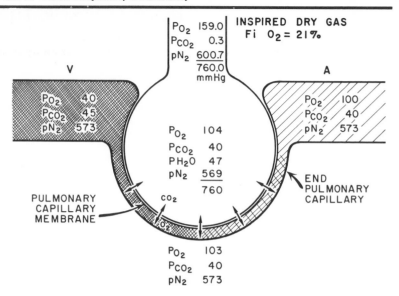

Figure 12-1. Diagram of gas exchange in the alveolus with 21% inspired oxygen concentration (F_{I_2}). Note that the final (Pa_{O_2}) is less than the initial Pa_{O_2}. This is the result of venous admixture from "normal" intrapulmonary shunting.

E. Arterial blood gases   Measurement of arterial blood gases (Fig. 12-1) is essential in the management of patients with acute respiratory insufficiency. A 10-ml syringe with a 22-gauge needle which has been rinsed with heparinized saline (1,000 u/100 ml) is used to obtain the arterial blood sample from the brachial, radial, or femoral artery. Only 2 ml of arterial blood is needed to complete all determinations. The sample should be placed in ice while being transported. For convenience and when frequent blood gas samples are needed, an indwelling catheter can be placed percutaneously into the radial artery and kept patent by flushing with heparinized saline.

1. **Pa_{O_2} is the partial pressure (tension) of oxygen** contained in arterial blood and is normally 90-100 mm Hg at sea level. The Pa_{O_2} is 5-10 mm Hg lower than the oxygen tension in the average alveolus (Pa_{O_2}).

2. **Pa_{CO_2} is the partial pressure of carbon dioxide** physically dissolved in arterial blood. The normal carbon dioxide tension is 36-40 mm Hg. If allowed only one blood gas determination, the Pa_{CO_2} is the most important single measurement to guide the adequacy of ventilation.

3. **Arterial pH** is an expression of hydrogen ion concentration in blood and relates directly to the ratio of bicarbonate to carbonic acid. The normal range is 7.36-7.44.

4. **Oxygen saturation** is the percent of oxygen (actual/theoretical) present in blood. The majority of oxygen in blood is carried by hemoglobin. One gram of hemoglobin carries 1.39 ml of oxygen when fully saturated.

When the Pa_{O_2} is 100 mm Hg, only 0.3 ml of oxygen is physically dissolved in each 100 ml of plasma. In a person with a hemoglobin level of 15 gm/100 ml, the total oxygen content of arterial blood is about 20 ml/100 ml of blood.

F. **Fractional inspired oxygen concentration (FI_{O_2})** is the percentage of oxygen in the inspired gases. The aim of therapeutically manipulating inspired oxygen concentration (FI_{O_2}) is to maintain the arterial oxygen between 70-80 mm Hg in normal patients. In chronic obstructive lung disease, a Pa_{O_2} of 50-60 mm Hg may be adequate.

G. **Alveolar-arterial oxygen difference ($D(A-a)O_2$)** is a measure of the effectiveness of arterial oxygen uptake from the lungs (diffusion) and of the degree of intrapulmonary shunting (venous admixture resulting from perfusion of nonventilated alveoli). The $D(A-a)O_2$ normally is 75-100 mm Hg.

1. **Calculation of $D(A-a)O_2$**   Assume that barometric pressure (ATM) reported by the weather bureau is 29 in. Hg, or 736.6 mm Hg (29 × 25.4 mm/in. = 736.6). The alveolar oxygen tension (Pa_{O_2}) after nitrogen washout while breathing 100% oxygen will be equal to barometric pressure minus corrections for alveolar water vapor (PA_{H_2O}) and carbon dioxide (PA_{CO_2}). PA_{H_2O} varies little, and for all calculations can be assumed to equal 47 mm Hg. PA_{CO_2}, because it diffuses so easily, will equal Pa_{CO_2} which is measured directly in arterial blood. Pa_{O_2} also is measured directly in an arterial blood sample. Thus,

$$D(A-a)O_2 = ATM - (PA_{H_2O} + Pa_{CO_2}) - Pa_{O_2}$$
$$= 736.6 - (47 + 40) - 560$$
$$= 89.6 \text{ mm Hg}$$

2. **The inspired oxygen concentration (FI_{O_2}) needed to achieve a desired Pa_{O_2}** can be calculated using $D(A-a)O_2$ in the formula:

$$FI_{O_2} \text{ needed} = [(D(A-a)O_2 + Pa_{O_2} \text{ desired}) \div ATM] \times 100$$

Example:
a. Pa_{O_2} desired = 70 mm Hg.
b. Blood gases measured after 15 min breathing 100% oxygen are Pa_{O_2} = 200 mm Hg, Pa_{CO_2} = 40 mm Hg.
c. ATM (weather bureau) = 737 mm Hg.
d. $D(A-a)O_2$ calculated as: 737 − (47 + 40) − 200 = 450 mm Hg.
e. Needed FI_{O_2} calculated as: [(450 + 70) ÷ 737] × 100 = 71% oxygen.

H. **Diffusion block** (alveolar-capillary block) refers to relative inability of oxygen to diffuse across the alveolar wall and into the pulmonary capillary. Diffusion of oxygen from gas to liquid phase across the alveolar-capillary membrane depends on the length of the diffusion path, the total area of diffusion, and the characteristics of the alveolar, capillary, and erythrocyte membranes. The presence of interstitial edema or fibrosis is associated with hypoxemia secondary to an increased diffusion path. Hyaline membrane formation and pulmonary edema act in a similar manner within the alveolus.

I. Respiratory acidosis is characterized by an increase in Pa_{CO_2} and results when tissue production of carbon dioxide exceeds removal by the lung. Patients with chronic obstructive lung disease who retain carbon dioxide become compensated and will not become acidotic unless Pa_{CO_2} acutely rises further. Respiratory acidosis is treated by increasing alveolar ventilation.

J. Respiratory alkalosis is characterized by a decrease in Pa_{CO_2}. Correction, if required, is made by decreasing the minute ventilation or increasing the dead space.

K. Oxygen toxicity   Use of oxygen tensions (FI_{O_2}) greater than 50% in the inspired gas mixture for more than short periods of time initiates progressive deterioration of lung function that may be manifest as hypoxemia. A decreased duration of administration is required as the FI_{O_2} is increased.

1. In animal experiments, interstitial and alveolar edema, as well as the development of hyaline membranes within the alveoli, have resulted from 72 hours exposure to high oxygen concentrations. These pathological changes imply primary capillary injury and an increased diffusion path for oxygen resulting in hypoxemia even though high concentrations of alveolar oxygen are present.

2. It is difficult to be so exact in humans because other complicating events causing deteriorating pulmonary function usually are present. There are some studies in normal volunteers that suggest that pathological changes are related directly to high FI_{O_2}. The aim should be to lower FI_{O_2} as soon as possible to 50% or less. Levels of FI_{O_2} of less than 50% are well tolerated for prolonged periods of time.

II. ETIOLOGY AND PATHOGENESIS OF ACUTE RESPIRATORY INSUFFICIENCY   The Pa_{O_2} always is low in acute respiratory insufficiency; the Pa_{CO_2} may be low, normal, or elevated.

A. The presence of a **low Pa_{O_2} with a low or normal Pa_{CO_2}** is seen in the following:

1. Atelectasis or collapse of alveoli may affect segments or entire lobes of the lung and generally follows obstruction of the tracheobronchial tree. In a postoperative patient, inability to clear secretions or poor expansion secondary to splinting results in atelectasis. Increased shunting is reflected by an increased $D(A-a)O_2$. The uninvolved areas of the lung are hyperventilated and hypocapnia may result.

2. Pneumonia or pulmonary edema results in fluid-filled alveoli accompanied by an interstitial inflammatory response which results in diffusion block and increased shunting.

3. **Pulmonary embolus**   Lung distal to a large embolus is not perfused; other areas of the lung are poorly ventilated secondary to bronchospasm. The net result is hypoxemia, initially primarily due to underventilation (increased shunting) and later, when bronchospasm relents, due to increased dead space (excess alveolar ventilation).

4. **Pneumothorax** results in collapse of lung tissue resulting in atelectasis and marked shunting.

5. **Respiratory distress syndrome** (white lung, shock lung, wet lung, etc.) follows critical surgical illness or major trauma. It develops slowly over 24-48 hr and is associated with an increase in pulmonary compliance, decrease in lung volume, and progressively increased shunting.

   Respiratory distress syndrome frequently is associated with fluid overload. Less common causes are fibrin and platelet microemboli in massive transfusion, pulmonary contusion associated with flail chest, fat emboli, shock, oxygen toxicity, sepsis, and amniotic fluid emboli.

B. A low Pa_{O_2} and an elevated Pa_{CO_2} usually indicates the presence of underlying chronic lung disease on which acute respiratory insufficiency is superimposed.

1. **Acute exacerbation of chronic obstructive pulmonary disease** (COPD) may follow an operation because of accumulation of secretions, bronchitis, or pneumonia. Poor diffusion because of interstitial fibrosis is present. Bronchospasm leads to air trapping in emphysematous segments, along with carbon dioxide retention and decreased alveolar ventilation.

2. **Hypoventilation** in a patient recovering from an anesthetic or in a heavily sedated patient leads to decreased Pa_{O_2} and carbon dioxide retention.

III. TREATMENT OF ACUTE RESPIRATORY INSUFFICIENCY

A. **Prophylaxis**   Simple treatment measures aimed at maintaining normal respiratory function and preventing development of postoperative respiratory insufficiency are discussed in Chapter 8. The importance of coughing, deep breathing, vigorous percussion of the chest wall, and use of blow bottles, combined with tracheal aspiration when indicated, cannot be overemphasized.

B. **Supplemental oxygen** can be delivered with one of several devices. A face mask, nasal cannula, or oxygen tent can deliver 40-50% humidified oxygen. Hypoxemia due to hypoventilation, ventilation-perfusion inequality, or diffusion block often can be corrected by inhalation of 35-50% oxygen. If a higher Fl_{O_2} is desired, a tight-fitting mask or endotracheal intubation will be necessary. Patients with COPD often are on an anoxic respiratory drive and a Venturi mask is required. The side vents in this mask mix oxygen with room air to deliver concentrations of 24-34%. Higher oxygen concentrations are avoided since they may depress the respiratory drive, leading to increasing hypercapnia and death.

C. **Intermittent positive pressure breathing** (IPPB) is used far more often than it needs to be. IPPB is an adjuvant form of therapy only and not a replacement for good trachobroncheal toilet, coughing, deep breathing, and use of blow bottles. IPPB may be of help in patients who have developed severe atelectasis with evidence of early pneumonia, i.e., persistent fever and a pulmonary infiltrate. If bronchospasm is present, application of a bronchodilator by means of this technique may be used.

D. **Intubation and respirator support**   If one is unable to maintain adequate ventilation and Pa_{O_2} minimally sufficient to maintain normal tissue oxygenation by means of supplemental oxygen using a face mask or nasal catheter, then it is necessary to proceed with tubation and possible ventilatory assistance with a respirator.

   1. **Indications** for intubation or tracheostomy and use of ventilatory assistance are summarized in Table 12-1.

      a. **A progressively rising Pa_{CO_2}** beyond 50 mm Hg in a patient who had normal pulmonary function prior to disability. Patients with COPD present an added set of problems: the Pa_{CO_2} ordinarily may be above 50 mm Hg. Ventilatory assistance should be used in COPD only when there is a rapid rise in Pa_{CO_2} producing acute respiratory acidosis.

      b. **The Pa_{O_2} is less than 70 mm Hg** in a normal patient breathing 100% oxygen. In the patient with COPD, a Pa_{O_2} of 50-60 mm Hg is generally adequate.

      c. **An arterial pH of 7.35 or below due to acute respiratory insufficiency.**

      d. A $D(A-a)O_2$ greater than 400 mm Hg.

      e. A respiratory rate over 35/min.

      f. A tidal volume of less than 3 ml/kg. In a 70-kg patient this would be a tidal volume of less than 210 ml per breath.

      g. Need to adequately suction copious secretions.

TABLE 12-1. Guidelines for Initiating Respirator Support

Function	Normal	Intubate and Ventilate
Respiratory rate	12-20/min	35/min
Oxygenation		
Pa_{O_2}	75-100 mm Hg (breathing room air)	70 mm Hg (on 100% O_2 by mask)
$D(A-a)O_2$	25-65 mm Hg	400 mm Hg
Ventilation		
Pa_{CO_2}	35-45 mm Hg	50 mm Hg (except in COPD)
VD/VT ratio	20-40%	60%

h. The presence of a flail chest causes paradoxical respiratory effort and a decrease in ventilation of the lungs. To stabilize the chest wall, the best method is to intubate the patient and place him on a respirator.

2. Care of the endotracheal tube or tracheostomy

a. Inspired gas must be humidified, else severe drying of secretions will occur. Humidified gas will decrease insensible loss from the lung. Appropriate adjustments in fluid allowances must be made to avoid excess water retention. Between 300-500 ml/day can be added to a patient's fluid intake from a nebulizer.

b. Use of low-pressure, high-volume soft cuffs designed to avoid tracheal compression and necrosis (Lanz, Portex, Shiley) are mandatory. Periodic deflation of the cuff for 1-2 min/hr also will help prevent wall injury. The oropharynx must be aspirated before releasing the cuff.

c. If the respirator can deliver sufficient inspiratory volume to compensate for air leakage, the deliberate underinflation of the cuff to permit 100-200 ml of air per cycle to leak proximally around the cuff to escape via the larynx will help obviate tracheal necrosis and also will help clear secretions from the trachea. Frequent suctioning of secretions from the oropharynx may be required in patients with a deliberate leak.

d. If the patient cannot be weaned from the respirator within 4-5 days, it will be necessary to replace the endotracheal tube with a tracheostomy.

e. The tracheostomy tube is removed and replaced with a clean tube at least every 3 days, or more often as conditions dictate. The inner cannula of a metal tracheostomy tube should be cleaned or replaced three times daily.

3. Complications of endotracheal and tracheostomy tubes

a. Massive atelectasis related to improper insertion into one main stem bronchus, usually the right. This mishap can be detected by auscultating the chest and confirming the tube position on an immediate postintubation chest film.

b. Dislodgment, kinking, and obstruction of the tube are constant threats that can be obviated or corrected by:

(1) Properly anchoring the tube.

(2) Positioning the tube and supporting the arms and tubing of the respirator so that the tube will not kink.

(3) Adequately suctioning secretions to prevent obstruction.

c. Tracheal stenosis is a late complication really related to improper care of the cuff, permitting ischemic pressure injury to the trachea.

4. **Respirators** are devices that mechanically substitute for inadequate ventilation. The goal of ventilatory assistance is to treat hypoxemia as well as to decrease the mechanical work of breathing. There are **two major types of respirators**—volume-limited and pressure-limited.

   a. In **volume-limited** respirators (Emerson, Bennett MA-1, Engstrom) the end of inspiration is terminated by:

      (1) Completion of delivery of a preset tidal volume (volume-cycled), or

      (2) Completion of a preset time interval (time-cycled) during which a preset rate of inspiratory flow governs delivery of the tidal volume.

   b. **Volume-limited respirators are preferred in treating patients with acute respiratory insufficiency.** The limitations of decreased pulmonary compliance or increased airway resistance are more easily managed with a volume-limited respirator.

   c. In **pressure-limited** respirators (Bird Mark VII, Bennett), the end of inspiration is limited by a preset value for peak tracheal pressure. These respirators can be triggered by minimal inspiratory effort and, therefore, can be used to assist as well as control respiration. Pressure-limited respirators are helpful during recovery from anesthesia until the patient's tidal volume returns to normal. They are also used for IPPB therapy.

   d. **Pressure-limited respirators should not be used in the management of acute respiratory failure** because if the airway resistance increases or the pulmonary compliance decreases, the tidal volume delivered will vary and usually is inadequate.

5. **Placing the patient on a respirator**

   a. Start with an FI_{O_2} of 100% and a respiratory rate slightly above the patient's spontaneous rate.

   b. Set the tidal volume initially at 15–20 ml/kg; make sure that ventilation is occurring by noting movement of the chest wall and by auscultating the lungs. If pulmonary function continues to deteriorate, the minute volume will have to be increased by varying the tidal volume and respiratory rate.

   c. Most patients will fight the respirator, producing uncoordinated efforts. The physician and nursing personnel should spend time with the patient to relieve his apprehension and aid in his acceptance of the machine. If verbal assurances are unavailing, temporary sedation with 5-10 mg morphine sulfate IV may be required.

d. Blood gases are measured 15-30 min after instituting therapy. From these data the $D(A-a)O_2$ and FI_{O_2} needed can be calculated as described earlier, and the FI_{O_2} is reduced to the required percentage. The least concentration of oxygen necessary to achieve the desired Pa_{O_2} is used.

e. When the patient has accepted and no longer fights the respirator, the respiratory rate is reduced to 12-15 cycles/min and the tidal volume is adjusted to maintain a minute volume of 8-10 liters.

f. The ventilator should have a sigh hyperinflation of one and a half to two times the preset tidal volume every 5-10 min to prevent atelectasis.

g. If the Pa_{CO_2} decreases below 30 mm Hg and attempts to decrease the minute volume are followed by deteriorating Pa_{O_2}, additional dead space, such as a 6-in. piece of tubing, can be added between the endotracheal tube and the respirator. Attempt to maintain the Pa_{CO_2} between 30-40 mm Hg. Continued addition of dead space eventually will decrease alveolar ventilation; a minimal alkalosis of up to pH 7.5 may have to be accepted. Such patients are prone to hypokalemia owing to the renal potassium wastage induced by alkalosis.

h. After the patient's ventilatory problem has stabilized, attempt to reduce the FI_{O_2} in stepwise fashion to the minimal concentration that will maintain a PA_{O_2} of 70-100 mm Hg.

i. Blood gases should be measured 15-30 min after each change in FI_{O_2} or ventilatory settings. Blood gases also should be checked frequently even if no changes are necessary.

6. **Positive end expiratory pressure (PEEP)**   There are some patients who, even on a respirator with high minute volume, are inadequately ventilated. For example, patients with severe shunting may have a large $D(A-a)O_2$ that is not corrected by 100% FI_{O_2}. Such patients frequently can be benefited by the addition of PEEP. The Bennett MA-1, Ohio 500, and Engstrom ventilators can be adjusted to provide positive pressure throughout the expiratory phase. End expiratory pressure should be adjusted to 5-10 cm H_2O.

a. PEEP improves oxygenation by:

(1) Increasing the functional reserve capacity by opening collapsed alveoli, thereby improving alveolar minute ventilation.

(2) Decreasing the diffusion distance for oxygen since fluid occupying the alveolus is thinned out against the wall by pressure and there is increasing movement of fluid out of the alveolus and also out of the interstitial space.

b. The criteria for institution of PEEP are:

(1) Inability of the patient to maintain a Pa_{O_2} of 70 mm Hg with an $F_{I_{O_2}}$ of 50% (or more) on usual zero end expiratory pressure ventilation.

(2) Failure of other therapeutic measures to reduce intrapulmonary shunting (e.g., treatment of cardiac failure with digitalis and diuretics, prevention or correction of fluid overload).

c. An adequate blood volume is mandatory prior to instituting this therapy, since **PEEP decreases the cardiac output.** In order for the patient to compensate, a normal blood volume must be present.

d. In the face of a low compliance, institution of PEEP with the usual tidal volume results in tremendously elevated inspiratory pressures. A gradual reduction of tidal volume and a concomitant increase in respiratory rate will be necessary to correct this.

e. The level of PEEP necessary is dictated by the Pa_{O_2}, blood pressure, magnitude of the shunt, lung volume, and the change in compliance. PEEP as high as 20 cm H_2O sometimes may be indicated. Generally start with PEEP of 5 cm H_2O and gradually increase as necessary or tolerated by the patient.

f. Patients in shock tolerate PEEP poorly because of the already decreased cardiac output.

g. Complications   The use of PEEP is not without hazard. The decrease in cardiac output has been mentioned. A very serious complication is the increased tendency to develop pneumothorax or pneumomediastinum. Complications can be avoided by decreasing or terminating PEEP when conditions so indicate.

h. Terminating PEEP   When conditions are stable, the $F_{I_{O_2}}$ is reduced first in stepwise fashion to 40-50%. If the arterial blood gases remain in the accepted range, then PEEP is next reduced stepwise in 5-cm decrements.

7. Care of the patient on a respirator

a. Successful treatment of a patient with respiratory failure is largely due to the care given by competent and well-trained nurses.

b. The patient is never left unattended. Patients with endotracheal tubes or on a respirator are treated in the ICU.

c. A chest x-ray is obtained immediately after the patient is placed on a respirator and is repeated as often as the patient's condition dictates.

d. A tracheal aspirate is sent for culture as soon after intubation as possible; cultures are repeated at the time of extubation and at least every fifth day during intubation. Antibiotics are administered as indicated by sensitivity studies whenever signs of invasive respiratory infection are present.

e. The nebulizer and lines are checked frequently to maintain proper function.

f. The FI_{O_2} should be measured daily, more often when changing oxygen concentration.

g. The tidal volume, respiratory rate, and minute volume should be measured at least every 4 hr, depending on the patient's condition. The measurements also should be done whenever the patient is taken off the respirator, even if only for 1-2 min.

h. The physiological shunt and dead space to tidal volume ratio should be calculated at least daily, and more often if required. The calculations have been discussed previously.

i. All patients on a respirator should be monitored; cardiac rhythm, especially if arrhythmias are present, pulse rate, CVP, and blood pressure are recorded continuously.

j. Changes in body position should be made hourly while awake, or around the clock if the patient is comatose. Care of skin in areas where pressure necrosis may occur must be emphasized.

k. Fluid intake and output must be accurately recorded.

l. Weight must be recorded daily. Increased weight reflects water retention.

m. Diuretics are necessary where a flagrant fluid overload exists.

n. Salt-poor albumin (12.5 gm) followed in 1 hr by IV diuretics, together with fluid restriction, will decrease the interstitial edema seen in complicated cases of acute respiratory distress syndrome.

o. Early treatment with steroids in pharmacological doses may be of help in the adult respiratory distress syndrome. Methylated steroids, 30 mg/kg as an IV bolus, followed by 1 gm every 6 hr for 1-2 days, appear to stabilize lysosomes and other membranes and to aid in decreasing alveolar and interstitial fluid accumulation.

8. Weaning the patient off the respirator

a. The **criteria for weaning** a patient from a respirator are:

(1) Pa_{O_2} is greater than 70 mm Hg on 40-50% oxygen without PEEP.

(2) Tidal volume off the respirator is 400-500 ml (5-7 ml/kg).

(3) Respiratory rate is 12-20/min.

(4) $D(A-a)O_2$ is less than 300 mm Hg on 100% oxygen.

(5) Pulmonary infiltrates have cleared or there is clinically sufficient reversal of pulmonary failure.

b. The **method of weaning** is:

(1) The ventilator is disconnected.

(2) With the cuff inflated, tidal volume and spontaneous respiratory rate are determined.

(3) The cuff is deflated and the patient is placed on 100% supplemental oxygen for up to 15 min, if tolerated. Blood gases then are measured and the patient is reconnected to the respirator.

(4) If Pa_{CO_2} and Pa_{O_2} are adequate ($Pa_{CO_2} < 45$; $Pa_{O_2} > 70$), time off the respirator is increased progressively. If blood gases remain adequate after an hour and the patient is not tiring, the patient can be left off the respirator but initially on 100% supplemental oxygen. After several hours, FI_{O_2} is decreased stepwise to 40%. Patients may benefit during this time from IPPB every 1-4 hr.

(5) During weaning, a higher FI_{O_2} may be required during spontaneous breathing than while on the respirator in order to compensate for increased oxygen consumption due to increased work of breathing.

(6) Some patients may tire and require ventilatory support during the night or a return to continuous respirator therapy. Attempts at weaning should not be resumed until at least a further 24 hr have elapsed.

(7) If blood gases are adequate after 24 hr of continuous unassisted breathing, the patient is weaned and can be extubated.

(8) Following extubation, humidified 40% oxygen by mask should be instituted. Assisted ventilation every 1-4 hr with IPPB may be necessary for 24-48 hr.

SUGGESTED READING

Blaisdell, W. F.   The respiratory distress syndrome: A review. *Surgery* 74:251, 1973.

Comroe, J. H., Jr., Forster, R. E., II, Dubois, A. B., Briscoe, W. A., and Carlsen, E.   *The Lung: Clinical Physiology and Pulmonary Function Tests* (2nd ed.). Chicago: Year Book, 1962.

Heironimus, T. W., III   *Mechanical Artificial Ventilation: A Manual for Students and Practitioners* (2nd ed.). Springfield, Ill.: Thomas, 1972.

Moore, F. D.   *Post-traumatic Pulmonary Insufficiency.* Philadelphia: Saunders, 1969.

Shapiro, B.   *Clinical Application of Blood Gases.* Chicago: Year Book, 1973.

13. SURGICAL ENDOCRINOLOGY

I. THE DIABETIC PATIENT

A. General information

1. The stress of anesthesia and operation exacerbates the patient's glucose intolerance, and the frequent necessary modifications in food and fluid intake during this period further complicate management.

2. To maintain nutrition and prevent ketoacidosis and hypoglycemia, it is imperative that the patient receive a **minimum of 200 gm carbohydrate daily** and that **adequate insulin be continuously available** to promote utilization of these carbohydrate calories. It must never be forgotten that caloric intake and insulin availability must always be considered together. A liter of 5% dextrose in water contains 50 gm carbohydrate.

3. It is obviously important that the diabetic patient be in the best possible nutritional balance at the time of operation. Therefore, if the operative procedure is not urgent, it should be delayed until the following are evaluated and controlled: diabetic state, nutritional status, hydration, and electrolyte status.

4. During the operative and postoperative period, complete and persistent control of the blood sugar within the normal range is not feasible. Patients receiving IV glucose may have rather marked glycosuria with only moderate hyperglycemia. For this reason, **blood glucose and serum ketone concentrations should be checked at least twice daily for 1-3 days after operation** to correlate with the urine sugar and ketone concentration and to evaluate better the patient's diabetic control.

5. **Hypoglycemia is a more hazardous condition than hyperglycemia** When there is no hyperketonemia, moderate hyperglycemia (200-250 mg/100 ml) is not hazardous and should be expected and accepted during the early postoperative period. Some diabetic patients who have had neurosurgical procedures and those receiving steroids or hyperalimentation are prone to develop marked hyperglycemia and hyperosmolality. These conditions should be anticipated and treated with increased doses of insulin.

6. **Diabetic patients are particularly liable to staphylococcal and mixed gramnegative infections** Usual body antibacterial defense mechanisms may be insufficient to prevent a gross wound infection in a diabetic individual

which, for the same degree of contamination, would never be a clinically apparent infection in a nondiabetic person. Antibiotics should be given whenever gross contamination of the operative area has occurred. Any apparent infection should be culturally defined and vigorously treated with appropriate antibiotics.

B. Minor operation under local anesthesia   Generally no alteration in diabetic management is necessary here. If it is necessary for the patient to omit a meal for the procedure, however, the carbohydrate content of that meal (approximately 50 gm, or 1,000 ml 5% dextrose in water or saline solution) should be given IV.

C. Major operation

1. Diabetes adequately controlled with diet and NPH or lente insulin

    a. Prior to the operation   No change in insulin or diet regimen is necessary.

    b. Day of the operation   Management is most convenient if the procedure can be done in the forenoon, although adjustments in the following regimen can be made if this is not possible.

        (1) In early morning

            (a) Omit breakfast.

            (b) Start IV infusion of 1,000 ml 10% glucose in water or saline solution, to be infused over a 6–8 hr period.

            (c) Give approximately half of the patient's usual daily dose of NPH or lente insulin subcutaneously at the time the glucose infusion is begun.

        (2) On completion of operation

            (a) Give remaining half of the patient's usual daily dose of NPH or lente insulin subcutaneously.

            (b) Continue IV infusion of 5 or 10% glucose in water or saline solution (generally ¼–⅓ of total fluid as saline solution) so that the patient receives a total of approximately 200 gm of glucose in 2,000–3,000 ml of fluids in the first 24-hr period. Modifications, of course, may need to be made depending on the fluid and electrolyte needs of the patient; just be certain to include at least 200 gm glucose daily.

            (c) Give oral fluids and food as soon as patient's condition permits.

            (d) Check urine sugar and ketones every 4 hr postoperatively (if patient can void) and blood glucose and plasma ketones every

8-12 hr, obtaining the first determinations as soon as the patient returns from the operation. Do not attempt strict control of hyperglycemia or glucosuria. Generally, no crystalline insulin supplementation is needed with this regimen. However, if moderate or severe ketonuria is present, serum ketones become elevated, or the blood sugar exceeds 250-300 mg/100 ml, give 5-20 units of crystalline insulin subcutaneously.

c. On days following operation

(1) Give patient the previously determined usual dose of NPH or lente insulin. If patient is to be maintained entirely on continuous IV fluids for several days, the insulin should be given as two equal doses 12 hr apart.

(2) Resume usual preoperative diet or a diet comparable in calories as soon as postoperative condition permits.

(3) If patient is unable to be fed orally or oral intake is inadequate, give IV infusion of 5 or 10% dextrose in water to total of approximately 200 gm carbohydrate/24 hr until patient's condition permits return to his usual diet.

2. Diabetes poorly controlled but without ketosis; operative procedure can be delayed at least 2-6 days

a. Preparation for operation

(1) Diet: Provide 200-300 gm carbohydrate, and at least 5 calories/kg of ideal body weight, with the diet divided into four equal portions and given every 6 hr.

(2) Crystalline insulin

(a) Injections should be given subcutaneously every 6 hr (½ hr before each meal). Initial basic dose of insulin should be approximately 10 units.

(b) Check fresh urine specimens for glucose and ketones 1 hr before each meal.

(c) Increase the basic insulin dose by approximately 10 units for 4+, and 5 units for 3+ glycosuria. A negative reaction indicates a need for a reduction of dose, but *not* omission of insulin so long as food or glucose is to follow the insulin injection.

(3) Blood glucose determinations just before meals may be used instead of urine sugar concentrations to adjust the subsequent dose of insulin if the patient is unable to void or is known to have a high renal threshold for glucose. If blood glucose exceeds 200 mg/100 ml, the next dose of crystalline insulin should be increased by 5 or

10 units for every 50 mg/100 ml glucose in excess of 200 mg/100 ml.

(4) When the patient's diabetes has been stabilized on this regimen (2-6 days), proceed with the elective operation.

b. On day of operation

(1) Omit breakfast.

(2) Start IV infusion of 5 or 10% glucose in water or saline solution and adjust rate (or start a new flask) so that the patient receives 750 ml containing 35-70 gm glucose every 6 hr. The patient should receive a total of approximately 200 gm glucose during the day of operation.

(3) Continue to administer crystalline insulin subcutaneously by the same regimen as when the patient was on oral feedings.

c. On days following operation

(1) Continue IV glucose and crystalline insulin regimen started on day of operation if patient cannot tolerate oral intake.

(2) Return to preoperative regimen of crystalline insulin and four oral feedings every 6 hr as quickly as patient can tolerate food.

(3) After several days, divide patient's total calories into three meals and a bedtime snack and start NPH or lente insulin each morning, the initial dose being about two thirds of the total daily dose of crystalline insulin.

3. Diabetes poorly controlled but with minimal or no ketosis; operation is urgent within a day

a. Preparation and during operation

(1) Give IV infusions of 5 or 10% glucose in water or saline solution at rate of 750 ml every 6 hr. Additional fluid and electrolyte replacement may be necessary prior to operation to correct deficits.

(2) Give crystalline insulin subcutaneously every 6 hr, starting with 10 units. Check blood or urine for sugar and ketones. Increase the insulin dose by 5-10 units for each 50 mg/100 ml blood glucose in excess of 200 mg/100 ml or for each 3+ or 4+ urine sugar reaction. Negative urine reaction for glucose may indicate a need for reduction in the dose (check blood sugar) but insulin should not be omitted completely so long as IV glucose is being given.

b. On days following operation   Continue the postoperative regimen outlined above [c(1)-(3)].

4. Severe ketoacidosis

   a. The patient in severe ketoacidosis is a very poor risk for any operation except an incision and drainage of an abscess or similar urgent procedure.

   b. A delay of 4-6 hr is imperative (much longer if possible) to initiate correction of ketoacidosis and fluid and electrolyte imbalance. Frequent and large doses of crystalline insulin should be given. Further details of management of severe ketoacidosis are beyond the scope of this discussion; consultation usually should be obtained.

   c. As soon as severe ketoacidosis has improved, the patient should be managed as outlined under **3** (p. 248).

5. Diabetes well controlled with an oral hypoglycemic agent

   a. This condition generally requires insulin during the stress of the surgical period.

   b. Continue the oral hypoglycemic agent but omit the evening dose just prior to the day of operation.

   c. On the day of the operation follow the procedure outlined under **b(1)-(3)** on page 248, initiating crystalline insulin therapy as outlined under **2(2)** on page 247.

   d. When the stress of the surgical period is over, the patient may be returned to his previous oral regimen.

6. Diabetes adequately controlled with diet and NPH or lente insulin—alternative method to C.1 (p. 246).   The method outlined under **C.1** is preferable and simpler. However, because some surgeons prefer to use crystalline insulin exclusively during the operative period, the following alternative regimen is given:

   a. Prior to operation   No change in insulin or diet regimen is necessary.

   b. Day of operation

   (1) Omit breakfast and NPH or lente insulin.

   (2) Administer IV glucose as outlined under **b(2)** on page 248.

   (3) Administer crystalline insulin every 6 hr, giving $\frac{1}{4}$ the units of the patient's prior total daily NPH or lente insulin dose. Adjust subsequent insulin doses as indicated by urine sugar and ketones, as outlined above.

c. Days following operation   Continue above regimen until oral feedings are tolerated. Then resume prior diet and NPH or lente insulin.

SUGGESTED READING

Marble, A., and Steinke, J.   Physiology and pharmacology in diabetes mellitus: Guiding the diabetic patient through the surgical period. *Anesthesiology* 24:442, 1963.

Steinke, J.   Management of diabetes mellitus and surgery. *N. Engl. J. Med.* 282:1472, 1970.

II. THE PATIENT ON STEROIDS

A. General information

1. Normal adrenal cortices secrete about 20 mg of hydrocortisone daily.

2. A patient's ability to withstand stress, surgical or otherwise, depends on the ability of his adrenals to respond by markedly increasing the output of hydrocortisone (up to 10 times the basal amount).

3. A patient who is receiving adrenal steroids currently, or who has received steroids for more than 1 or 2 wk within the 6- to 12-mo period prior to the operation, has an unpredictable degree of functional adrenocortical suppression. These patients should be considered to have iatrogenic adrenocortical insufficiency at the time of operation and they should be managed accordingly.

4. The same type of management should be employed for (a) previously adrenalectomized patients or patients with spontaneous adrenal insufficiency and (b) patients who are to undergo adrenalectomy.

5. It is important to recognize (a) that these patients will need large amounts of hydrocortisone or cortisone readily available to all tissues at all times during the stress of the surgical period and (b) that short-term excess of glucocorticoids is relatively harmless, but short-term deficiency during stress can be fatal.

6. The following outline includes a planned excess of adrenal steroids given by more than one route to assure continuous availability during the period of maximal stress.

B. Schedule for patients with adrenal insufficiency undergoing operation or for patients undergoing adrenalectomy

1. **Day before operation**   12–16 hr preoperatively: cortisone acetate, 100 mg IM.

2. **Day of operation**

a. 2 hr preoperatively: cortisone acetate, 100 mg IM.

b. ½ hr preoperatively: hydrocortisone hemisuccinate or phosphate, 100 mg IM.

    c. ½ hr preoperatively: start hydrocortisone hemisuccinate by continuous IV drip, 100 mg every 8 hr for 24 hr.

    d. Immediately postoperatively: cortisone acetate, 50 mg IM every 4 hr.

3. Days following operation

    a. Days 1 and 2: cortisone acetate, 50 mg IM every 6 hr.

    b. Days 3 and 4: cortisone acetate, 50 mg IM every 8 hr.

    c. Days 5 and 6: cortisone acetate, 25 mg IM every 6 hr.

    d. Days 7 and 8: cortisone acetate, 25 mg IM every 8 hr.

    e. Days 9 and 10: cortisone acetate, 25 mg IM every 12 hr.

    f. Days 11 and 12: cortisone acetate, 12.5 mg IM every 8 hr.

    g. Day 13 and thereafter: maintenance dosage for patients with known adrenal insufficiency; discontinuance of cortisone in those patients minimally suspected of steroid-induced adrenocortical suppression and therefore treated only during surgical stress.

4. Modifications

    a. The above regimen of dose reduction is a general guide, to be modified to each patient's needs, as judged by his clinical status (especially the presence or absence of fever, pain, or other stress), blood pressure, serum electrolytes, and so forth.

    b. When the patient can tolerate and retain oral feedings without difficulty, medication can be given orally.

    c. Amounts of cortisone or hydrocortisone greater than 100 mg daily exert adequate mineralocorticoid effects. When the daily dose is reduced below 100 mg daily, 9α-fluorohydrocortisone, 0.1 mg orally daily, should be added to the regimen.

    d. The cortisone dose reduction regimen for patients who have undergone adrenalectomy for Cushing's syndrome generally must proceed more slowly and the dose often cannot be reduced below 50 mg daily for several weeks.

    e. Conversely, in patients with questionable adrenocortical suppression because of past steroid therapy, the postoperative steroid dosage may be reduced more rapidly and often may be discontinued within 4–7 days.

    f. The addition of potassium (40–80 mEq daily) to the IV fluids and later to the oral intake is helpful in preventing potassium depletion.

5. Minor procedures   Patients undergoing minor procedures, such as tooth extractions or biopsy, should receive 50-100 mg cortisone about 2 hr before the procedure and 50-100 mg about 4 hr after the procedure. Generally, the patient's maintenance regimen can be resumed the following day.

SUGGESTED READING

Cahill, G. F., and Thorn, G. W.   Preoperative and postoperative management of adrenal cortical hyperfunction. *Anesthesiology* 24:472, 1963.

Thorn, G. W., and Lauler, D. P.   Clinical therapeutics of adrenal disorders. *Am. J. Med.* 53:673, 1972.

III. ACUTE HYPERCALCEMIA (hypercalcemic crisis)

A. Recognition   Serum calcium levels normally are 8.5-10.5 mg/100 ml. Elevation of calcium to 11-13 mg may be associated with only vague symptoms: tiredness, easy fatigability, constipation, polyuria, nocturia, and polydipsia. As elevation of calcium progresses, more toxic symptoms and a life-threatening situation are present: anorexia, nausea and vomiting, dehydration and prerenal azotemia, and somnolence progressing to stupor and coma. Remember that 40-50% of serum calcium is bound to protein, primarily albumin. Patients with hypoalbuminemia and hypercalcemia may have a relatively lower total calcium but an elevated ionized fraction of calcium.

B. Diagnosis   Acute hypercalcemic crisis is a syndrome seen primarily in patients with (1) hyperparathyroidism and (2) neoplasms associated with bone metastases. Parathyroid hormone (PTH) levels usually are not elevated with bone metastases, although some neoplasms do produce excess PTH or a PTH-like hormone resulting in hypercalcemia without bone involvement. Rarely do the other causes of hypercalcemia listed below produce crises except when certain drugs are superimposed or when hypercalcemia is exacerbated by dehydration.

C. Major causes of hypercalcemia

1. Primary hyperparathyroidism (adenoma or hyperplasia).

2. Neoplasia associated with osteolytic lesions: breast, lung, kidney, ovary (PTH not elevated).

3. Neoplasia producing PTH or PTH-like hormone: renal cell, lung, ovary, pancreas, sarcoma.

4. Multiple myeloma.

5. Sarcoidosis.

6. Drugs: vitamin D intoxication, thiazides, estrogens (particularly when used in therapy of breast cancer), excess Ca^+ intake in combination with antacids (milk-alkali syndrome).

7. Immobilization.

8. Acute osteoporosis.

9. Idiopathic hypercalcemia of infancy.

10. Hyperthyroidism.

D. Treatment   Acute hypercalcemic crises can be fatal and must be treated promptly.

   1. Serum calcium can be decreased by (1) increased calcium excretion, (2) decreased bone resorption, and (3) decreased calcium intake. The most judicious and practical methods currently in use are listed in Table 13-1.

   2. Rehydration with saline infusion and **diuresis** with furosemide, accompanied by careful monitoring of CVP, body weight, urine output, and serum electrolytes (particularly K^+ and Mg^+), are the initial treatment of hypercalcemic crisis. Phosphate may be used if a response is not immediate. Mithramycin is reserved for patients with neoplasia.

TABLE 13-1. Preferred Methods of Treatment of Hypercalcemic Crises

Agent	Dosage and Route	Mechanism of Action	Complications, Remarks
0.9% saline	100-200 ml/hr IV	Rehydration; increased urinary CA excretion	Na and H_2O overload; congestive heart failure. Monitor CVP, body weight
Furosemide (Lasix)	50-100 mg/hr IV (must be given with 0.9% saline infusion)	Induced diuresis; increased urinary Ca excretion	Volume, K, and Mg depletion; renal failure if oliguria not responsive. Monitor weight, CVP, urine, electrolytes; replace appropriately
Inorganic phosphate Neutra-Phos	300-1000 mg/day (oral or through nasogastric tube)	Binds GI Ca	Monitor serum phosphorous, creatinine, and urine
Phosphate-phosphorous in glucose (Inphos)	50 millimols in 500-1000 ml 5% dextrose q 6-12 hr IV	? Deposition of Ca PO_4 salts	*Hazardous:* Avoid hyperphosphatemia >5 mg/100 ml because of possible soft tissue calcification. Limited usefulness in renal insufficiency
Corticosteroids[a] prednisone	40-80 mg/day starting dose	Increased bone resorption; ? anti-vitamin D	Delayed effect, reserved for vitamin D intoxication, lymphomas, sarcoidosis, myeloma, and breast carcinoma
Mithramycin[a] (reserve for patients with neoplasia)	25 μg/kg/day IV	? Antitumor or PTH antagonist; no increase in urinary calcium	Effect in 24-48 hr; may be given for 5 days. Hepatotoxic, nephrotoxic, thrombocytopenia

[a] Adjunctive therapy: Use after rehydration, furosemide, and possibly phosphate.

3. Other agents used to lower serum calcium:

   a. Corticosteroids may lower serum Ca^+ in some diseases, but the response is inconsistent and the onset slow. Patients with vitamin D intoxication, lymphomas, sarcoidosis, myeloma, or breast carcinoma in addition to hypercalcemia may be benefited by steroids.

   b. Edetic acid (EDTA) given IV lowers serum Ca^+, but the effect is transient, requiring administration of additional EDTA, and each dose increases the risk of renal tubular damage.

   c. Sodium sulfate infusion offers no advantage over phosphates and may be less effective.

IV. PARATHYROID INSUFFICIENCY

A. General comments

1. Parathyroid insufficiency following thyroidectomy occurs *transiently* in 8% of surgically treated patients; symptoms may persist for 3-6 mo but eventually clear completely. Symptomatic hypoparathyroidism occurs transiently in 70% of patients having excision of abnormal parathyroid glands. This state is probably a result of compromise of the blood supply of the remaining normal parathyroid glands.

2. If the operative procedure was a parathyroidectomy for hyperparathyroidism associated with an elevated alkaline phosphatase or with overt bone disease, postoperative hypocalcemic tetany may be particularly severe because of the rapid uptake of calcium by osteoblasts. Continual adjustment of postoperative calcium and vitamin D therapy in these patients is required until the alkaline phosphatase has returned to normal.

3. **Permanent hypoparathyroidism** or tetany as a complication of thyroid or parathyroid surgery is uncommon. The incidence following operations for benign thyroid disease is less than 1%; following operations for thyroid cancer, it is 5%.

4. **Symptoms** are related to neuromuscular irritability secondary to hypocalcemia. Initially, the patient may exhibit only nervousness, irritability and personality changes. Later, tingling of the extremities may appear, followed by parasthesias, muscle cramps, and numbness.

5. Chvostek's sign often is positive and tendon reflexes are hyperactive. Carpopedal spasms and a positive Trousseau's sign appear only later.

6. Laryngeal stridor or convulsions may supervene at any time, without marked warning symptoms.

7. There may be ECG evidence of hypocalcemia manifested by a prolonged Q-T interval.

8. The diagnosis is confirmed by determination of the serum calcium. Levels below 7 mg/100 ml (3.5 mEq/liter) in the absence of alkalosis are usually symptomatic and require treatment. Occasionally a patient may be seen with a low-normal serum calcium who still exhibits a positive Chvostek's sign.

B. Treatment

1. Blood for a serum calcium determination should be drawn before any therapy is given.

2. If symptoms are severe, 1 gm (10 ml) of 10% calcium gluconate should be given *slowly* IV with ECG control. Slow administration of calcium is emphasized, especially if the patient is receiving digitalis, so that acute hypercalcemic cardiac arrest will not ensue.

3. Oral calcium salts (calcium gluconate or lactate powder or wafers), 12 gm/day in divided doses, is the mainstay of therapy and all that will be required in the majority of patients.

4. Should signs of hypocalcemia persist after oral calcium therapy, vitamin D is indicated. The usual starting dose of calciferol (vitamin D_2) is 50,000 units daily. Occasionally doses of vitamin D up to 500,000 units/day may be required.

5. Oral antacids—such as magaldrate (Riopan) and magnesium-aluminum hydroxide (Maalox)—which bind phosphates will permit enhanced absorption of dietary calcium and should be given with meals.

V. THYROID STORM

A. Thyroid storm can be described as a marked augmentation of the symptoms of thyrotoxicosis. It is now thought to be due to markedly increased serum levels of triiodothyronine (T_3) and thyroxine (T_4) (singly or in combination), combined with hypersensitivity of beta-adrenergic receptors.

B. The **symptoms,** which may occur following any operation in the hyperthyroid patient and occasionally following operations in a euthyroid patient who has been pretreated with iodine, are:

1. Hyperpyrexia—may be severe, 41.6-42.2°C (107-108°F).

2. Tachycardia—160-200 beats/min.

3. Nervousness, irritability, frank psychosis.

4. Vomiting and diarrhea.

5. High output cardiac failure is the most common cause of death.

C. Treatment

1. Prevention is the cornerstone of therapy. Propylthiouracil is administered preoperatively to convert the toxic patient to euthyroidism. Beta-adrenergic blockade with propranolol, 20-40 mg tid, is more rapid-acting but does not treat the primary disease, only its effects.

2. When the syndrome has developed, immediate treatment consists of:

   a. Symptomatic therapy for hyperpyrexia: cooling mattresses and oxygen.

   b. Beta-adrenergic blockade with 1-2 mg of propranolol slowly IV as a test dose under cardiac monitor control after adequate volume restoration, followed by titration of the patient with an IV drip containing 1-200 mg of propranolol given at a rate that controls symptoms (usually 50-100 μg/min).

   c. Institution of long-term thyroid suppression with propylthiouracil and iodide therapy. This will not be effective alone in the acute stage but will allow orderly transfer to this regimen when acute symptoms subside, usually in 3-5 days.

   d. Digitalization if symptoms are severe.

   e. Both lithium acetate and plasmapheresis have been used in treatment of thyroid storm. Though promising, these treatments are unproved.

SUGGESTED READING

Lee, T. C., Coffee, R. J., Mackin, J., Cobb, M., Routon, J., and Canary, J. J. The use of propranolol in the surgical treatment of thyrotoxic patients. *Ann. Surg.* 173:643, 1973.

Parsons, V., and Jewitt, D. Beta-adrenergic blockade in management of acute thyrotoxic crisis, tachycardia, and arrhythmia. *Postgrad. Med. J.* 43:756, 1967.

14. SURGICAL INFECTIONS

I. DIAGNOSIS The early and accurate diagnosis of surgical infection is essential, for delayed or inadequate therapy can result in overwhelming sepsis in an already stressed postoperative patient. Surgical infection usually can be treated successfully with specific antibiotics in conjunction with proper surgical care.

    A. History and physical examination are still the surgeon's most important diagnostic tools. Although a number of surgical infections are present prior to operation, many occur in the postoperative period. Wound infections rarely occur before the third postoperative day. They manifest themselves by **induration** (the earliest sign), erythema, and pain. Excessive **wound pain** is a commonly overlooked early sign, particularly with wound infections caused by gram-negative organisms. **Auscultation of the chest** may reveal the presence of pneumonia before it is evident on x-ray. **Rectal examination** may show tenderness and induration as signs of a developing pelvic abscess. Inspection of the calves and IV cannula dressings may reveal thrombophlebitis. In general, *fever occurring within the first 24 hr suggests pulmonary atelectasis; within 48 hr, a urinary tract infection; and after 72 hr, a wound infection.*

    B. Tests

        1. Hematology and urinalysis Most bacterial infections produce an increase in the leukocyte count and a **shift to the left** in the differential count. This shift to the more immature forms of the polymorphonuclear leukocytes may signal infection before a rise in the total leukocyte count has occurred. The differential may also reveal lymphocytosis in viral infections, monocytosis in tuberculosis, eosinophilia in parasitic infections or hypersensitivity reactions (drug allergy), and toxic granulations of leukocytes in acute bacterial infections. A leukemoid response (total count over 25,000 cells/mm^3) may be seen in septicemia, pneumococcal infections, liver abscess or cholangitis, suppurative pancreatitis, necrotic bowel, and retroperitoneal phlegmon. Leukopenia is a sign of overwhelming bacterial infection, viral infection, or tuberculosis. Hemolytic anemia may be found with infections caused by *Clostridium perfringens* or group A streptococci.

        2. X-rays Chest films or a flat plate of the abdomen may confirm a clinical diagnosis or reveal unsuspected pneumonitis, small-bowel obstruction, or free air in the abdomen or chest.

3. Bacteriology

a. Observation of exudates and secretions (wound drainage, urine, sputum, etc.) for odor, color, and consistency may be helpful. Sweet, grape-like odors occur with *Pseudomonas,* urea odors with *Proteus,* and feculent odors with anaerobic organisms (bacteroides, fusiforms, and clostridia).

b. A **Gram stain** offers the earliest clues to the etiology of an infection. Note should be taken of the polymorphonuclear leukocytes on the slide (few, many, loaded) and whether organisms can be seen inside them. Acid-fast and fungus stains can be used if these are in question.

c. **Culture and sensitivity** tests are essential. Both aerobic and anaerobic cultures should be requested. Ideally, anaerobic specimens should be transported immediately in a CO_2-filled tube and plated within 1 hr (otherwise the organism will die, and the culture report will be negative). If the specimen must be held overnight, it should be placed in cooked meat broth and left at room temperature. Under no circumstances should an anaerobic specimen be refrigerated.

d. **Blood cultures** are indicated in all serious infections. Careful cleansing of the venipuncture site with an iodine preparation should be followed by an alcohol swab. Blood should never be drawn for culture through an existing IV needle or catheter. It is important to obtain a number of blood cultures at different times. If possible, they should be obtained at the start of a chill or the beginning of a fever spike. Both aerobic and anaerobic cultures should be obtained.

e. **Biopsy** of skin lesions and lymph nodes may be helpful. Avoid lymph node biopsy of the inguinal region. If no nodes are palpable, a scalene (fat-pad) node biopsy may be productive. Specimens should be sent for routine bacterial, acid-fast bacillus (AFB), and fungal cultures as well as to the pathology department for histological examination. With the exception of tuberculosis, skin tests have a limited usefulness. Serological tests are more reliable in diagnosis of fungal diseases.

II. GENERAL PRINCIPLES OF THERAPY

A. Nosocomial infections   Up to 15% of patients entering a general hospital will acquire an infection. Most of these will be caused by gram-negative bacilli. Even in units in which the risks of infection are stressed, breaks in technique occur.

1. One third of **IV catheters** become colonized with bacteria within 2 days. Bacteremia will occur in 1% of patients with an IV catheter in place longer than 48 hr, and the risk of sepsis increases to 4-5% as the length of time the catheter remains in place increases. Since the advent of hyperalimentation, the figures are higher. IV catheters always should be cultured, especially when bacteremia is suspected.

2. **Foley catheters** should be connected to closed drainage systems. A uro-sheath is a preferable alternative in male patients; drainage should be used only if they are incontinent.

3. The nebulizers and tubing of **respirators** often become colonized with bacteria and can lead to bacterial pneumonia.

4. Breaks of **technique** in the operating room, such as failure to cover the exposed hair of the surgical team, inadequate preparation of the incision site, and failure to redrape and to use a second set of instruments following colon operations have all been responsible for postoperative wound infections.

B. Treatment

1. Make a **diagnosis** (see Sect. I).

2. Select the proper **antibiotic** as determined by the bacterial etiology and the following factors:

   a. **Effectiveness**   Gram-positive organisms are usually sensitive to penicillin and related compounds. Gram-negative aerobic organisms are likely to be sensitive to aminoglycosides. Anaerobic organisms may be sensitive to chloramphenicol, clindamycin, erythromycin, lincomycin, or tetracycline. Other factors to consider are the penetration of the antibiotic into infected areas and whether the drug is bactericidal or bacteriostatic.

   b. **Side effects and toxicity.**

   c. **Route of excretion**   The penicillins and aminoglycosides are excreted by the kidneys. Of the tetracyclines, chlortetracycline is the safest to use in the presence of renal failure. The drugs metabolized primarily by the liver include chloramphenicol, erythromycin, and chlortetracycline.

   d. In general, use **one antibiotic** rather than two.

   e. When there is no response to treatment by the end of 48 hr, the adequacy of antibiotic therapy should be **reevaluated.** Preliminary culture and disk sensitivities should be available by this time. In difficult cases, the bacteriology laboratory can provide precise antibiotic sensitivity levels by determining the minimal inhibitory concentration (MIC) and the minimal bactericidal concentration (MBC). Serum antibiotic levels and serum "killing power" also can be measured.

C. Treatment of severe infection with unidentified bacteria

1. **No infection is so severe as to be treated without first culturing the patient** A Gram stain will prove especially useful in selecting the proper antibiotic. In patients with IV catheters, Gram stain and culture of the catheter

tip can often provide an early diagnosis. Gram stains of an unspun urine specimen may give a clue to the presence of infecting organisms. In septicemia, microorganisms may be seen in Gram stain preparations of the buffy coat of centrifuged blood.

2. In critically ill patients with suspected sepsis, antibiotics have to be administered in advance of bacteriological confirmation. Many regimens are used, depending on the **most likely source of infection:** cephalothin and gentamicin; kanamycin and clindamycin; clindamycin and gentamicin; or cephalothin and kanamycin are combinations often prescribed. It is obvious that no combination will include all potential pathogens; therefore, some clinical judgment is necessary in selecting the most appropriate regimen.

D. **Gram-negative septicemia**   Clinical findings include disturbed sensorium, tachypnea, tachycardia, hypotension, fever, oliguria, and heart failure. In postoperative patients, the sudden appearance of tachypnea and hypotension suggests gram-negative septicemia. This condition has a 30-50% mortality; early diagnosis and treatment improve chance of survival. **Important procedures in successful therapy** include:

1. Ensure adequate **airway.**

2. Monitor **CVP.**

3. Maintain adequate circulatory volume with **IV fluids and blood** on basis of CVP values.

4. If CVP is elevated in the presence of hypotension, use **digitalis.** Give multiple small doses of digoxin or lanatoside C IV until digitalizing dose is reached.

5. If there is no response to volume replacement and urine output is still diminished, use small doses of **isoproterenol.**

6. Avoid methoxamine and use only small doses of **norepinephrine** (Levophed) with adequate volume replacement.

7. Monitor **urine output** hourly.

8. Use of **steroids** is controversial; many authorities do recommend steroids in gram-negative sepsis. When employed they should be given early as a single IV bolus of dexamethasone phosphate, 3-5 mg/kg, or methylprednisolone succinate, 20-40 mg/kg, over a 5-10-min period along with IV fluids.

9. If the identity of the organism is unknown, treat as outlined above for unidentified organism until the results of the **blood cultures** are known. The most important part of therapy is control of the infection.

E. **Bacteriological versus clinical suprainfection**   Changes in the microbial flora of the skin, respiratory tract, and GI tract are seen in most seriously ill patients, regardless of the underlying disease. Resistant gram-negative organisms, staphylococci, and fungi usually colonize such patients shortly after admission to the hospital. Factors increasing the incidence of colonization are antibiotic administration, use of inhalation therapy equipment, immunosuppressive or irradiation therapy, and depressed neurological status. The dilemma for the surgeon is to decide when bacteriological suprainfection becomes clinically significant or is associated with tissue-penetrating disease. One must use clinical parameters such as fever, leukocytosis, purulent sputum or wound discharge, deteriorating status, etc., to make this decision. However, it should be emphasized that *the bacteriology report must be judged in the total clinical setting;* reflex and uncritical use of antimicrobials on the basis of a positive sputum or wound culture is to be avoided.

F. **Antibiotic prophylaxis**   The use of antibiotics for prophylaxis should be directed against specific microorganisms for a limited period. The "umbrella" of antibiotic protection is now recognized to be a myth in routine surgical cases and in uncomplicated deliveries. Attempts to prepare operative sites by prophylactic use of antibiotics often only result in altered flora and bacterial resistance. Similar undesirable effects are produced by injudicious postoperative use of antibiotics.

1. **Patients with valvular or congenital heart disease**   Dental extraction, operations on the GI or genitourinary systems, pregnancy with prolonged labor, and cardiac surgery are known to be associated with bacteremia. In such situations, short-term prophylaxis has been recommended for patients with valvular or congenital heart disease. The following regimens can be used:

   a. **Dental manipulation** and ear, nose, and throat procedures

   (1) 600,000 units procaine penicillin 1 hr prior to procedure. Repeat on each of the next 2 days.

   (2) 600,000 units procaine penicillin 1 hr prior to procedure and an oral penicillin, 400,000 units qid, for 3 days.

   b. **GI and genitourinary system operations**   Administer 1,200,000 units procaine penicillin and 1 gm streptomycin 1 hr prior to procedure and repeat at 12-hr intervals for 3 days.

2. **Cardiac and vascular operations; operations in which a prosthesis or other foreign body is implanted**   There is reasonably good evidence that short-term prophylaxis directed against gram-positive cocci, especially staphylococci, prevents postoperative infection of the prosthesis or the suture line. Cephalothin may be given 1 hr preoperatively (1-2 gm IV) and subsequently every 6 hr during the next 18-24 hr. It is also important to culture the nose and throat preoperatively to detect carriers of staphylococci, pneumococci, and group A streptococci.

3. **Infection-prone patients**   There is no evidence that prophylactic antibiotics alter the incidence of wound infections in patients with diabetes,

malnutrition, cancer, or other causes of diminished bacterial defense mechanisms.

III. SPECIFIC MICROORGANISMS

A. Gram-positive cocci

1. **Staphylococcal** infections are often localized **abscesses** containing creamy, yellow, odorless pus. This organism may also cause **cellulitis** with accompanying lymphangitis. Multiple small pustules suggest staphylococcal bacteremia. Treatment of localized lesions consists of rest, heat, and elevation of the infected area. Incision and drainage are indicated in large localized abscesses or carbuncles. Hospital-acquired staphylococci are almost invariably resistant to penicillin. Staphylococci outside the hospital also have a high incidence of resistance, in some series up to 70%. For this reason, *all staphylococcal infections must be treated with semisynthetic, penicillinase-resistant penicillins* (methicillin, oxacillin, nafcillin, cloxacillin) *or a cephalosporin* until antibiotic sensitivity is determined. Some hospitals have encountered virulent staphylococci resistant to all penicillins and cephalosporins; vancomycin may be useful in treatment of these organisms. Clindamycin, erythromycin, or lincomycin can be employed in patients with penicillin allergy. Staphylococcal wound infections should be treated with antibiotics until purulent drainage has ceased and the patient has become afebrile. Pneumonia or septicemia resulting from staphylococci requires 4 wk of parenteral antibiotic therapy because of the high risk of coexistent endocarditis. When prosthetic devices such as heart valves, neurosurgical drainage valves, or orthopedic pins become infected with staphylococci, antibiotics usually fail to cure the infection and removal of the prosthesis is required.

2. **Streptococci**   Group A streptococci may cause **cellulitis** and erysipelas. Because of the involvement of lymphatics, there is often elevation and edema of the area with red streaking of the skin. **Fasciitis** involves the fascial tissue of wounds; the infection undermines the skin, often resulting in necrosis. These infections spread extremely rapidly and must be treated with large doses of parenteral penicillin (20 million units/day). Drainage and wide debridement also may be indicated. **Burrowing ulcers** are caused by microaerophilic streptococci and coexisting staphylococci (Meleney's ulcer). Such lesions have a characteristic metallic sheen, cause necrosis of large areas of skin, and may produce sinus tracts in the underlying tissue. These should be incised, drained, and treated with large doses of penicillin. **Subacute bacterial endocarditis** is usually caused by *Streptococcus viridans* (70%) or *S. faecalis* (25%). All *S. viridans* are sensitive to penicillin. Six million units/24 hr given parenterally for 4 wk will usually be curative. *S. faecalis* (enterococci) vary in their sensitivity patterns; most strains will be inhibited by penicillin (20 million units/24 hr) in combination with streptomycin (1-2 gm/24 hr) for 4-6 wk. Anaerobic streptococci are normal flora in the mouth and GI tract. In contrast with other streptococcal wound infections, these organisms produce a thin brown discharge, often with crepitation in the infected tissues **(anaerobic celluli-**

tis). Treatment consists of appropriate incision and drainage and parenteral penicillin G, 10–20 million units/24 hr. Other antibiotics which may be effective are cephalosporin, lincomycin, and erythromycin, but not tetracycline.

3. **Pneumococci** are the most common cause of bacterial pneumonia. A Gram stain of the sputum will show numerous gram-positive diplococci, often encapsulated or phagocytosed by polymorphonuclear leukocytes. Pneumococci usually produce **lobar pneumonia,** although bronchopneumonia may occasionally be seen. Complications include empyema, lung abscess, endocarditis, and septic arthritis. **Septicemia** is seen in 25% of cases of pneumococcal pneumonia. Patients may develop toxic encephalitis or pancreatitis. All strains of pneumococci are sensitive to penicillin G. Recommended therapy for pneumonia is 1–2 million units of penicillin/24 hr parenterally in four divided doses. There is no evidence that larger doses of penicillin reduce mortality. Alternative agents are cephalosporin, erythromycin, and lincomycin. Tetracycline-resistant pneumococci have been reported, so that this agent is not generally recommended. The outcome of pneumococcal infections depends on host factors: in many series, the mortality is still 30% despite antibiotic treatment.

B. Gram-positive rods

1. **Clostridia** species are ubiquitous in nature and are present in the GI tract of man and animals. Several species are associated with gas gangrene or anaerobic cellulitis. Clostridial septicemia or intra-abdominal abscess may be found with carcinoma of the large bowel or with traumatic injuries. Many clostridial septicemias are unexplained and the patient may have a benign course even without therapy. Toxin production requires anaerobic conditions such as necrotic and devitalized tissue. All strains of clostridia are sensitive to penicillin. Tetracycline and chloramphenicol are satisfactory alternative drugs. During treatment attempt to alter the anaerobic environment necessary for the growth of these organisms either by surgical debridement or by the use of a hyperbaric oxygen chamber.

2. **Diphtheroids** are the most common organisms present on skin. They are usually contaminants in wounds, but occasionally they may cause septicemia and infections of prosthetic cardiac valves.

3. *Listeria* may cause meningitis or septicemia in patients with cancer or those being treated with immunosuppressive drugs and in whom bacterial defense mechanisms are inhibited or compromised. Most strains of *Listeria monocytogenes* are sensitive to a variety of antibiotics: tetracyclines, penicillins, or aminoglycosides.

C. Gram-negative cocci

1. **Gonococci** most frequently cause genital infections, symptomatic in men, often asymptomatic in women. These organisms also may cause arthritis, meningitis, pharyngitis, ophthalmitis, and endocarditis. Septicemia is

found more frequently with extragenital infections and may be associated with the finding of blood-filled vesicles in the skin.

2. **Meningococci** are introduced through the nasopharynx, producing initial septicemia and then settling out in the meninges, joints, or skin. The Waterhaus-Friderichsen syndrome is an overwhelming meningococcal infection presenting with shock. There is virtually a 100% mortality; patients show hemorrhage of the adrenal glands and evidence of a generalized Shwartzman reaction.

D. **Gram-negative rods**   These organisms are widespread in the GI tract of man and animals and are present everywhere in the hospital environment. Some species are inherently pathogenic, such as *Salmonella* and *Pseudomonas,* while others have little potential for penetrating tissue. However, we have come to recognize that under appropriate circumstances any microorganism can cause disease in man.

1. *Escherichia coli* is the major coliform species in the GI tract. While most strains are sensitive to the majority of antibiotics, those associated with prolonged infections may become highly resistant. *E. coli* is the most common cause of acute urinary tract infections. It is also the major cause of septicemia.

2. *Klebsiella-Enterobacter (Aerobacter)* species are present in the GI tract, in contaminated food, and in the hospital environment. *Klebsiella* are generally sensitive to cephalosporin and resistant to carbenicillin, while enterobacter species show the reverse pattern. Thickly encapsulated *Klebsiella* (types 1-6) may cause Friedländer's pneumonia. Other strains cause urinary tract infections, intra-abdominal infections, and gram-negative pneumonia.

3. *Proteus* species may be inhabitants of the GI tract and are found in the hospital environment, especially in moist crevices. Indole-negative strains *(mirabilis)* are the most common cause of genitourinary infections and are usually sensitive to penicillins. Indole-positive strains (*rettgeri, morganii,* and *vulgaris*) cause more stubborn infections, resistant to many antimicrobial agents. Gentamicin and carbenicillin may be effective antibiotics against these species. Because of the urea-splitting properties of *Proteus* strains, discharges from these infections are generally alkaline and have an ammonia smell.

4. *Pseudomonas* has become the most common gram-negative suprainfecting organism in many hospitals. These bacteria thrive in a moist environment and often contaminate respiratory equipment, soap dishes, and improperly dried instruments. *Pseudomonas* cause necrotizing wound and pulmonary infections, with invasion of blood vessels. Discharges are often green with a distinctive odor from pyocine production. Most *Pseudomonas* strains currently are sensitive to gentamicin, but there has been an alarming increase of resistant strains. More resistance is seen to carbenicillin, and strains may acquire resistance to this antibiotic during a single course of therapy. It is advisable to use gentamicin and carbenicillin in combination for serious *Pseudomonas* infections.

5. **Serratia** species were formerly considered to be nonpathogenic. Recently, they have been associated with infections resulting from IV catheters. They may produce septicemia, endocarditis, and genitourinary infections. Approximately 20% of pathogenic strains are pigmented, and discharges may show a characteristic red color. *Serratia* are resistant to the majority of antibiotics; gentamicin or kanamycin is recommended for these infections.

6. **Salmonellae** are present in animal or bird products or may be transmitted by human carriers. These organisms usually cause **mild gastroenteritis.** Antibiotic treatment of gastroenteritis is not advised, since it does not reduce the severity of clinical symptoms and may only prolong the carrier state. Antibiotic therapy is recommended for **septicemia, typhoidal symptoms, osteomyelitis, and localized abscesses.** For serious salmonellae infections, chloramphenicol is the drug of choice. Ampicillin may be used in milder cases. Antibiotics usually fail to eradicate the carrier state. In patients who are food handlers or who work in a hospital, cholecystectomy may be the only method of eradicating the carrier state of these organisms. Salmonellae may also cause food-borne epidemics within a hospital.

7. **Herrella-mimae** is a mixed group of gram-negative rods and cocci inhabiting the mouth and GI tract. They may cause infection in a compromised host. These organisms are generally resistant to penicillin but sensitive to most broad-spectrum antibiotics.

E. **Anaerobic bacteria**   This diverse group of fastidious microorganisms includes both gram-negative and gram-positive rods and cocci. They are the predominant members of the endogenous microflora of the human mouth, colon, and vagina and are found in high concentrations in other GI organs. Since the advent of improved anaerobic bacteriological collection and isolation techniques, obligate anaerobes have been isolated with increasing frequency from widely varied clinical infections. The critical factor necessary for the growth of anerobes is an environment with decreased oxygen content such as that found in abscesses, empyemas, and necrotizing infections.

1. **Oral anaeobes** include *Bacteroides, Peptostreptococcus, Bifidobacteria, Fusobacterium,* and *Actinomyces.* These anerobes are isolated in high concentrations particularly in dental plaque and around the periodontal membrane. They are noted to increase in patients with poor dental hygiene. These organisms result in local sepsis following head and neck surgery. If aspirated, they can result in lung abscess, putrid empyema, and necrotizing pneumonitis. These microorganisms are generally highly sensitive to penicillin and the cephalosporins. Treatment of actinomycosis requires long-term, high-dose penicillin therapy.

2. **Intestinal anaerobes** include the oral anaerobes swallowed with saliva and food that transiently inhabit the upper GI tract in low numbers ($<10^4$). In the distal ileum and colon, however, a resident anaerobic microflora of high concentrations (10^4-10^{10}) exists. *B. fragilis* and *Clostridium* are major members of this flora along with *Peptostreptococcus* and *Fusobacterium.* These colonic anaerobes frequently are associated with intra-ab-

dominal and pelvic abscess, wound abscess, septicemia, and septic thrombophlebitis following colonic resection, penetrating traumatic colon injuries, or perforated appendicitis or diverticulitis. Treatment of these complications should include drainage, where indicated, in addition to parenteral antibiotics.

B. fragilis, the anaerobe most commonly implicated in these infections, is resistant to penicillin and should be treated parenterally with either clindamycin or chloramphenicol. Less desirable alternatives are lincomycin, erythromycin, or tetracycline. Currently 30-40% of these organisms are resistant to tetracyclines.

3. **Vaginal anaerobes** include the same organisms mentioned under intestinal anaerobes. Vaginal cuff or pelvic abscess following hysterectomy, and septic endometritis following childbirth or abortion, frequently are due to these organisms either alone or in combination with aerobic coliforms. When *B. fragilis* is suspected or isolated, treatment should include parenteral clindamycin or chloramphenicol.

F. Fungi

1. *Candida albicans* is the most frequent fungus infection complicating surgical therapy. Oral thrush may be treated with general mouth care and nystatin gargles. Candidal septicemia usually is caused by an indwelling IV catheter, especially when the patient is being hyperalimented. In most cases, removal of the catheter will abort the disease. Persistent fungemia or endocarditis requires intensive amphotericin B therapy. Compromised hosts are particularly susceptible to generalized candidiasis.

2. **Histoplasmosis, coccidioidomycosis, and blastomycosis** are generalized fungal infections less commonly seen in surgical practice. These infections are treated with amphotericin B and, in selected cases, with surgical excision of the infective focus. **Sporotrichosis** presents as a localized lesion of the extremity with lymphangitic spread; occasionally, generalized infections involving the lung and bone may occur. *Cryptococcus* usually causes meningitis or pulmonary infections.

G. **Viruses**   The role of viral infections in the surgical patient is generally not well understood owing primarily to the difficulty of the techniques necessary for investigation of these organisms. Many types of viruses have been implicated in appendicitis and intussusception in children as well as in pancreatitis in adults. Viral infections due to cytomegalovirus have been observed in immunologically impaired patients with malignancy or after renal transplantation.

IV. ANTIBIOTICS

A. Penicillin

1. **Crystalline benzyl penicillin,** sodium or potassium salt, aqueous (penicillin G)

   a. **Highly effective against many species of gram-positive and some gram-negative microorganisms**   All group A, beta-hemolytic streptococci,

S. viridans, and pneumococci are sensitive, but group D strains (enterococcus) are variably sensitive. First choice for sensitive staphylococci, but ineffective against penicillinase-producing strains. Gonococci and meningococci are sensitive, as are *Corynebacterium diphtheriae, Listeria monocytogenes, Treponema pallidum,* clostridia, and *Actinomyces.* Some species of gram-negative enteric bacteria are affected by penicillin in high concentrations. This group includes *E. coli, P. mirabilis,* and many strains of salmonellae and shigellae.

b. Mechanism of action   Interferes with cell wall formation by inhibiting synthesis of muramic acid. Active mainly against rapidly growing organisms.

c. Absorption   Orally one third to one half is absorbed; drug is destroyed by gastric acid. Peak plasma level in 1-2 hr. Parenterally, peak blood level in 15-30 min, with effect lasting 3-4 hr, depending on renal function.

d. Distribution   Low concentrations (one tenth of serum) in meningeal, pericardial, and pleural spaces; significant concentrations in joints and bile; and very high concentrations in kidney. When meninges are inflamed, penicillin penetrates into spinal fluid more readily.

e. Excretion   From 60-90% of dose excreted in urine, 90% by tubular excretion. Probenecid (0.5 gm/6 hr) will block tubular excretion and raise serum levels.

f. Preparations

(1) Aqueous (crystalline) penicillin

(a) Oral potassium penicillin G or sodium penicillin G in tablets of 50,000-500,000 units. Given every 6 hr, either ½ hr before or 2 hr after meals.

(b) Parenteral   Buffered or unbuffered potassium penicillin G in ampules of 1, 5, or 20 million units. Given every 4-6 hr by IM or IV injection. Available as a potassium or sodium salt (1.5 mEq/million units). Advantage: high peak levels. Disadvantages: rapid excretion, painful injection.

(2) Procaine penicillin   For IM use only. Procaine penicillin and procaine penicillin with aluminum monostearate suspension available in 1-ml cartridges and 10-ml vials, 300,000 units/ml. Limit dose in single site to 2 ml. Advantages: prolonged serum levels (24-36 hr), painless injections. Disadvantage: low serum (<1 mg/ml) and tissue levels.

(3) Benzathine penicillin G (Bicillin)   IM use only. Same spectrum and action as crystalline penicillin. Low concentrations in blood are present for 20-30 days. Recommended for rheumatic fever prophylaxis.

2. **Phenoxymethyl penicillin**   Is more stable in gastric acid than penicillin G and is better absorbed after an oral dose. Available as Pen-Vee, Compocillin-VK, Pen-Vee K, and V-Cillin K in tablets of 125, 250, and 500 mg (125 mg equals 200,000 units). **Phenoxyethyl penicillin** may produce slightly higher blood levels than phynoxymethyl penicillin. Available as Syncillin and Maxipen in tablets of 125 mg and 250 mg.

3. **Ampicillin**   Less effective than penicillin G against sensitive gram-positive cocci, but more active against *Hemophilus influenzae, E. coli*, and some strains of *Proteus, Enterobacter, Salmonella*, and *Shigella*. Ineffective against *Pseudomonas* species. It is destroyed by penicillinase. Well absorbed after oral administration, with peak blood level reached in 1–2 hr. Excreted in urine and bile. Ampicillin (Penbritin, Polycillin) is available orally as 250- and 500-mg capsules; for parenteral use in vials of 250 mg–2.0 gm.

4. **Penicillinase-resistant penicillins**

   a. **Indicated** for treatment of infections caused by penicillinase-producing *Staphylococcus aureus*. These drugs are not as effective as penicillin G against other gram-positive organisms and have little effect on gram-negative bacteria. Mode of action is interference with cell wall synthesis.

   b. **Excreted** unchanged in the urine in the same manner as penicillin G.

   c. **Preparations**

      (1) Methicillin sodium (Staphcillin). Ampules of 1, 4, or 6 gm. Inactivated by gastric acid and is only available for parenteral use. Dose is 3–4 gm/6 hr IV or IM.

      (2) Oxacillin sodium (Prostaphlin). 250 or 500 mg capsules. Also available in parenteral form.

      (3) Cloxacillin sodium (Tegopen). Resembles oxacillin.

      (4) Nafcillin sodium (Unipen). Available as 250-mg capsules or 500-mg ampules. Higher excretion in bile.

5. **Carbenicillin** is semisynthetic benzyl penicillin with good activity against gram-negative organisms but relatively poor activity against gram-positive strains. It is destroyed by penicillinase and should not be used in staphylococcal infections. Sensitive organisms include *Pseudomonas, Proteus* (both indole-positive and -negative), *Enterobacter* (but not *Klebsiella*), and *E. coli*. IV dose for serious illnesses is 6–8 gm/6 hr. Smaller doses (1–2 gm/6 hr IV) can be used in urinary tract infections. Oral preparations are available, but absorption is poor, resulting in low blood levels. Oral carbenicillin should not be used in serious infections.

6. **Reactions to penicillin** and its analogs

    a. **Hypersensitivity effects**   Skin rashes, glossitis, stomatitis, fever, eosinophilia, angioneurotic edema, serum sickness, anaphylaxis, and Arthus reaction. These reactions may occur in 10-15% of patients treated with a penicillin preparation. However, a penicillin reaction does not necessarily render the patient sensitive to penicillin for life; most patients lose their hypersensitivity to the drug after some months or years. Before treating any patient with penicillin who has a questionable history of allergy, a skin test is mandatory. Penicillin G is diluted to a concentration of 1,000 units/ml. A superficial scratch is made with a needle in the anterior forearm and 1 drop of the penicillin solution is placed in the scratch. A positive wheal-flare reaction will occur within 15-20 min. If the scratch test is negative, an intradermal injection of the dilute penicillin solution should be attempted. Negative reactions to these tests give reasonable assurance that an anaphylactic reaction will not occur. It should be stressed that there is cross-sensitization among all penicillin preparations. The least sensitizing route is oral, followed by intradermal, IM, and, the most challenging, IV.

    b. **Renal insufficiency** has been reported with use of the semisynthetic compounds and rarely with penicillin G.

    c. **Bone marrow depression** is a rare complication of therapy with semisynthetic penicillins.

    d. **CNS toxicity** is seen with all penicillins after very high doses, i.e., 40-80 million units of penicillin G, or with smaller doses of penicillins in the presence of renal insufficiency. The reaction begins with myoclonic twitching, proceeding to generalized seizures. Reducing the dose of penicillin will terminate the reaction; no sequelae have been reported.

    e. **Irritative effects**   Epigastric distress and diarrhea may occur.

B. **Cephalosporin**

1. **The cephalosporins have a structure similar to that of the penicillins;** hence, there is some cross-allergenicity. They are effective against gram-positive organisms, including penicillin-sensitive and resistant staphylococci, streptococci, *Neisseria, Salmonella, P. mirabilis,* and most *E. coli* and *Klebsiella.* They are not effective against *Pseudomonas, Serratia,* indole-positive *Proteus,* enterococci, and *Enterobacter.*

2. **Mechanism of action**   Interference with cell wall synthesis.

3. **Absorption**   IM or IV injection gives peak blood levels in 30 min. Cephalexin is 50% absorbed when given orally; low blood levels are achieved with oral preparations. Cephalosporins penetrate poorly into the meninges and should not be used in CNS infections.

4. Excretion   From 70–80% excreted unchanged in the urine by glomerular filtration and some tubular excretion.

5. Preparations   Cephalothin (Keflin) is available as 10- and 50-ml ampules containing 1 and 4 gm of antibiotic, respectively, for IM or IV injection. Special IV ampules of 2 or 4 gm are available for dilution with 50–100 ml of 5% dextrose in water. Cephaloridine (Loridine) is available for parenteral administration as a dry powder for reconstitution with sterile water in 5- and 10-ml ampules containing 0.5 and 1.0 gm of antibiotic, respectively. Cephalexin (Keflex) is supplied in 250-mg capsules for oral administration.

6. Reactions to the cephalosporins

   a. Hypersensitivity effects   Eosinophilia, fever, skin rashes, and serum sickness are reported. An increased incidence of reactions has occurred in penicillin-sensitive individuals.

   b. Toxic effects   Cases of neutropenia and depressed leukopoiesis have been reported. Cephaloridine is a frequent cause of renal insufficiency; the dose of this drug should never exceed 4 gm/24 hr.

   c. Irritative effects   Thrombophlebitis and pain on IM injection are frequently seen with cephalothin.

C. Tetracycline

1. The first broad-spectrum antibiotics, the tetracyclines, are **effective** against many gram-positive and gram-negative organisms, as well as inhibiting growth of rickettsiae, amebas, *Mycoplasma,* and agents of the psittacosis and lymphogranuloma venereum group. Nearly all strains of *Proteus* and *Pseudomonas* and many staphylococci and enterococci are resistant. Strains of *E. coli, Klebsiella,* and *Enterobacter* vary widely in sensitivity. Anaerobic streptococci and 30–50% of *B. fragilis* strains are resistant.

2. Mechanism of action   Inhibition of protein synthesis; these drugs are bacteriostatic.

3. Absorption   Incompletely absorbed after oral administration. Most active in the stomach and upper small bowel. Absorption decreased by milk products and antacids as a result of chelating effect. After oral doses, peak levels in 2–4 hr, lasting 6 or more hr. Demethylchlortetracycline and doxycyline produce significant blood levels for 12–24 hr.

4. The tetracyclines are widely **distributed** in tissues. Diffusion across the blood-brain barrier is good, even with noninflamed meninges. High concentrations are found in bile.

5. Excretion   From 20–60% of IV dose excreted in urine in first 24 hr; a high proportion is protein-bound. Demethylchlortetracycline and doxycycline are longer-acting, owing to a decreased rate of renal excretion.

6. Preparations

a. Oral use Chlortetracycline hydrochloride, oxytetracycline, and tetracycline hydrochloride are available as 250-mg capsules. Demethylchlortetracycline is available as 75-, 150-, and 300-mg capsules. Doxycycline is prepared in 50-mg capsules.

b. Parenteral use Tetracycline preparations are supplied in 100-, 250-, or 500-mg vials. Parenteral doses are half those used orally.

c. Ophthalmic preparations are available for local application.

7. Reactions to tetracyclines

a. Hypersensitivity effects Cheilosis, brown or black coating of the tongue, glossitis, vaginitis, and pruritus ani are relatively frequent side effects. Morbilliform rashes, dermatitis, angioneurotic edema, eosinophilia, and anaphlyaxis occur, but are rare.

b. Toxic effects Patients receiving large doses of tetracycline may develop jaundice and fatty liver. Pregnant women are especially prone to the development of hepatotoxicity. Other effects include delay in blood coagulation, brown discoloration of teeth (in infants), increased intracranial pressure, and azotemia. Outdated drug may produce the Fanconi syndrome.

c. Irritative effects GI irritation manifested by epigastric burning, nausea, emesis, and diarrhea. IV administration frequently followed by thrombophlebitis. IM use can lead to suppurative myositis. Photosensitivity of skin occurs with demethylchlortetracycline.

d. Suprainfection Overgrowth of resistant microorganisms can cause staphylococcal enterocolitis, pseudomembranous colitis, and intestinal candidiasis.

D. Chloramphenicol

1. Primarily bacteriostatic, chloramphenicol has a wide spectrum of activity. It has an **inhibitory effect** against *E. coli, K. pneumoniae, H. influenzae, Sal. typhosa,* certain strains of *Proteus, Shigella,* and *Brucella,* some streptococci and staphylococci, the rickettsiae, and the psittacosis-lymphogranuloma groups of organisms. Most anaerobes (*Bacteroides,* fusiforms, streptococci) are sensitive.

2. **Mechanism of action** Inhibition of protein synthesis.

3. **Absorption** Rapidly absorbed after oral administration.

4. **Distribution** Present in bile and CSF in high concentration. Penetrates tissues in high levels.

5. **Excretion** Excreted in the urine (80-90%), but only 5-10% is in biologically active form.

6. **Preparation**   Chloramphenicol is available as capsules of 50, 100, and 250 mg. Parenteral and ophthalmic forms are also available. IM route should not be used because of poor absorption.

7. **Reactions to chloramphenicol**

   a. **Hypersensitivity effects**   Agranulocytosis occurs in one in 30,000 administrations of this drug. This reaction is not dose-related. It usually follows a previous sensitizing dose. Most fatal cases are associated with inappropriate use for trivial viral infections. Bone marrow shows maturation arrest with vacuolization of granulocyte precursors. Skin rashes, fever, stomatitis, and anaphylaxis are rarely seen.

   b. **Toxic effects**   Anemia with a low reticulocyte count and increased serum iron is a dose-related, reversible effect. The "gray syndrome" is seen in premature infants and neonates who are unable to excrete chloramphenicol, producing cyanosis, tachypnea, circulatory collapse, emesis, and diarrhea.

   c. **Irritative effects**   GI disturbances are seen with oral therapy.

   d. **Suprainfection** may occur, especially with *Candida* or staphylococci.

8. **Indications for chloramphenicol therapy**   Typhoid fever, rickettsial infections, and serious *Salmonella* infections should be treated with chloramphenicol. Bacterial meningitis in a penicillin-sensitive patient can be treated with chloramphenicol. *Bacteroides* infections and anaerobic abscesses also are indications for use of this drug.

E. **Erythromycin**

1. This drug belongs to the macrolide class of antibiotics. It is **effective** against gram-positive cocci, i.e., group A streptococci, pneumococci, and 95% of staphylococci, including penicillinase-producers. Some strains of *H. influenzae, Listeria, Brucella,* and *Treponema* are also sensitive. Anaerobic microorganisms such as *Bacteroides, Peptostreptococci,* and *Clostridium* also usually are sensitive. *Proteus, E. coli, Enterobacter, Klebsiella,* and *Pseudomonas* are resistant.

2. **Mechanism of action**   Interference with protein synthesis.

3. **Absorption**   From 40-70% is absorbed in the upper small bowel. Peak plasma levels appear in 1-4 hr.

4. **Distribution**   Diffuses readily into body fluids. CSF levels are low.

5. **Excretion**   Excreted by the liver and pancreas. From 5-15% is excreted in the urine.

6. **Preparations**

   a. **Oral**   Erythromycin and erythromycin stearate (Erythrocin stearate) are available as 125- and 250-mg capsules. Dose is 250 mg-1 gm/6 hr.

Where utilized in preoperative bowel preparation, erythromycin base should be used because this drug is in the active form in the intestinal lumen, not first requiring absorption and biochemical alteration for its activity.

b. Parenteral use is not recommended. IM injections are painful and cause myositis.

7. Toxic effects

a. Hypersensitivity effects Skin rashes, angioneurotic edema, serum sickness, and anaphylaxis. Cholestatic jaundice may occur with the estolate preparation. Liver biopsy shows periportal infiltration, mostly with eosinophils.

b. Irritative effects GI upset, vaginitis, and pruritus have been noted. Severe diarrhea may occur.

F. Lincomycin

1. This drug resembles erythromycin and can be used in place of it when parenteral therapy is needed in penicillin-sensitive patients who harbor gram-positive coccal infections. It has good **activity** against group A streptococci, pneumococci, and 95% of staphylococci. Anaerobic infections with *Bacteroides* and anaerobic streptococci are successfully treated with lincomycin.

2. Absorption Absorbed soon after oral administration; peak blood levels are obtained in 2-4 hr. IM and IV absorption is also good, with peak levels in 30 min, persisting for 8-12 hr.

3. Distribution CSF penetration is poor; otherwise distributes readily in most body tissues.

4. Excretion Up to 25% is excreted by kidney in urine.

5. Preparations Available in capsules of 250 and 500 mg and vials of 600 mg. Usual adult IM or IV dose is 600 mg/8 hr.

6. Side effects Diarrhea in most patients is a dose-related phenomenon with oral therapy. Diarrhea may be severe in 10% of patients, occasionally being associated with passage of blood and on rare occasions leading to a clinical picture similar to ulcerative colitis. Skin rashes have been reported. Liver toxicity is occasionally seen with high doses.

G. Clindamycin

1. This drug is a derivative of lincomycin differing only by the substitution of a chloride for a hydroxyl group on the lincomycin molecule. This change has resulted in better absorption and greater potency against anaerobic *B. fragilis* organisms. This drug also has increased activity against group A streptococci, pneumococci, and staphylococci.

2. **Absorption**   Absorbed rapidly after oral administration; peak blood levels are obtained within 1-2 hr. Parenteral absorption takes place rapidly, with peak serum levels occurring at about 10 min after IV administration and about 3 hr after IM administration.

3. **Distribution**   CSF penetration is poor; otherwise this agent distributes readily in most body tissues.

4. **Excretion**   Mainly in the bile, with from 5-25% appearing in the urine.

5. **Preparations**   Available in 75- and 150-mg capsules and in vials of 300, 600, 900 mg. Usual adult IV dose is 600 mg q6-8h.

6. **Side effects**   Fewer GI complaints than with lincomycin; otherwise very similar side effects. Diarrhea, occasionally of severe nature, primarily follows oral administration. Discontinuing this agent usually results in alleviation of diarrheal symptoms. Antidiarrheal medications should be avoided for fear of increasing toxicity.

H. Streptomycin

1. Because of high incidence of bacterial resistance, the indications for streptomycin are relatively limited. It is combined with penicillin in treating enterococcal or *H. influenzae* infections, brucellosis, tularemia, and plague, and combined with INH (isoniazid) in treating tuberculosis.

2. **Resistant bacteria**   Exposure to the drug may convert highly sensitive strains to resistant ones in as short as 48 hr. Delay in emergence of bacterial resistance is achieved by combination with other antibiotics.

3. **Mechanism of action**   Interference with protein synthesis.

4. **Absorption**   Poorly absorbed orally. IM and subcutaneous injections are well absorbed.

5. **Distribution**   Streptomycin is distributed in the extracellular fluids, especially in the pericardial and peritoneal cavities. Pleural and synovial fluids also contain appreciable drug activity. With normal meninges, CSF penetration is poor.

6. **Excretion**   From 50-60% is excreted unchanged in urine in the first 24 hr. A small portion is excreted in the bile. The feces contain a small amount.

7. **Preparation**   Streptomycin sulfate is available for parenteral injection in vials containing 0.5, 1, or 5 gm. Dose of 1 gm/24 hr IM may be given for 30-45 days. For tuberculosis therapy, 1 gm three times a week is used.

8. **Reactions to streptomycin**

   a. **Hypersensitivity effects**   Skin rashes, fever, blood dyscrasias, stomatitis, anaphylaxis, exfoliative dermatitis, and eosinophilia.

      b. Toxic effects   Most important effects involve the eighth nerve. Patients receiving 2 gm or more per 24 hr for more than 1–2 wk may manifest vestibular disturbance; recovery may require 12–18 mo. Neural disturbances in hearing also occur; a high-pitched tinnitus is often the first sign of toxicity; nerve deafness often is not reversible. Scotomas, peripheral neuritis, apnea, and encephalopathy also are reported. Toxic renal effects are manifested by proteinuria and reduced volume of urine flow.

      c. Irritative effects   Pain at site of injection; sterile abscesses.

I. Kanamycin

1. Kanamycin is **effective** against *E. coli, Enterobacter, Klebsiella, Salmonella, Shigella, Neisseria,* and *S. aureus.* Most strains of *Proteus, Bacteroides,* and *Pseudomonas* are resistant.

2. **Mechanism of action**   Causes incorrect transcription of messenger RNA within bacteria.

3. **Absorption**   Poorly absorbed orally. IM injection produces peak levels in 1 hr.

4. **Distribution**   Diffuses into most body fluids in significant concentrations. CSF penetration is poor.

5. **Excretion**   From 50–80% is recovered in the urine.

6. **Preparation**   Kanamycin sulfate (Kantrex) is available in vials of 250 and 500 mg and as oral capsules of 0.5 gm. The IM or IV dosage in adults with normal renal function is 15 mg/kg/24 hr in two divided doses.

7. **Side effects**

      a. Hypersensitivity effects   These include eosinophilia fever, rashes, and pruritus.

      b. Toxic effects   Ototoxicity (damage to both the cochlear and vestibular parts) and nephrotoxicity (hematuria, proteinuria, and cylindruria) are the most important effects. Nephrotoxicity is reversible on cessation of treatment. Kanamycin has a curare-like action on neuromuscular transmission; paralysis of respiration has been reported following intraperitoneal instillation of the drug.

      c. Irritative effects   These include GI distress, stomatitis, proctitis.

J. Gentamicin

1. Gentamicin is an aminoglycoside with good **activity** against *Pseudomonas,* indole-positive *Proteus, Enterobacter, Klebsiella, E. coli, Serratia,* and *Staphylococcus.* It is the preferred treatment for *Pseudomonas* infections and resistant gram-negative infections acquired in the hospital.

2. Mechanism of action   Interference with protein synthesis.

3. Absorption   Poorly absorbed orally. IM injection gives peak levels in 30–60 min, which persist for 8–12 hr.

4. Excretion   Mainly by glomerular filtration.

5. Preparation   Gentamicin is available in single-use vials (40 mg/cc) or in multiple-dose vials. Approved for IM and IV use. Initial dose in serious infections is 5 mg/kg/24 hr in three divided doses; thereafter, 1–3 mg/kg/24 hr in three divided doses. In renal insufficiency the same initial 24-hr dose is used but subsequent dosage is reduced (see Chap. 11).

6. Toxic effects   These occur primarily in the renal systems and the eighth nerve (usually vestibular). The renal deficits are usually reversible; auditory losses are usually permanent. Toxicity of gentamicin is similar to other aminoglycosides and the effects are additive.

K. Polymyxins

1. The polymyxins are bactericidal against gram-negative bacteria, including many strains of *Pseudomonas. Proteus* species are usually resistant.

2. Mechanism of action   Interference with lipoprotein in cell membranes, causing permeability changes in bacterial cell wall.

3. Absorption   Not absorbed orally. After parenteral administration, peak levels are reached in 1–2 hr.

4. Distribution   CSF penetration is poor even in the face of meningitis.

5. Excretion   Via kidney, although excretion is delayed.

6. Preparations   Polymyxin B (Aerosporin) is available in vials of 20 and 50 mg for parenteral injection; the usual adult dose is 2.5 mg/kg/24 hr in four divided doses. Colistin (Coly-Mycin) (Polymyxin E) is marketed for IM use in vials of 150 mg. The average adult dose is 5 mg/kg/24 hr in three divided doses. The dose of either drug should be reduced in the presence of renal insufficiency.

7. Reactions to the polymyxins

a. Hypersensitivity effects   Drug fever, skin rashes, pruritus, dizziness, and transient paresthesias.

b. Toxic effects   Severe ataxia, leukopenia, and granulocytopenia. A curare-like effect leading to respiratory arrest has been reported with colistin.

c. Irritative effects   GI disturbances; pain at injection sites.

SUGGESTED READING
Gorbach, S. L., Bartlett, J. G., and Nichols, R. L. *Management of Surgical Infections.* Boston: Little, Brown. To be published.

V. PROPHYLACTIC USE OF ANTIBIOTICS

A. Parenteral preoperative antibiotics

1. Much controversy exists concerning the use and value of prophylactic parenteral antibiotics. There appears to be no value in their use in clean operative procedures such as hernia repair or thyroidectomy. In clean-contaminated and contaminated cases, antibiotics appear to be of value if appropriate agents are started early and continued only for short periods of time (2-4 days).

2. Experimental and clinical studies have shown that if antibiotics are to prevent formation of a primary infection, they must be given within 3 hr of tissue contamination. Practically speaking, this means that antibiotics should be started during the immediate preoperative period in cases in which bacterial contamination is highly likely or known to be present. This will provide tissue levels of the antibiotic at the time the bacterial invasion occurs.

3. The choice of antibiotics depends on a knowledge of the nature of the offending microflora and on the expected antibiotic sensitivies of these microorganisms. When the GI tract is the source of the bacterial contamination, antibiotics that suppress both the aerobic coliforms and anaerobic bacteroides should be given. When the operating room environment and the patient's skin are the source of contamination, as in most cardiovascular and orthopedic cases, antibiotics active against aerobic streptococci and staphylococci should be employed.

4. The **prophylactic use of antibiotics appears to be indicated** in the following types of operative procedures:

   a. Cases where the **host resistance is altered,** such as metabolic derangements, agammaglobulinemia, anemia, and chronic corticosteroid or immunosuppressive therapy.

   b. Orthopedic procedures involving **fixation of open fractures** or **implantation of large foreign bodies,** such as total hip replacement.

   c. Operative procedures (including dental work) done in **patients with valvular heart disease or indwelling cardiac prosthetic valves.**

   d. Operative procedures done with **extracorporeal heart-lung bypass.**

   e. Peripheral vascular procedures that include the use of **prosthetic grafts.**

f. Soft tissue traumatic injuries where there has been a delay in surgical debridement or where tissue of questionable viability has been left behind.

g. Penetrating traumatic injuries of the chest or abdominal cavity.

h. Cases where emergency operation is necessary in the face of an **active infection elsewhere in the body.**

i. GI procedures where **heavy contamination** is present, as in gangrenous cholecystitis, perforated appendicitis, or diverticulitis, and also in cases where bowel resection with open anastomosis is done in the face of an unprepared bowel.

B. Preoperative bowel preparation

1. **Nonintestinal operations**   If a patient is to have a general anesthetic, the colon should be evacuated the night before the operation. An empty colon may be an aid in exposure, but the principal reason for emptying the colon is to avert uncontrolled defecation with its hazard of contamination. Colonic evacuation is promoted by enemas in patients who cannot defecate spontaneously.

2. **Small-bowel operations**   As the small-bowel content is liquid and transit time is rapid, preparation usually is unnecessary. Restricting alimentation 8–12 hr prior to operation usually will suffice. Preoperative antibiotic preparation should be employed, however, when distal ileal operations are planned because of the resident bacterial microflora present at this level of the intestine.

3. **Colon operations**

   a. The **objectives** of preparation of the large bowel are removal of the feces from the bowel lumen and reduction of the bacterial population.

   b. Methods used to accomplish preparation of the colon are (a) reduction in residue content of the diet, (b) chemical and mechanical stimulation and evacuation of the bowel, and (c) administration of antibiotics.

   c. Mechanical cleansing of the colon is the most important single element in preparation. Properly done, mechanical cleansing alone will remove all feces and reduce the numbers of bacteria in the bowel.

   d. Antibiotic bowel preparation is ineffective if mechanical cleansing has not been accomplished.

   e. Stimulant cathartics act by increasing peristalsis, either by irritating the mucosa or by acting on the autonomic intramural plexuses in the bowel wall. In this group of agents, bisacodyl (Dulcolax) or dioctyl calcium sulfosuccinate (Surfak) is preferred. Do not use castor oil; it is unnecessarily unpleasant.

f. Saline cathartics are slowly absorbed salts that act osmotically to increase the volume of bowel content and stimulate peristalsis. Because they bring fluid into the bowel lumen, saline cathartics help keep feces in a more fluid state, thereby promoting evacuation. In this group of agents, magnesium sulfate is the agent of choice.

g. Nonabsorbable sulfonamides require several days to accomplish a maximal reduction in colonic bacterial flora. During this period, overgrowth of yeasts and other organisms causes diarrhea, which is undesirable. Therefore, sulfonamides are not used in antibiotic preparation of the colon.

h. Neomycin and kanamycin are effective in 24-36 hr in reducing the aerobic colonic microflora. Both agents afford only irregular suppression of the fecal anaerobes, including *Bacteroides,* the most numerous fecal bacteria.

i. Neomycin in combination with erythromycin base has been found to suppress adequately the entire colonic microflora, and is the combination of choice for bowel preparation. Erythromycin base is used because this form of the drug is active in the intestinal lumen, not first requiring absorption and metabolism for activity against the colonic anaerobes. The following is recommended for colon preparation:

Day 1: Low-residue diet.
        Bisacodyl, 1 capsule at 6 P.M.
Day 2: Continue low-residue diet.
        Magnesium sulfate, 30 ml of 50% solution (15 gm) at 10 A.M., 2 P.M., and 6 P.M.
Day 3: Neomycin, 1 gm, and erythromycin base, 1 gm, orally at 1 P.M., 2 P.M., and 11 P.M.
        Clear liquid diet.
        Magnesium sulfate, 30 ml of 50% solution at 10 A.M. and 2 P.M.
        No enemas.
        IV maintenance fluids started if clinically indicated.
Day 4: Operation at 8 A.M.

j. Complications

(1) Dehydration can be prevented by maintaining oral or IV fluid intake at 3,000 ml/day during the mechanical and antibiotic preparation of the colon.

(2) Enterocolitis resulting from overgrowth of yeasts or resistant staphylococci is now uncommon; the first clue is passage of a small diarrheal stool through the anus or colostomy early in the postoperative period. Gram stain a smear of the first postoperative stool; if predominant gram-positive cocci are seen, start treatment. Staphylococcal overgrowth requires a systemic antibiotic such as dimethoxyphenyl penicillin (methicillin), 1 gm every 4 hr IM or IV. In addition, give vancomycin, 2 gm stat, then 1 gm every 6 hr orally, which will be effective against staphylococci within the bowel. If the overgrowth is of yeasts, resumption of oral intake is the best measure; repopulation of the bowel with *Lact. acidophilus* (Bacid or Lactinex, 2 capsules bid) may be of limited help.

SUGGESTED READING

Burke, J. F.   The effective period of preventive antibiotic action in experimental incisions and dermal lesions. *Surgery* 50:161, 1961.

Fullen, W. D., Hunt, J., and Altemeier, W. A.   Prophylactic antibiotics in penetrating wounds of the abdomen. *J. Trauma* 12:282, 1972.

Nichols, R. L., Broido, P., Condon, R. E., Gorbach, S. L., and Nyhus, L. M.   Effect of preoperative neomycin-erythromycin intestinal preparation on the incidence of infectious complications following colon surgery. *Ann. Surg.* 178:453, 1973.

Polk, H. C., Jr., and Lopez-Mayor, J. F.   Postoperative wound infection: A prospective study of determinant factors and prevention. *Surgery* 66:97, 1969.

VI. WOUND AND SOFT TISSUE INFECTIONS

A. Prevention

1. All wounds, including those made at the operating table as well as those resulting from civil or military trauma, provide a perfect environment for bacterial growth.

2. **Infections can be minimized** if wound management follows these principles:

    a. Minimize contamination by use of aseptic techniques.

    b. Remove all debris, devitalized tissue, and foreign bodies.

    c. Achieve complete hemostasis.

    d. Preserve blood supply.

    e. Handle tissue gently to keep operative trauma at a minimum.

    f. Avoid and eliminate dead space during closure.

    g. Close the wound with careful layer-to-layer approximation without tension.

    h. Keep operative time at a minimum to reduce numbers of bacteria in wound.

    i. Lavage the wound with liberal amounts of sterile saline before closure of the skin and subcutaneous tissue.

3. **Do not depend on antibiotics to make up for errors or carelessness in wound management.**

B. Therapy of established infections

1. Treatment measures available

   a. Local moist heat relieves pain and increases blood and lymph flow. Heat is best applied by intermittent moist compresses; this hastens localization, whereas prolonged heat encourages edema and satellite infection.

   b. Incision and drainage are indicated whenever infection is localized or occurs in a closed space or viscus. Fluctuance signals the appropriate time for drainage of most superficial abscesses. When in doubt, needle aspiration may be diagnostic, especially in deeper infections. The incision must be large and must be in the most dependent area of the wound. Superficial wound abscesses should be packed lightly with gauze after drainage, while deeper abscesses are kept open by the use of rubber drains or sump tubes.

   c. Systemic antibiotics usually are not indicated for uncomplicated wound abscesses Incision and drainage are the essential treatment.

   d. Appropriate parenteral antibiotics are required, in addition to incision and drainage, when there is evidence of **septicemia** (systemic toxicity, high fever) or **progression of infection** despite adequate drainage. Systemic antibiotics also are indicated in conjunction with surgical drainage in all cases of intra-abdominal abscess. Choose antibiotics initially on the basis of the Gram stain and clinical information.

   Purulent material from the deepest aspect of the wound should be sent for aerobic and anaerobic culture and sensitivity studies. Generally speaking, *E. coli* (aerobe) and *B. fragilis* (anaerobe) are the usual causes of wound sepsis following GI or gynecological surgery, while *Staphylococcus* and *Pseudomonas* are the usual causative organisms when intra-abdominal viscera have not been resected or opened. The organisms causing surgical infections, as well as the antibiotics which prove most effective, are listed in Table 14-1.

2. General guidelines for the management of soft tissue infections

   a. Unlocalized infections No pus under pressure (cellulitis, lymphangitis). Treat with antibiotics, local heat, rest, and elevation. Surgical incision and drainage not indicated.

   b. Unlocalized early infection in closed space Pus under pressure (tendon sheath, fascial space, hollow viscus infections). Treat with antibiotics; incise and drain; then rest, elevation, and local heat.

   c. Localized acute infection (abscess) Incise and drain; give antibiotics only if patient has systemic symptoms or there are local signs of progression of the bacterial invasion.

TABLE 14-1. Antibiotic Treatment of Common Organisms Causing Wound Infections

Organism	Drug(s) of Choice	Daily Dose and Route (adults)[a]	Alternative Drugs
Escherichia coli	Gentamicin[b] or Kanamycin	240–300 mg IM or IV 1 gm IM	[c]
Proteus mirabilis	Ampicillin	2 gm IV or IM	Kanamycin, gentamicin[b]
Proteus, indole-positive	Kanamycin or Gentamicin[b]	1–2 gm IM 240–300 mg IM or IV	[c]
Klebsiella	Gentamicin[b]	240–300 mg IM or IV	Kanamycin, cephalosporin
Enterobacter (Aerobacter)	Kanamycin or Gentamicin[b]	1–2 gm IM 240–300 mg IM or IV	[c]
Pseudomonas	Gentamicin[b,e] and Carbenicillin[e]	300 mg IM or IV 20 gm IV	Polymyxin B
Serratia[d]	Kanamycin or Gentamicin[b]	1–2 gm IM 240–300 mg IM or IV	[c]
Staphylococcus, penicillin-resistant	Oxacillin or Methicillin[f]	4 gm PO 4 gm IV or IM	Cephalosporin, clindamycin
penicillin-sensitive	Penicillin	4.8 million units IV or IM	Cephalosporin, clindamycin
Streptococcus, Group A	Penicillin	2.4 million units IV or IM	Erythromycin, clindamycin
Enterococcus (*S. faecalis*)	Ampicillin and Gentamicin[b]	2–4 gm IV or IM 240–300 mg IM or IV	[c]
Anaerobic (*Peptostreptococcus*)	Penicillin	6.0 million units IV or IM	Cephalosporin, clindamycin, erythromycin
Pneumoccus	Penicillin	2.4 million units IV or IM	Cephalosporin, clindamycin, erythromycin
Bacteroides Oral strains (lung, head, neck infections)	Penicillin	6.0 million units IV or IM	Ampicillin, cephalosporin, clindamycin, erythromycin
Intestinal strains (*B. fragilis*)	Clindamycin	600 mg IV q6h	Chloramphenicol
Clostridium	Penicillin	20 million units IV or IM	Erythromycin, tetracycline, clindamycin
Actinomyces	Penicillin	20 million units IV or IM	Tetracycline

[a] Usually divide into two or four equal doses administered every 6 or 12 hr.
[b] Dose is calculated according to body weight.
[c] Choose drugs according to sensitivity tests.
[d] Many strains are resistant to many antibiotics; therapy should be guided by sensitivity tests of the specific infecting organism.
[e] Often used in combination to prevent emergence of resistant organisms and to enhance efficacy.
[f] Methicillin-resistant strains should be treated with vancomycin.

C. Special types of surgical infections

1. **Necrotizing fasciitis** is a serious infection caused by hemolytic streptococci or staphylococci. It involves the epifascial tissues of an operative wound, laceration, abrasion, or puncture. It may be fulminant or remain dormant 6 or more days before beginning its rapid spread. Subcutaneous and fascial necrosis accompanies extensive undermining of the skin and results in gangrene. Treatment is excision of the entire area of fascial involvement, administration of large doses of penicillin (12-20 million units/day), and appropriate systemic support.

2. **Chronic progressive bacterial synergistic gangrene** (Meleney's synergistic gangrene) is caused by the synergistic action of microaerophilic nonhemolytic streptococci and aerobic hemolytic staphylococci. The incubation period is 7-14 days. Cellulitis is followed by gangrenous ulceration which is progressive unless treated. Radical excision of the ulcerated lesion and its gangrenous borders is imperative, along with large systemic doses of penicillin.

3. **Human bite wounds** are contaminated with a combination of aerobic nonhemolytic streptococci, anaerobic streptococci, *B. melaninogenicus*, spirochetes, and staphylococci. The original wound must be treated by debridement, thorough cleansing with irrigation, and immobilization; systemic antibiotics, usually penicillin, must be used. When infection has become established, radical debridement of the infected area is imperative, and must be accompanied by antibiotic therapy.

4. **Nonclostridial gangrenous cellulitis** caused by *B. melaninogenicus* and anaerobic streptococci is typified by a progressive gangrenous infection of the skin, areolar, and fascial tissues. Prompt incision and drainage and large doses of penicillin are necessary. Supportive treatment is imperative, as toxemia with dehydration, fever, and prostration rapidly develops.

5. **Clostridial cellulitis** is a serosanguineous, crepitant, septic process of subcutaneous, retroperitoneal, or other areolar tissue caused principally by *C. perfringens* (also known as *C. welchii*). It differs from gas gangrene in that the infection does not involve muscle. The infection spreads rapidly via fascial planes. Extensive gangrene results from vascular thrombosis. Systemic effects are moderate if the infection is treated promptly. Early surgical debridement and penicillin therapy are necessary.

6. **Clostridial myonecrosis (gas gangrene)** is an anaerobic infection of muscle characterized by profound toxemia, extensive local edema, massive necrosis of tissue, and a variable degree of gas production. The causative organisms are the clostridia, which abound in soil, dust, and the alimentary tract of most animals, and which usually are saprophytic. *C. perfringens* is the most common organism causing gas gangrene. All clostridia owe their pathogenicity to soluble exotoxins which destroy tissue and blood cells. Clostridia enter a wound, multiply in the presence of devitalized muscle, and elaborate necrotizing exotoxins. Disruption and frag-

mentation of normal, nontraumatized muscle cells and capillaries result in massive necrosis, hemorrhage, and edema. There is no fibrin formation or polymorphonuclear leukocytic reaction. The affected muscles are first red and friable, but progress to a purplish black, stringy, pulpy mass. The presence of gas is variable. The affected area swells and discharges a brownish malodorous fluid. The overlying skin initially shows blotchy ecchymoses (marbling), then blackens, and finally sloughs. The diagnosis of gas gangrene is almost entirely clinical. Fever is seldom marked.

Treatment of gas gangrene   Immediate removal of involved muscle groups is necessary. Amputation is employed if the remaining muscles are insufficient for useful function. High doses of IV penicillin and whole blood are given preoperatively and postoperatively. Multiple treatments with hyperbaric oxygen (oxygen at three times atmospheric pressure) may reduce the amount of debridement necessary and lower the mortality. Untreated gas gangrene is fatal in all cases. The fatality rate of treated cases varies from 25-40%.

7. **Tetanus** is caused by a spore-forming obligate anaerobe, *C. tetani*, occurring in feces of man and animals and capable of long survival in soil. Two **exotoxins** are produced: tetanospasmin, a neurotoxin, and tetanolysin, a hemolysin. The optimal culture medium for germination of tetanus spores is provided by dead muscle and clotted blood. Traumatic injuries with compound fractures and devitalization of muscle are very susceptible to tetanus infection. Equally vulnerable are small puncture wounds harboring a clot deep in the tissues.

Locally produced tetanolysin contributes to optimal growth conditions through its lecithinase, gelatinase, esterase, and lipase activity. Tetanospasmin, the neurotoxin responsible for the clinical features of the disease, does not act peripherally or locally but is carried to the CNS and acts centrally. In order to neutralize blood-borne toxin, antitoxin must be present before tetanospasmin becomes fixed by nerve cells. Hence, antitoxin therapy given at the time symptoms are apparent only limits further intoxication of nerve cells and cannot reverse developing symptoms.

There is considerable variability in progression of the disease from onset. There may be a prodromal period of headache, stiff jaw muscles, restlessness, yawning, and wound pain beginning 6-15 days after a traumatic wound. The active stage follows in 12-24 hr, with trismus, facial distortion, opisthotonos, pain, clonic spasms, and seizures. Acute asphyxia is a major hazard and may result from either spasm of the respiratory muscles or aspiration. The shorter the incubation period, the poorer the prognosis.

Treatment of established tetanus involves:
a. Tetanus human immune globulin (Hyper-Tet), 3,000 units IM, is given immediately to neutralize circulating toxins. An additional 1,000 units can be injected into and immediately proximal to the wound. Widely debride and drain the contaminated wound at least 1 hr after administration of immune globulin. Then give 500 units immune globulin IM daily. If symptoms persist longer than 2 wk, repeat administration of the large initial doses of the immune globulin.

b. Establish and maintain an airway; use respirator support and oxygen as needed. Tracheostomy will be needed in every patient with more than prodromal symptoms and should be done before the situation becomes urgent.

c. Control muscular spasms with IM meprobamate or chlorpromazine. If spasms persist, curare should be given.

d. Maintain sedation with IM barbiturate. Place the patient in a quiet, dark room and keep environmental stimulation at a minimum to avoid triggering seizures. Control convulsions with IV Pentothal.

e. Give penicillin in high doses.

f. Maintain nutrition parenterally or feed via a gastrostomy.

g. Sphincter spasm will prevent voluntary urination; drain the bladder via an indwelling catheter to a closed system.

h. Actively immunize the tetanus toxoid after patient has recovered. With appropriate early care, 75% of patients survive. There is no neurological residual in patients who survive.

Tetanus prophylaxis principles are:

a. Tetanus is absolutely preventable by prior active immunization. Effective active immunization (not associated with a fresh wound) is accomplished by injection of alum-precipitated toxoid, 0.5 ml; repeat this dose at 1 and 6 mo.

b. Immediate meticulous surgical care of the fresh wound is of prime importance. Removal of devitalized tissue, blood clot, and foreign bodies, obliteration of dead space, and prevention of tissue ischemia in the wound are the objectives of initial treatment. Wounds that are seen late or that are grossly contaminated may be left unsutured after debridement, protected by a sterile dressing for 3–5 days, and then closed by delayed primary suture if the tissues appear clean and healthy.

c. Patients previously immunized (including reinforcing doses) within the past 10 yr should be given 0.5 ml fluid tetanus toxoid booster.

d. Patients immunized more than 10 years previously should be treated as follows:

(1) Uncontaminated wound: 0.5 ml fluid tetanus toxoid.

(2) Grossly contaminated wound: 0.5 ml fluid tetanus toxoid and 250 units tetanus human immune globulin; start penicillin therapy.

e. Patients not previously immunized should be treated as follows:

(1) Clean minor wound: Immunize with alum-precipated tetanus toxoid; give 0.5 ml alum-precipitated toxoid now and repeat at 1, 2, and 6 mo.

(2) Contaminated wound: Start active immunization with 0.5 ml alum-precipitated toxoid and repeat at 1, 2, and 6 mo in addition to passive immunization with 250 units human immune globulin; start penicillin therapy.

VII. SEPTICEMIA   This is a severe form of infection characterized by invasion and multiplication in the bloodstream of large numbers of bacteria. Fever usually is high, spiking, and accompanied by chills. Tachycardia accompanies or precedes fever and is proportional to it. Leukocyte counts may not show much abnormality in sepsis. The differential count is more reliable. Nearly always there is a shift to the left. Petechialike lesions may be seen in the skin or conjunctivae in septicemia caused by streptococci, meningococci, or *Pseudomonas*. Anemia secondary to hemolysis may appear rapidly in septicemia due to staphylococci, *Pseudomonas, E. coli,* and *Clostridium*. Shock is frequent in gram-negative septicemia, but occurs less often with gram-positive sepsis. Metastatic abscesses, especially involving bone, brain, or spleen, are not unusual after septicemia. Any injured tissue is easily infected during septicemia. Diagnosis is aided by a high index of suspicion.

A. The **etiology of septicemia** is an infection somewhere in the body which is seeding the bloodstream. The type of bacteria causing sepsis usually can be identified from the source of the infection:

1. Wound or intra-abdominal infection: coliforms, *Bacteroides,* or *Staphylococcus*.

2. Burns: *Pseudomonas, Serratia,* or *Staphylococcus*.

3. IV site: *Serratia, Klebsiella, Bacteroides,* or *Staphylococcus*.

4. Lung: *Pneumococcus, Streptococcus, Staphylococcus, Klebsiella,* or *Pseudomonas*.

5. Urinary tract: usually *E. coli* or *Proteus*.

6. CNS: *Pneumococcus* or *Meningococcus*.

B. Management of septicemia

1. Establish an etiological diagnosis

a. Septicemia rarely develops early in the postoperative period unless the operation was in or through infected tissues or the patient had a preexisting infection.

b. Examine the patient for clues to the source of infection. Is there pain or redness in the surgical wound or at an IV infusion site? Does the patient have purulent sputum, cough, pleuritic pain, rales, or dullness? Is there diarrhea? Is there dysuria, or flank pain? Is there pain in the shoulder and an immobile diaphragm, suggesting a subphrenic abscess? Is there a pelvis or prostatic mass on rectal examination? Is there headache or nuchal rigidity?

c. Carry out appropriate laboratory studies: blood count; urinalysis; Gram stain of any discharge or of sputum or urine; chest x-ray; and fluoroscopy for diaphragm motion.

2. Take appropriate cultures: blood (50 ml from single or multiple sites), urine, sputum, wound or other drainage, stool if diarrhea is present, and CSF if there is headache or nuchal rigidity. *Always obtain cultures prior to starting antibiotics.*

3. Antibiotics should be started immediately after the physical examination has been completed and cultures have been taken. Antibiotics are given in high doses by the IV route and, when possible, should be bactericidal in action and as specific as possible. The choice of antibiotic is based on the probable source of infection, the most likely bacteria found in that area, and information gained from Gram stains of material obtained from the infected area (Table 14-1). If the infection is not responding readily to the agents being used, the antibiotics should be changed in accordance with the results of cultures and sensitivity studies when these become available.

4. Drainage   When a collection of pus is sealed off, forming an abscess, it is difficult for antibiotics to penetrate the area. An abscess should be drained as soon as its presence and location are determined and the patient's overall condition permits. Drainage is done only after large doses of antibiotics have been given.

VIII. ISOLATION PROCEDURES

A. General comments

1. Isolation procedures are a prime source of frustration, wasted time, and wasted facilities in most hospitals.

2. The unnecessary use of strict isolation procedures is harmful, since an unneeded barrier is placed between the patient and his nurses and physicians. The isolation barrier tends to interfere with observation and care of the patient and is damaging to patient morale.

3. Failure to use appropriate isolation procedures also is harmful since a patient with a communicable infection then may become a threat to all patients and staff in the hospital.

4. Reasonable isolation procedures have as their objective the **interruption of pathways of transmission of communicable infections** either from an infected patient to others or from the environment to a highly susceptible patient.

5. Isolation should be discontinued as soon as the infection hazard is minimal.

6. To isolate a patient, all that is required is a room containing a sink and a closed soap dispenser. **Outside** the room place a table or cart containing gowns, masks, gloves, dressings, and any other materials needed repeatedly. **Inside** the room place a commode for the patient's use if the room has no bathroom, a linen hamper to receive contaminated linen, and plastic bags in which to discard disposable items.

7. Hand-washing before and after attending each patient is aesthetically and professionally proper behavior. As a matter of isolation technique, however, thorough hand-washing is carried out either on leaving or on entering the isolation room, depending on the objectives being sought by isolation. Hands are washed on leaving in most isolation situations, but are washed on entering the room of a patient in protective isolation.

8. It is pointless to isolate patients with minor wound infections caused by common fecal organisms, since these organisms are ubiquitous in the hospital. This does not mean that careless dressing technique is condoned; such wounds must always be covered with an adequate dry dressing.

B. Strict isolation

1. **Indications**   Infections at any site with staphylococci, group A streptococci, meningococci; open cavitary tuberculosis; clostridial myonecrosis; "traditional" communicable infections such as smallpox and diphtheria, hepatitis.

2. **Technique**

   a. Gown: put on outside room on entering and discard inside room when leaving.

   b. Mask: put on when entering room, discard when leaving.

   c. Gloves: wear if in contact with patient.

   d. Hand-washing: on leaving room.

   e. Linen, equipment: discard when possible; place linen in marked bags and autoclave before routine laundering, or use an inner plastic bag that is soluble in hot water; dressings should be placed in impervious bags for incineration; disinfect equipment before removing from room or remove wrapped for autoclaving.

    f. Terminal cleaning: Air the room for 2 hr with windows open and doors closed. Furniture, floors, and soiled walls then should be washed with a germicidal solution.

C. Wound isolation

    1. Indications Grossly infected or copiously draining wounds infected with organisms other than those requiring strict isolation.

    2. Technique

        a. Gown: wear if in direct contact with patient.

        b. Mask: wear if in close contact with patient.

        c. Gloves: wear if in direct contact with patient or during dressing changes using forceps (no touch) technique.

        d. Hand-washing: on leaving room.

        e. Linen, equipment: discard when possible; linen in marked bags for routine laundering, contaminated dressings in an impervious bag for incineration; disinfect equipment before removing from room or remove wrapped for autoclaving.

D. Stool precautions

    1. Indications Patients with enteric infections in which viable organisms are passed in the feces—amebiasis, salmonellosis, shigellosis, and similar infections.

    2. Technique

        a. Gown: wear if in direct contact with patient.

        b. Mask: not necessary.

        c. Gloves: wear if in direct contact with patient or when handling material contaminated by feces.

        d. Hand-washing: on leaving room.

        e. Linen, equipment: discard when possible; place linen in marked bags for routine laundering; disinfect equipment before removing from room or remove wrapped for autoclaving.

        f. Stools: passed or discarded directly into sewage system; if patient uses bedpan or if laboratory stool specimen is removed from room, wrap and treat containers as contaminated.

E. Urine precautions

1. Indications   Patients with infections in which viable organisms are passed in the urine—leptospirosis, certain cases of genitourinary tuberculosis.

2. Technique

  a. Gown: wear if in direct contact with patient.

  b. Mask: not necessary.

  c. Gloves: wear if in direct contact with patient.

  d. Hand-washing: on leaving room.

  e. Linen, equipment: no special precautions unless patient is incontinent.

  f. Urine: passed or discarded directly into sewage system; if patient uses bed urinal or bedpan or if laboratory urine specimen is removed from room, wrap and treat containers as contaminated.

F. Protective (reverse) isolation

1. Indications   Premature and newborn infants, patients with reduced resistance to bacterial infections—acute burns, exfoliative dermatitis, agranulocytosis, and similar acutely ill patients.

2. Technique

  a. Gown: put on outside room on entering and discard outside room on leaving.

  b. Mask: put on when entering room, discard after leaving.

  c. Gloves: not necessary.

  d. Hand-washing: on entering room.

  e. Linen, equipment: no special precautions.

G. Infections not requiring isolation

1. Peritonitis or empyema.

2. Wound infections which are not draining copiously.

3. Pneumonia.

4. Tetanus.

5. Animal bites.

6. Food poisoning.

7. Any infection requiring an animal or arthropod vector or intermediate host, if the vector or host can be excluded.

8. Infections limited to the bloodstream, such as subacute bacterial endocarditis or septicemia.

15. BLOOD TRANSFUSION REACTIONS

Untoward reactions to transfusion may occur at any time during or after the administration of whole blood, cells, or other blood components. Immediate reactions occur during or shortly after transfusion; delayed reactions occur from 10 days to several months after transfusion.

I. **IMMEDIATE TRANSFUSION REACTIONS** (Table 15-1) Transfusion should be stopped by clamping the IV tubing at the first sign of any untoward reaction so that the nature of the transfusion reaction can be determined. In most cases, the transfusion reaction will be found to be minor and to respond to treatment. In such cases, administration of the involved unit of blood may be continued, or it may be discarded. Reactions due to bacterial contamination or to incompatible blood make mandatory not only cessation of transfusion of that unit of blood but also investigation of the source of the problem, as well as the immediate treatment outlined below.

A. **Reactions in which blood may be continued**

1. **Allergic reactions** have been reported in 4% of recipients of whole blood, packed cells, or, less often, fresh-frozen plasma. Rarely, severe reactions may involve bronchospasm or laryngospasm.

a. Usual **symptoms** are flushing, chills, fever, and urticaria, with or without subjective complaints of itching. **Itching and hives occur only in allergic reactions, not in other varieties of transfusion reaction.**

TABLE 15-1. Acute Transfusion Reactions

Reaction	Frequency	Components Involved
Allergic reaction	4% of all recipients; 50% of recipients with prior history of atopy	Whole blood, packed cells, occasionally plasma
Febrile (minor) reaction	2% of recipients	Whole blood, occasionally packed cells or plasma
Acute hemolytic reaction	0.03% of recipients	Whole blood, packed cells
Bacteremia (severe febrile reaction)	0.01% (or less) of recipients	Usually whole blood
Circulatory overload	Unknown	Any
Delayed hemolysis	Unknown, probably frequent	Whole blood, packed cells

b. The **etiology** of allergic transfusion reactions is passive transfer of donor antigen to the sensitive recipient. The antigen generally has been ingested by the donor just prior to donation of the unit of blood.

c. Allergic reactions may occur in at least 50% of patients with a previous history of atopy, hay fever, or bronchial asthma. Such patients should be transfused with packed, washed plasma-free erythrocytes, if possible.

d. Allergic reactions do not occur until the patient has received ½ unit of whole blood (250 ml) or ½ unit of packed cells (125 ml). If symptoms of chills and fever develop in a patient early in the course of transfusion (less than 50 ml), the reaction is more likely a hemolytic reaction or due to bacterial contamination rather than an allergic reaction. It is imperative that the volume of blood, packed cells, or plasma already infused be documented at the time of onset of symptoms.

e. As a rule, it is not desirable to stop the transfusion if a patient has an allergic reaction, unless symptoms fail to respond to treatment. In some instances, symptoms do not develop until after the transfusion has been completed.

f. In most circumstances, administration of an **antihistaminic,** diphenhydramine (Benadryl), 50 mg, is the treatment for patients who develop symptoms of allergic reaction. Prophylactic administration of an antihistaminic should be reserved for patients with known allergies, or patients who have had previous transfusion reactions of the allergic type.

2. Febrile reactions   In some instances during a transfusion, a patient will experience fever, sometimes accompanied by flushing, headache, or chills. The fever rarely exceeds 39.4°C (103°F); the patient is not toxic and may be unaware of any untoward happening. Febrile reactions usually are caused by leukoagglutinins or platelet agglutinins present in the recipient; less often, they are due to transfusion of antibody. **Transfusion of more than ½ unit of infused blood or cells is required to cause symptoms. Aspirin** may be administered orally or rectally to reduce the fever; diphenhydramine is of some benefit if fever persists longer than 2-3 hr.

3. Circulatory overload   This is not really a transfusion reaction, but is an error in administering an excessive volume of blood or other colloid at a more rapid rate than the circulatory system can tolerate. CVP always should be monitored if the patient has a history of heart disease or, as with major hemorrhage, it is important to keep CVP below 15 cm H_2O during the course of rapid transfusion. If the patient continues to have a volume or red cell deficit, circulatory overload frequently can be handled by reducing the rate of infusion, administering rapid-acting digitalis IV, and, if necessary, giving 60 mg of furosemide IV.

B. Reactions in which blood must be stopped

1. **Severe febrile reactions, bacterial contamination**   Approximately 0.1% of all units of whole blood are contaminated with **cold-growing organisms.** Transfusion of the bacteria and toxins in the blood results in a fever over 39.4°C (103°F), intense flushing, headache, vomiting, diarrhea, and hypotension. The rapidity of onset and the severity of the reaction varies considerably, but typically, the patient appears acutely ill and frequently will develop shock. The bacteria usually are gram-negative (occasionally gram-positive) facultatively anaerobic, cold-growing organisms. Contamination of a unit of blood by bacteria can be suspected if the **supernatant plasma is turbid,** has a brownish or brownish purple discoloration, or does not display a sharp line of demarcation at the interface between red cells and plasma following 12-18 hr of refrigeration in an undisturbed state. **Whenever bacterial contamination is suspected, the transfusion must be stopped;** samples of the donor unit and of the recipient's blood are incubated at incubator temperature, at refrigerator temperature, and at room temperature in both aerobic and anaerobic environments. Septicemia is treated, as in any such instance, with **IV fluids, antibiotics, steroids, and transfusion of fresh uncontaminated blood,** if indicated.

2. **Hemolytic transfusion reactions**   Administration of grossly incompatible blood occurs once in 3,000 transfusions. In order for this reaction to occur, whole blood or packed cells must be administered; major hemolytic reactions do not occur when plasma, platelet-rich plasma, or similar blood components are given. The mismatch resulting in this reaction may be a result of faulty blood-bank technique or, equally, the result of an error by the treating physician in failing to identify correctly the patient and the unit of blood. It should be routine practice to match the label on the unit with the patient's wrist identification tag; the name and hospital number on both must be identical.

   When a hemolytic reaction occurs, the incompatible donor cells are agglutinated by preexisting antibodies in the receipient's plasma. Much less commonly, donor plasma antibody may react with the cells of the recipient; such plasma incompatibility rarely results in a serious reaction.

   A hemolytic transfusion reaction may be characterized as either the **slowly developing type,** with jaundice appearing hours or days after the transfusion, or the much more dramatic but less common **fulminant type,** with immediate appearance of symptoms due to rapid cell agglutination in the recipient. The symptoms of the fulminant reaction are the result of disseminated intravascular coagulation (DIC) and consist of chills and fever, tachypnea, tachycardia, flank pain, constriction in the chest or back, pain in the extremities, and occipital headache. The patient may vomit. Symptoms progress to oliguria, hemoglobinuria, and jaundice. If the reaction occurs during operation, the patient exhibits sudden unexpected bleeding and severe hypotension leading to shock. **The signs of a serious hemolytic transfusion reaction always occur during transfusion of the first 100 ml of blood or cells.** The patient always should be under close observation during the early part of a transfusion of whole blood or packed cells. It is helpful to monitor the pulse rate, to observe any wounds or incisions for signs of abnormal bleeding, and to watch both blood pressure and respiration to detect transfusion reaction in the sedated or anesthetized patient.

If a hemolytic transfusion reaction is suspected, the transfusion must be stopped at once. Residual donor blood, together with a sample of recipient blood and urine, is sent to the laboratory. Regrouping of the donor and recipient blood, repeat cross matching, and an indirect Coombs test should reveal any significant incompatibility. It is also necessary to check the recipient's blood sample for irregular antibodies; a cell panel is used for this purpose. Increased free plasma hemoglobin, methemoglobinemia, and hemoglobinuria will help to confirm the diagnosis. Schumm's test for methemoglobin is helpful if the investigation is delayed for more than 6 hr.

Blood also should be drawn for a platelet count, and measurement of fibrinogen and fibrin split products. If platelets are below 75,000 per mm^3, fibrinogen is below 100 mg/100 ml, and fibrin split products are markedly elevated, the patient should receive IV **heparin** immediately. The usual dose is 200 mg (20,000 IU). Hypotension also must be treated; if it is the result of hypovolemia, another transfusion of compatible (freshly cross-matched) blood or serum albumin must be administered rapidly. If blood volume is deemed to be normal and hypotension persists, vasopressors may be required. Oxygen administration is useful support. Fibrinogen and ε-aminocaproic acid (EACA) should not be given to a patient with a hemolytic transfusion reaction.

Steroids have been advocated, and it is not harmful to administer 100 mg of hydrocortisone IV. Attempt to promote **diuresis** by rapid infusion of 100 ml of 20% mannitol. At the same time, an infusion of 40 mEq of **sodium bicarbonate** is given along with rapid administration of 1,000 ml of Ringer's lactate solution. The purpose of the Ringer's lactate infusion and the alkalization of the urine with bicarbonate is to attempt to wash through any free hemoglobin present in the tubules and, hopefully, to reduce the degree of tubular damage. The patient should be observed carefully for development of acute renal failure. Depending on the degree of tubular damage, hemolytic transfusion reactions are followed either by frank renal failure or by a diuretic episode.

3. **Delayed hemolytic reactions**   These reactions occur from one to several days after transfusion of apparently compatible blood and are characterized by the appearance of jaundice and hemoglobinuria. They are considered to be caused by an anamnestic response to a previous transfusion or pregnancy. The patient is treated as described for immediate hemolytic reactions.

II. LATE TRANSFUSION REACTIONS

A. **Isosensitization**   This is not strictly a transfusion reaction, but a consequence of the infusion of large numbers of unidentified antigens attached to red cells. When a patient is given a unit of blood or a unit of packed cells, there is a possibility that a factor carried on the red cells will sensitize the recipient whose red cells do not contain such a factor. From 10-21 days is required for antibody to develop to the infused antigen or antigens, so the possibility of an isosensitization reaction is not of consequence until after 2 wk following transfusion. However, if such a patient later were to be given universal donor blood (type O, Rh-negative) or were to become pregnant, the possibility exists that a serious recipient reaction to the newly transfused blood, or even erythroblastosis in the pregnant female, could occur. Unfortunately, there is no way to predict the occurrence of isosensitization nor can it be prevented. The occurrence of such incidents reemphasizes the need to be circumspect about administering whole blood or packed cells, using these materials only when they are necessary.

B. **Disease transmission**   Three diseases may be transmitted by blood transfusion: serum hepatitis, brucellosis, and malaria. Syphilis will not be transmitted in bank blood which has been cooled to refrigerator temperature 4-7°C (39-45°F) for 12 hr or longer.

1. **Serum hepatitis**   The incidence of serum hepatitis varies according to the source of donor blood and the number of units transfused, but occurs in 0.1-0.3% of patients receiving blood. If blood is obtained from voluntary or "family" donors, the incidence is lower. If the blood is commercially purchased from "professionals" paid for their donation, the risk is much greater. Testing of bank blood for hepatitis associated antigen (HAA) has decreased the frequency of serum hepatitis transmission, although it has not eliminated this possibility.

The mortality rate of serum hepatitis in a transfusion recipient is 12%, the majority of those succumbing being under the age of 5 or over the age of 65. The incubation period of serum hepatitis is 35-120 days. Some recipients undoubtedly have anicteric hepatitis and only mild or transient hepatic dysfunction. In others, the disease may be extremely severe; it is rare for very elderly patients to survive an attack of serum hepatitis. The use of hyperimmune globulin may modify the disease in susceptible patients, but probably does not prevent infection. Within 1 wk of transfusion, 3 ml can be given IM and a similar dose should be administered 1 and 3 mo later.

When serum hepatitis occurs, it is important to test the patient for HAA—tests are positive in 80% of these patients. At that time, it is also necessary to trace the donors who contributed the blood and to eliminate them from the donor pool.

The use of frozen red blood cells has been shown to diminish the incidence of serum hepatitis. The use of packed cells, especially washed cells, also has been associated with a decrease in the incidence of serum hepatitis. It is not clear why freezing cells or washing cells diminishes the incidence of hepatitis, but it is assumed that the concentration of virus in the plasma of transfused material is diminished.

2. **Brucellosis**   Although rarely transmitted by transfusion, brucellosis may occur if a person donates blood during the 10-day prodromal stage of clinical infection, thus transmitting viable *Brucella* organisms to the recipient. Chills, fever, myalgia, and an erythematous skin eruption are common symptoms, ordinarily occurring 7-14 days after the transfusion. Treatment with tetracycline or chloramphenicol is specific.

3. **Malaria** is a rare complication of blood transfusion. The occurrence of a spiking fever 1-10 days after transfusion always should arouse a suspicion that *Plasmodium* organisms have been transmitted by transfusion. Blood smears should be done on repeated occasions to detect the infecting organisms. Treatment with antimalarial drugs should be started promptly.

III. MASSIVE TRANSFUSION

A. **The rapid administration of large quantities** of ACD- or CPD-preserved banked blood (one half of the circulating blood volume or more) is likely to result in one of several problems unless the patient is carefully monitored and certain preventive measures are undertaken.

1. **Hypothermia** is common if blood is administered rapidly through a central venous catheter, or through a peripheral vein under pressure. Transfusion within 1-2 hr of 3-5 units of bank blood at refrigerator temperature may lower the recipient's body temperature by 3-4°C (5-7°F), resulting in diminished cardiac output and metabolic acidosis. In this state, certain drugs, a change in ventilation, and other usual pathophysiological phenomena may trigger cardiac arrest.

   Blood should be prewarmed when it has to be given rapidly in large volume. Warming should never be attempted by placing the blood container in warm water; rather, a long coil of tubing in the infusion line is immersed in a water bath at 35°C (95°F).

2. **Citrate intoxication, fall in ionized calcium**   Citrate is present in excess in both ACD- and CPD-preserved bank blood. When citrate is infused into a normal recipient, binding of ionized calcium is not important as there is rapid mobilization of calcium from bone. *An adult ordinarily can tolerate the administration of the amount of excess citrate in a unit of bank blood every 10 min (6 units/hr) without undue symptoms.* Patients in whom inadequate stores of bone calcium may permit a citrate-induced ionized calcium deficit to develop during massive transfusion are small children, elderly or osteoporotic patients, especially if there is metastatic replacement of bone by tumor, and patients who have been bedridden for 8-10 wk or more. *When citrate intoxication occurs, it does not lead to abnormal bleeding as is commonly supposed, but rather affects myocardial function,* causing bradycardia, arrhythmias, and hypotension. If the presence of citrate intoxication is suspected, give the patient 1 gm of calcium chloride for every 2 units of whole blood infused. Excess citrate infusion initially results in acidosis, but as the liver metabolizes the citrate to bicarbonate, metabolic alkalosis develops. It is rarely necessary to treat either the acidosis or the alkalosis.

3. **Hyperkalemia**   When blood is banked, potassium continuously leaks from the erythrocytes into the surrounding plasma. The plasma potassium concentration may approach 25 mEq/liter after 21 days. This leakage of potassium is related to loss of cell membrane integrity resulting from hypoxia, as well as to phosphate enzyme deterioration during stor-

age. When the cells are infused into the recipient and are reoxygenated, the leaked potassium is taken up again, reducing the plasma concentration of potassium in the recipient. However, hyperkalemia can be a problem if extremely rapid transfusion transiently raises the venous concentration of potassium. Although rare, this factor has been implicated in sudden cardiac arrest and should be kept in mind if the blood administered is more than 10 days old. It is always wise to intersperse fresh units of blood with others during transfusion of large volumes.

4. **Acidosis**   The pH of 2-week-old bank blood is 6.5 owing to leakage of lactate and pyruvate into the surrounding plasma due to red cell hypoxia during storage. If aged blood is transfused rapidly, development of acidosis is theoretically possible. However, plasma buffers will handle large amounts of hydrogen ion provided the patient was not acidotic prior to transfusion. Effective treatment of shock with transfused blood usually results in clearing of the associated acidosis when shock is the only cause of acidosis; administration of buffers such as sodium bicarbonate or THAM may not be necessary. In patients with preexisting acidosis and who are to receive 1 unit of blood every 20 min or more rapidly, transfused blood should be buffered with IV sodium bicarbonate, 20 mEq for each unit transfused.

5. **Hyperammonemia**   The concentration of ammonia in bank blood begins to rise after 5-7 days and reaches high levels after 2-3 wk of storage. In normal patients, this is unimportant, but in patients with severe liver disease, especially those with preexisting hyperammonemia, it is important that administered blood not be more than 5-7 days old.

6. **Coagulation defects**   When massive transfusions are given, representing one half of the patient's blood volume or more (roughly 2,500 ml) in 12 hr or less, bleeding may occur. Bleeding is said to be the result of dilutional decreases in platelets and other labile clotting factors. In most patients, however, platelet counts are not reduced to critically low levels (less than 75,000/mm^3), as marrow replacement of platelets is extremely rapid. Unless the volume transfused in a 12-hr period exceeds the patient's own blood volume, some explanation other than dilution must account for rare true coagulation defects. Prevention of coagulation defects can be accomplished if every fifth unit transfused is less than 36-hr old. In addition, if more than 10 units of whole blood are given in a 24-hr period, it is probably wise to administer 1 unit of fresh-frozen plasma for every 5 units of whole blood.

B. **Post-transfusion lung syndrome** and other pulmonary complications. Most lung problems (hypoxia) that develop following transfusion are caused by circulatory overload or by reactions to transfusion of multiple units. The administration of large volumes of bank blood through a standard nylon mesh filter permits enormous amounts of microaggregated cells and fibrin to enter the pulmonary and other circuits, causing DIC. To prevent this complication, whenever more than 4 units of whole blood are to be administered in 1 day, the blood is given through a micropore filter effective in removing microaggregates.

SUGGESTED READING

Baker, R. J., and Nyhus, L. M.   Diagnosis and treatment of immediate transfusion reaction. *Surg. Gynecol. Obstet.* 130:665, 1970.

Mollison, P. L.   *Blood Transfusion in Clinical Medicine.* Oxford: Blackwell, 1972.

16. ACUTE COAGULATION DISORDERS

I. MECHANISMS OF HEMOSTASIS

A. Hemostasis involves a series of reactions that serve to prevent excessive blood loss following injury to blood vessels, and also to maintain intravascular blood in the fluid state. Normal intima prevents fibrin formation and probably is essential to maintain the fluid state of blood. When fibrin does form intravascularly, the fibrinolytic system immediately digests the fibrin to keep the vessel open.

B. Following injury, a series of reactions (Fig. 16-1) occur rapidly.

1. Vascular response Reflex contraction of smooth muscle of the blood vessel wall occurs in the region of injury. Smaller blood vessels may close completely.

2. Platelet response Platelets begin aggregating when they come in contact with collagen at the point of injury. Then the platelets undergo a release reaction, emitting adenosine diphosphate and serotonin. This is followed by further aggregation.

3. Formation of fibrin (intrinsic system) For maintenance of vessel closure, a series of protein and phospholipid reactions leading to thrombin and fibrin formation must occur. Most of the required proteins are carried adsorbed on the surface of platelets and are readily available for the required interaction at the site of vessel injury.

4. Formation of fibrin (extrinsic system) At the site of vascular injury, the tissues supply a thromboplastic material that interacts with coagulation factor VII to initiate further fibrin formation. Both the extrinsic and the intrinsic pathways are required for adequate fibrin formation. Deficiency of proteins in either pathway or of lipo-protein from platelets can result in excessive blood loss.

II. DIAGNOSIS OF ABNORMAL BLEEDING

A. Clues from the history and physical examination are of great help in identifying preoperatively the patient with possible coagulopathy.

1. Bleeding after dental extractions or previous operations is suggestive of a hemostatic defect, but is not specific.

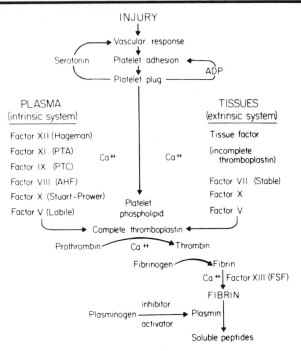

Figure 16-1. Current concept of hemostatic process. (Courtesy of Dr. Irving Schulman.)

2. Sudden onset of bleeding from multiple sites suggests DIC.

3. Epistaxis suggests abnormal capillaries, as in hereditary telangiectasia, but also can be seen with platelet disorders.

4. Petechiae indicate a possible platelet disorder or, less frequently, the presence of acute, severe stasis.

5. Purpura and menorrhagia suggest von Willebrand's disease, platelet decrease or dysfunction, or sensitivity to aspirin or other medication.

6. Hemarthrosis and deep muscle hematomas suggest hemophilia.

7. Inheritance history can be helpful.

    a. Sex-linked recessive inheritance is seen with hemophilia A and B and with a rare form of thrombocytopenia.

    b. Autosomal dominant inheritance characterizes the most common bleeding disorders: von Willebrand's disease, thrombopathy (platelet dysfunction), thrombocytopenia, and hereditary telangiectasia.

    c. Autosomal recessive inheritance is seen with plasma coagulation factor abnormalities. These conditions are rare.

B. Types of acute coagulation disorders   The acquired coagulopathies most frequently encountered in surgical patients are (1) platelet disorders, (2) plasma factor deficiencies, (3) DIC, (4) primary fibrinolysis, and (5) exogenous anticoagulants. The clinical situations commonly associated with acute coagulation disorders are listed in Table 16-1.

1. Platelet disorders

   a. Thrombocytopenia can result from "wash out" when multiple transfusions of bank blood are required, from excess protamine sulfate administered to neutralize heparin, during DIC, or from decreased marrow production as a consequence of replacement by tumor cells, of radiotherapy, or in chronic idiopathic thrombocytopenia.

   b. Thrombopathia, or abnormal platelet function, is seen in acute or chronic renal disease and as an idiopathic acquired disorder.

   c. Thrombocythemia is present if the platelet count is over 1 million. This is a myeloproliferative disorder. It is seen frequently with polycythemia vera and, transiently, occasionally after splenectomy.

TABLE 16-1. Clinical Setting of Coagulopathy

Clinical Setting	Platelet Disorder	Plasma Factor Deficiency[a]	Disseminated Intravascular Coagulation	Primary Fibrinolysin
Acute problem				
Multiple transfusions	X	X	X	
Incompatible transfusion			X	
Shock			X	
Cardiac arrest			X	
Multiple trauma			X	
Chronic disease				
Liver disease	X	X	X	X
Renal disease	X	X		
Collagen disease	X		X	
Polycythemia	X			
Leukemia	X		X	X
Chronic idiopathic thrombocytopenic purpura	X			
Metastatic cancer	X	X	X	X
Surgery				
Open-heart	X		X	X
Vascular	X			
Prostatic			X	X
Medication				
Warfarin (Coumadin)		X		
Long-term antibiotics		X		
Aspirin	X			

[a] Plasma factor deficiency without DIC or primary fibrinolysin.

2. Plasma factor deficiencies

    a. Vitamin K-related factor deficiency involves **factors II, VII, IX, and X.** Long-term antibiotic therapy, biliary obstruction, dietary deficiency, and acute stress are etiological factors.

    b. Liver disease also results in deficiency of factors II, VII, IX, and X, but **deficiency of factor V also is present.**

3. DIC

    a. This is a syndrome of thrombocytopenia, multiple plasma coagulation deficiencies, and secondary fibrinolysis resulting from activation of the coagulation systems and platelet aggregation within the vascular system (Fig. 16-2).

    b. Causes

        (1) Hypoxia with endothelial damage, shock, cardiac arrest, septicemia, viremia, heat stroke.

        (2) Multiple trauma, fat emboli, crush injuries, tissue necrosis, burns.

        (3) Intravascular hemolysis, extracorporeal circulation, incompatible blood transfusion, acquired hemolytic anemia, sickle cell anemia, paroxysmal nocturnal hemoglobinemia.

        (4) Metastatic carcinoma.

        (5) Obstetrical problems (abruptio placentae, amniotic fluid embolus, retained dead fetus).

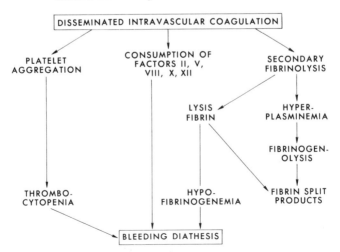

Figure 16-2. Pathophysiological mechanisms in disseminated intravascular coagulation.

(6) Giant hemangioma.

(7) Antigen-antibody reactions.

4. **Primary fibrinolysis** must be carefully distinguished from the secondary fibrinolysis of DIC.

   a. Primary fibrinolysis is seen in liver disease, in metastatic carcinoma, and in association with open-heart surgery.

   b. Hyperfibrinolysis may be produced from excess activators, resulting in lysis of all clots and excessive bleeding. The activators may be generalized, i.e., liver disease, or localized, e.g., in prostatic surgery. Decreased fibrinogen and increased fibrin split products are present in the plasma (Fig. 16-3).

5. **Exogenous anticoagulants**

   a. Heparin. Unless the clotting time is extremely prolonged, bleeding as a rule occurs with some other underlying abnormality or at the site of operation.

   b. Warfarin (Coumadin). In the therapeutic range (up to 2.5 times control), bleeding may be enhanced following trauma or when medications such as aspirin have been used. With warfarin excess, deficiencies of factors II, VII, IX, and X are extreme. Bleeding can be spontaneous or can follow minimal trauma.

C. **Coagulation tests and their interpretation** (Tables 16-2 and 16-3).

1. **Bleeding time**

   a. Measured as the time for bleeding to stop when a cut 2–4 mm in depth is made in the earlobe or forearm.

   b. Normal value for the Duke bleeding time done on an earlobe is 1–3 min, and for the Ivy bleeding time done on a forearm with pressure cuff maintained at 40 mm Hg is 2–6 min.

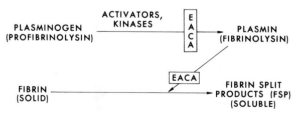

Figure 16-3. In primary fibrinolysis, ε-aminocaproic acid (EACA) blocks activation of plasmin and plasmin effect on fibrinogen.

TABLE 16-2. Differential Diagnosis of Acute Coagulation Disorders

	Bleeding Time	Platelet Count	Prothrombin Time	Thrombin Time	Factor V Assay	Partial Thromboplastin Time	Fibrinogen	Fibrin Split Products	Euglobulin Lysis Time	Prothrombin Consumption Time
Platelet disorders										
Thrombocytopenia	Long	Low	Normal			Normal				Long
Thrombopathy	Normal or long	Normal	Normal			Normal				Long
Thrombocythemia		Increased	Normal			Normal				
Disseminated Intravascular Coagulation	Long	Low	Long	Long	Low	Long	Low	Increased	Normal or short	
Primary fibrinolysis		Normal	Normal or long	Normal or long	Normal or low		Low	Slight increase	Short	
Anticoagulants										
Heparin			Normal or long	Long		Long				
Warfarin (Coumadin)			Long		Normal	Long				
Medications										
Antibiotics			Long							
Aspirin	Long		Normal or long			Long				

306

TABLE 16-3. Coagulation Tests in Plasma Factor Deficiency

	Coagulation Tests				
Factor Deficiency	Prothrombin Time	Partial Thrombo-plastin Time	Prothrombin Consumption Time	Factor V Assay	Fibrinogen
I	A	A	N		A
II	A	A		N	
V	A	A	A	A	
VII	A	N	N	N	
VIII[a]	N	A	A		
IX	N	A	A		
X	A	A	A	N	
XI	N	A	A		
XII	N	A	A		

N = normal; A = abnormal. Results indicated are for single deficiency states; with multiple abnormalities, individual assays may be required.
[a] Factor VIII deficiency occurs in both hemophilia A and von Willebrand's disease.

    c. Normal results depend on adequate numbers of platelets, adequate platelet function, and a normal reflex vascular contractile response.

    d. Since access to either the patient's earlobe or forearm is required, this test cannot be done readily in the operating room.

    e. Prolonged bleeding time may occur with thrombocytopenia and von Willebrand's disease and following ingestion of aspirin. In the presence of an underlying coagulation deficiency or stress, any patient may have a prolonged bleeding time after ingestion of aspirin.

2. Platelet count

    a. Normal quantitative platelet count is 150,000-350,000/mm^3.

    b. A quantitative count is preferable, but examination of a blood smear allows an estimate of platelet numbers. The presence of 5 or more platelets per high-power field (approximately 75,000/mm^3) in a blood smear indicates that adequate numbers of platelets are present for hemostasis if they are of normal function.

    c. Thrombocytopenia capable of causing bleeding is present if the platelet count is 50,000/mm^3 or less.

3. Prothrombin time (PT)

    a. Normal is 12 ± 0.5 sec.

    b. PT is influenced by plasma factors I, II, V, VII, and X.

c. Vitamin K deficiency or vitamin K antagonist drugs result in a prolonged PT owing to deficiencies of factors II, VII, and X. Factor IX deficiency also occurs but is not detectable by the PT.

d. In liver disease, the PT is prolonged owing to deficiencies of factors II, V, VII, and X. The **deficiency of factor V differentiates liver disease from vitamin K deficiency in the absence of DIC.** Normal factor V is 80–100%.

4. Partial thromboplastin time (PTT)

   a. Normal is less than 45 sec.

   b. This test is sensitive to levels below 30% of factors I, II, V, IX, X, XI, and XII.

   c. If the PT is normal but the PTT is abnormal, the deficiency is limited to factors VIII, IX, XI, and XII.

5. Fibrinogen (factor I)

   a. Normal is 150–400 mg/100 ml.

   b. Mild deficiency, in the range of 100–150 mg/100 ml, occurs in liver disease and with primary fibrinolysis.

   c. Levels of less than 100 mg/100 ml are seen in DIC.

   d. If DIC occurs in patients with septicemia but without the stress of operation, fibrinogen levels usually are above 100 mg/100 ml.

6. Fibrin split products result from the action of plasmin on fibrin and, sometimes, fibrinogen.

   a. Fibrin split products contain the same antigenic sites as fibrinogen, so they can be assayed using antifibrinogen serums. Using the tanned red cell inhibition immunoassay, normal is 0–10 μg/ml.

   b. With primary fibrinolysis, fibrin split product levels are 0–50 μg/ml.

   c. In DIC, fibrin split products levels over 80 μg/ml are seen.

7. Thrombin time (TT) is a measure of the rate of fibrin formation when thrombin is added to oxalated plasma.

   a. Normal TT is within 10 sec of control using 1 unit/ml of thrombin.

   b. Abnormal when low concentrations of fibrinogen or certain fibrin split products are present. Heparin effect can be differentiated from fibrin split products with use of a snake venom extract that acts on fibrinogen.

8. Euglobulin lysis time (ELT) is a relatively rapid method of detecting increased fibrinolytic activator in the plasma and increased circulating fibrinolysin (plasmin).

    a. Normal lysis of clot from the euglobulin fraction of plasma requires 5-18 hr. Lysis is more rapid (frequently less than 1 hr) as the level of activator or fibrinolysis increases.

    b. The ELT is always abnormal with primary fibrinolysis and may be abnormal in DIC. Frequently, the secondary fibrinolysis in DIC is localized in small vessels and is not reflected in the ELT.

9. Prothrombin consumption time (PCT) is a sensitive means of measuring platelet function.

    a. Normal PCT is 17-35 sec.

    b. With platelets numbering less than $50,000/mm^3$, or adequate numbers but poor platelet function, the PCT is abnormal, in the range of 8-15 sec.

    c. By adding sources of various factors, the deficient factor can be identified. For platelet abnormalities, an abnormal PCT will be corrected only by platelets or a platelet substitute.

    d. The PCT can also be used to measure plasma coagulation factors acting in the intrinsic coagulation mechanism.

III. MANAGING THE SURGICAL PATIENT WITH SUSPECTED ACUTE COAGULOPATHY

A. Initial diagnostic maneuvers

    1. Draw blood for platelet count, fibrinogen, PT, factor V, PTT, TT, ELT.

    2. Until laboratory results are obtained, use **fresh-frozen plasma** and **packed red cells.**

    3. On the basis of laboratory results, give **definitive treatment** as outlined in Table 16-4.

B. Simple thrombocytopenia is present if platelet count is $50,000/mm^3$ or less without other plasma factor deficiencies. Give platelet concentrates.

C. DIC is indicated by a platelet count of less than $50,000/mm^3$, factor V less than 20%, PT more than 16 sec, PTT more than 50 sec, and fibrinogen less than 100 mg/100 ml. Heparin therapy is used unless the cause of DIC can be eliminated, e.g., open-heart surgical patient taken off pump.

D. Plasma factor deficiency without thrombocytopenia or increased fibrinolysin will be reflected by abnormal values of either PT or PTT, or both. Use fresh-frozen plasma or, if available, concentrate of the specific deficient factor.

TABLE 16-4. Treatment of Acute Coagulation Disorders

Abnormality	Therapy
Thrombocytopenia (platelets <50,000/mm³)	Platelet concentrate transfusions
Thrombopathy (platelet dysfunction)	Platelet concentrate transfusions; fresh unrefrigerated whole blood (<2-3 hr old)
Plasma factor deficiency	Fresh-frozen plasma, with packed cells if needed, or fresh whole blood (<5 days old)
	Factor concentrates are commercially available for factors II, VII, IX, X (Konyne) and for factor VIII (antihemophilic factor). Total units of factor concentrates to be given a patient = weight (kg) × 60 × increase (units/ml plasma) needed by patient. Fibrinogen is also readily available commercially; usually 1-2 gm is administered as needed.
Disseminated intravascular coagulation	First, restore normal condition, i.e., blood volume, capillary flow, pH; evacuate abruptio placentae
	If DIC persists: heparin, 2,000 units q4h
	EACA (Amicar) if fibrinolytic activity excessive, but only after DIC completely controlled
Primary fibrinolysis	First, rule out "secondary" fibrinolysis, i.e., DIC
	Amicar (EACA), 5-10 gm IV, then 2 gm/hr IV for next 2-3 hr, then 1 gm/4 hr orally or IV as needed
Anticoagulants	
Heparin	Protamine sulfate—1 mg neutralizes 100 units heparin
Warfarin (Coumadin)	Replace factor deficiency by transfusion (immediate) and administer vitamin K (effective in 18-24 hr)

E. **Primary fibrinolysis** can be diagnosed if the platelet count is over 100,000/mm³, there is mild deficiency of factor V and fibrinogen as compared with DIC, but the TT is prolonged and the ELT is short. Amicar, 5 gm is given immediately (see Table 16-4). Follow the progress of the patient's coagulopathy by means of TT and ELT. When bleeding is controlled, lower doses of Amicar are administered.

F. **Residual heparin** present in a patient having open-heart or vascular surgery causes prolonged thrombin time (Table 16-2). Give 25-50 mg protamine sulfate and repeat the TT.

SUGGESTED READING

Quick, A. J.   *The Hemorrhagic Diseases and the Pathology of Hemostasis.* Springfield, Ill.: Thomas, 1974.

Rossi, E. C. (Ed.)   Symposium on hemorrhagic disorders. *Med. Clin. North Am.* 56:1, 1972.

Silver, D., and McGregor, F. H.   Non-mechanical causes of surgical bleeding. *Curr. Probl. Surg.* January 1970.

17. PULMONARY EMBOLUS

Pulmonary emboli usually originate from occult thrombi in the venous circulation. The less common varieties of pulmonary emboli—septic and fat emboli—are discussed separately.

I. CAUSES AND EFFECTS

A. Factors predisposing to pulmonary emboli

1. Lower extremity trauma.

2. Visceral cancer.

3. Heart failure.

4. Immobility.

5. Obesity.

6. Advanced (+70) age.

7. History of venous thrombosis or pulmonary embolism.

B. Sources of fatal pulmonary emboli are indicated in Table 17-1. *In surgical patients most emboli originate in the legs or pelvis*, while on a medical service the heart also is an important source of emboli.

C. The immediate consequences of a pulmonary embolus are related to both mechanical effects and humoral-reflex effects.

TABLE 17-1. Sources of Fatal Pulmonary Emboli (%)

Source	Surgical Service[a]	Medical Service[b]
Right side of heart	0	25
Inferior vena cava	10	18
Pelvic veins	15	15
Iliofemoral and leg veins	40	42
Calf veins	17	

[a] Adapted from Crane, *N. Engl. J. Med.* 257:147, 1957.
[b] Adapted from Smith, Dexter, and Dammin, in A. A. Sasahara and M. Stein (eds.), *Pulmonary Embolic Disease,* New York: Grune & Stratton, 1965. P. 126.

1. **Mechanical effects** resulting from passage and lodgment of the clot are relatively insignificant until more than 25% of the pulmonary artery circulation is occluded. With 25–30% blockage, **pulmonary artery mean pressure begins to rise.** As pulmonary artery occlusion approaches 35%, the pulmonary artery mean pressure exceeds 30 mm Hg and right atrial mean pressure also rises. Cardiac output remains normal or increased until pulmonary artery occlusion exceeds 50% (massive embolism). Underlying cardiac or respiratory insufficiency contributes significantly to premature failure of cardiac output. The mechanical effects of a pulmonary embolus also result in:

   a. Arrhythmia, as the clot traverses the right atrium and ventricle.

   b. Dilation of bronchial arteries, which serve as collateral vessels to the distal pulmonary arterial tree.

   c. Decreased pulmonary blood flow results in:

      (1) Decreased cardiac output, systemic hypotension, shock.

      (2) High ventilation-perfusion ratio resulting from decreased pulmonary arteriolar circulation in areas of normal alveolar ventilation and leading to arterial hypoxemia and a high arterial-alveolar gradient for carbon dioxide.

      (3) Myocardial hypoxia, ectopic irritable foci, arrhythmia.

   d. Infarction occurs in less than 10% of pulmonary emboli. The development of an infarct depends on:

      (1) Completeness of occlusion.

      (2) Effectiveness of collateral circulation.

      (3) Condition of lung; congestion or infection increases the likelihood of infarction.

2. **Humoral reflex effects,** although less significant than mechanical effects, probably are due in most instances to the release of biologically active amines (e.g., histamine and serotonin) from platelets. Humoral reflex effects include:

   a. Increased pulmonary artery resistance and pressure; decreased pulmonary blood flow.

   b. Bronchoconstriction causing increased airway resistance and resulting in decreased compliance, decreased alveolar ventilation, hypoxemia, and tachypnea.

   c. Systemic hypotension not related to alterations in pulmonary blood flow.

II. CLINICAL FEATURES

A. **The first sign of pulmonary embolus in 70% of patients is the embolus itself** ! Less than one third of patients exhibit even minimal clinical signs of venous disease before their embolus. But, of patients with fatal pulmonary embolus, 85% have had some warning sign—a prior minor embolus or symptomatic venous disease.

B. **Signs and symptoms** are listed in Table 17-2. Note that dyspnea, tachypnea, and a loud second pulmonic sound are common. The "classic" signs of pleuritis, hemoptysis, and a pleural friction rub are not common; they are not really signs of pulmonary embolus but of infarction.

C. **Unexplained asthma or heart failure** appearing in a hospitalized patient is very suggestive of pulmonary embolus.

D. The most common incorrect diagnoses in patients having pulmonary emboli are congestive heart failure, pneumonia, and myocardial infarction.

E. **Leukocytosis** of greater than $15,000/mm^3$ is unusual with pulmonary embolus; if the leukocyte count is high, pneumonia is more likely.

F. The **"diagnostic enzyme pattern"** of elevated lactic dehydrogenase and bilirubin with normal serum glutamic oxaloacetic transaminase values is found in only 12% of patients. Although elevation of LDH is common ($>80\%$), it is of no value in differentiating pulmonary embolus from pneumonia. Elevation of bilirubin is related to heart failure resulting from the pulmonary embolus, rather than to any direct effect of the embolus.

TABLE 17-2. Clinical Signs and Symptoms of Pulmonary Embolus

Signs and Symptoms	Frequency (%)
Dyspnea	100
Tachypnea ($+20$/min)	95
Loud P_2	95
Tachycardia ($+90$/min)	70
Fever	55
Rales	55
Cough	50
Pleuritic pain	35
Phlebitis	30
Hemoptysis	25
Pleural friction rub	20
Cyanosis	15
Gallop rhythm	15
X-ray infiltrate	15
Substernal pain	10
Syncope	5
Shock	5

G. Blood gases   The most consistent finding is Pa_{O_2} <80 mm Hg; Pa_{CO_2} values remain normal.

H. The **ECG is neither a sensitive nor a specific diagnostic aid** in cases of pulmonary embolus. Many patients have a preexisting abnormal ECG and most of these show no change. Only one fourth of patients with a pulmonary embolus will show abnormal ECG changes; 80% of these changes will be rhythm disturbances. The classic ECG changes of pulmonary embolus— large P-waves, right axis deviation, S-T segment depression, T-wave inversion, etc.,—are uncommon and are found in only 5% of all patients with a proved pulmonary embolus. The major value of an ECG is differentiation of a pulmonary embolus from a myocardial infarction.

I. Tests designed to **detect occult deep venous thrombosis** may be helpful. These are phlebography, impedance plethysmography, Doppler ultrasound, and ^{125}I-fibrinogen scans.

1. Phlebography and iliofemoral venography are excellent methods of visualizing clots in the deep venous system, but they fail to demonstrate the age, i.e., adherence and clinical significance, of these thrombi.

2. Impedance plethysmography is a rapid, noninvasive method for detecting deep venous thrombosis. However, the test is less accurate than venography and there are significant numbers of false-negative tests.

3. Doppler ultrasound flow studies accurately detect femoral and popliteal thromboses but cannot be used to detect infrapopliteal venous thrombosis.

4. ^{125}I-fibrinogen uptake studies are very sensitive and probably detect clinically insignificant thrombi as well as significant ones. In order to be positive, the test must be performed while the thrombi are developing.

J. Chest x-rays may be entirely normal (50%) or may show the following:

1. Prominent pulmonary artery (hilar) shadows.

2. Diminished vascular markings in the area of embolization.

3. Enlarged right ventricle or widening of superior mediastinum.

4. Small pleural effusion or elevation of diaphragm.

5. Cone, hump-shaped, or other nondescript densities based on the pleural surface usually in the lower lobes and suggestive of pulmonary infarction (15% of patients).

K. Pulmonary angiography is the definitive diagnostic examination in cases of suspected pulmonary embolus. Visualization of **an intraluminal filling defect, an abrupt vessel cutoff, or loss of side branches (pruning) are diagnostic signs.** Delayed filling of the pulmonary artery and a delayed venous phase are suggestive angiographic signs, but are not diagnostic of pulmonary embolus. Contrast media should be injected through a catheter selectively placed into the main pulmonary artery; this catheter subsequently can be retracted and used to measure right ventricular pressure (see below). Pulmonary cineangiography details flow and vascular motion and is a valuable study if the results of routine pulmonary angiography are equivocal. Pulmonary angiography is dangerous if the patient is in shock or in marked heart failure; if the examination is to be done in such patients, partial bypass should be established first.

Although formal pulmonary angiograms are desirable, acceptable substitutes may be obtained by rapid injection of 50 ml of contrast media from a hand-held syringe. The injection is made through a large-bore (16-gauge) catheter, placed in the right side of the heart, during exposure of a chest film. This method will demonstrate only large emboli, but those are the only ones likely to require this emergency procedure.

The major complications of angiography include transient hypotension and arrhythmias, which can be reduced by avoiding injections directly into the right heart. Vessels 2 mm or smaller cannot be visualized on angiography, so microemboli may be overlooked with this technique.

L. **Pulmonary scanning** following injection of radioiodinated macroaggregated serum albumin, ^{51}Cr, or ^{99m}Tc also is an excellent diagnostic measure and is simple to perform. The lung scan is **particularly useful in differentiating a major pulmonary embolus from acute myocardial infarction.** A lung scan is not as specific as angiography in diagnosis of a pulmonary embolus. The scan really demonstrates diminished blood flow in the lung; a picture similar to that of pulmonary embolus also can be produced by neoplasm, atelectasis, pneumonia, and emphysematous bullae. In the case of neoplasm, atelectasis, or pneumonia, the chest x-ray will be grossly abnormal, whereas with pulmonary embolus, the chest x-ray is likely to be normal or to show only subtle changes. The differentiation between an emphysematous bleb and a pulmonary embolus can be made with the addition of a ^{133}Xe ventilation scan; an emphysematous bulla produces a hypoventilated area as opposed to the normally ventilated area seen in pulmonary embolism.

M. **Catheterization of the right side of the heart** and measurement of pulmonary artery and right ventricular end diastolic pressure are important adjuncts to pulmonary angiography and provide useful prognostic data which aid in making critical therapeutic decisions.

III. THERAPEUTIC MEASURES

A. Anticoagulation

1. Indications

a. **Prophylactic**   Any patient who has a high risk of developing a pulmonary embolus, e.g., patient over 50 years of age with a fracture of the pelvis, hip, or lower extremities; bed-ridden patients who are obese, in congestive heart failure, or who have a prior history of venous thrombosis or pulmonary embolus, or both.

b. Therapeutic   Suspected pulmonary embolus or deep venous thrombosis.

2. Contraindications

a. Absolute

(1) Trauma to or recent operation on brain or spinal cord.

(2) Clotting disorder (blood dyscrasia, liver disease).

(3) Septic phlebitis.

(4) Subacute or acute bacterial endocarditis.

b. Relative

(1) Major visceral injury.

(2) Acute fractures.

(3) Recent operation in thorax, abdomen, or retroperitoneum which could lead to concealed bleeding.

(4) History of cerebral hemorrhage.

(5) Hypertension (diastolic >120 mm Hg).

(6) Gross hematuria, melena, or other present evidence of bleeding.

(7) History of presence of GI cancer, ulcer, or other bleeding lesion.

3. Heparin schedule

a. All heparin is given IV; absorption of Depo-Heparin or heparin given subcutaneously is erratic and unreliable; in addition, IM or subcutaneous administration of heparin produces local ecchymoses, fat necrosis, and pain.

b. Heparin therapy should be monitored with either the PTT (partial thromboplastin time) or the Lee-White clotting time. Careful monitoring to assure heparin effect will not decrease the incidence of bleeding (8%) but will reduce the incidence of recurrent thromboembolism during anticoagulation. PTT is more reproducible and therefore preferable. Clotting time has the advantage of being available at the bedside.

c. Clotting time or PTT is drawn prior to therapy and redrawn 30 min prior to the next heparin dose (twice on day 1, daily thereafter). Clotting time should be maintained at two to three times normal (20-35 min), or PTT at one and a half to two times normal (50-80 seconds).

d. Heparin may be given either by intermittent IV injection or continuous IV infusion. The latter method requires closer supervision and the use of a constant controlled infusion pump.

(1) Intermittent method: 10,000-15,000 units of sodium heparin initially, followed by 5,000-10,000 units every 4 hr thereafter (minimum dose, 60,000 units in first 24 hr).

(2) Continuous method: 5,000-unit bolus, followed by 1,000 units/hr thereafter.

e. Continue therapy unless major bleeding occurs; heparin treatment is not interrupted because of microscopic hematuria, minor epistaxis, appearance of guaiac-positive stools, or similar evidence of minor and tolerable blood loss.

f. Heparin is usually continued for 8-10 days (the approximate time for venous thrombi to become firmly adherent to the vein walls) or until all acute symptoms have subsided and the patient is fully ambulatory.

4. Warfarin schedule (oral or parenteral)

a. The antithrombin effect of warfarin is negligible until after 5-7 days of therapy; therefore, warfarin is started 2-3 days after the onset of heparin therapy, continued concomitantly with heparin for 5-7 days, and then continued after heparin has been discontinued.

b. Blood samples for prothrombin time are obtained immediately prior to the next heparin dose to minimize the effect of heparin on that determination. Prothrombin time should be obtained daily during the first week; twice weekly during the second week, and weekly to twice monthly thereafter.

c. When warfarin is given along with heparin for 5-7 days, a loading dose of warfarin is unnecessary; simply give 10-15 mg daily, adjusting the dose subsequently according to the prothrombin values. Prothrombin time should be kept at two to three times normal.

d. Following a documented episode of pulmonary embolism, oral anticoagulation should be continued for a minimum of 4 mo, longer if the threat of recurrent embolism is great.

e. Warfarin should be avoided in pregnant patients since it crosses the placental barrier and may cause cerebral hemorrhage in the infant. Heparin, which does not cross the placenta, is used in place of warfarin and, if being used at the time of delivery, can be reversed with protamine sulfate and reinstituted 4 days later.

f. When the patient has been maintained within the therapeutic range for 1 wk, total the week's dose of warfarin and divide by 7; the result is a satisfactory daily dose for future maintenance.

5. Management of bleeding in anticoagulated patients

a. If bleeding is minimal, simply reduce the amount of anticoagulant given.

b. If bleeding is massive during heparin anticoagulation, the heparin effect can be neutralized rapidly with protamine sulfate (each mg of protamine sulfate neutralizes approximately 100 USP units of sodium heparin). Protamine is itself an anticoagulant and further bleeding will occur with larger doses. Transfusion does not correct the clotting abnormality produced by heparin.

c. If bleeding is massive during warfarin anticoagulation, this can be reversed with vitamin K_1, 10–25 mg parenterally, as well as by transfusion of fresh whole blood. Some effect of vitamin K_1 is noted at 2 hr, but complete warfarin reversal takes 6–24 hr.

B. Venous interruption operations

1. Objective Immediate prevention of recurrent pulmonary embolus. Because collateral circulation develops around any venous obstruction, late recurrence of emboli from or via collateral venous channels still may occur after venous interruption.

2. Indications

a. When anticoagulant therapy is contraindicated.

b. When anticoagulant therapy fails (major bleeding complication, recurrent pulmonary embolus).

c. First pulmonary embolus in high-risk patient.

d. History of recurrent pulmonary emboli.

e. Septic phlebitis.

f. Septic pulmonary embolus.

g. Following pulmonary embolectomy.

3. Contraindications In the presence of marked heart failure (pulmonary artery pressure >35 mm Hg), the mortality of caval ligation approaches 50%.

4. Complications

a. Acute volume sequestration in legs with transient decreased cardiac output.

b. Acute and chronic venous insufficiency of the legs.

    c. Recurrent pulmonary emboli via large collateral veins (10-20%).

    d. Specific complications attend the use of an intracaval umbrella, i.e., caval thrombosis, erosion into the intestine or aorta, retroperitoneal bleeding, and umbrella embolus.

5. Choice of operation

    a. Insertion below the renal veins via the internal jugular vein of an **intracaval umbrella** device is the method of choice in poor-risk patients who are in need of caval interruption.

    b. Caval interruption may be accomplished by ligation, plication, silk screen, plastic clip, or stapling techniques. Caval interruption usually is performed through a retroperitoneal approach. The vena cava is ligated just below the left renal vein. If gonadal vein ligation seems advisable as well, an intraperitoneal approach is used.

    c. Significant differences between caval ligation and caval plication have not been demonstrated in either incidence of recurrent embolus or leg sequellae. Caval plication frequently results in complete interruption, as the channels through the plication or umbrella quickly occlude with either newly formed thrombus or small recurrent emboli.

    d. Femoral vein ligation is indicated only when the source of embolus clearly has been demonstrated by phlebography and iliofemoral venography to arise from the lower extremity. This may be the procedure of choice in poor-risk patients, but the incidence of recurrent embolism is greater than that following caval ligation.

    e. Anticoagulation should be instituted or reinstituted 24 hr postoperatively after caval interruption and continued for 4-6 mo.

    f. Routine use of elevation and elastic stockings will reduce the degree of postoperative edema of the legs. Edema eventually will clear completely in half of these patients as venous collaterals develop. Persisting edema probably is due to underlying venous disease in the legs.

C. Thrombolytic agents

1. Objective   To speed natural processes of clot dissolution. Two thrombolysins, urokinase and streptokinase, have been studied extensively. Both act by enhancing the fibrinolytic system.

2. Indication   Massive pulmonary embolism which initially appears to require pulmonary embolectomy.

3. Choice of agent

    a. Urokinase   A natural fibrinolysin recovered from human urine. Administration is not associated with fever or allergic reactions, and effective blood levels can be achieved. The chief objection to urokinase is its great expense and the high incidence of abnormal bleeding attending its use. The drug currently is under trial and appears to be effective although improvement in mortality from pulmonary embolism has not been demonstrated.

b. Streptolysin Unsatisfactory because administration produces fever and it is associated with a high incidence of allergic reactions; also, it is difficult to maintain blood concentrations that are high enough to alter the rate of clot lysis.

c. Widespread use of thrombolysins awaits the development of a readily available, safe, synthetic agent.

D. Pulmonary embolectomy

1. Objective Mechanical removal of clot from the pulmonary arteries.

2. Indications

a. Persistent and progressive shock in a patient with massive pulmonary embolism documented by angiography.

b. Chronic pulmonary hypertension in a patient with angiographic evidence of right or left main pulmonary artery occlusion.

3. Techniques

a. Pulmonary embolectomy under direct vision through **pulmonary arteriotomy** accompanied by cardiopulmonary bypass. This is the usual method and carries a 33% mortality risk.

b. Pulmonary embolectomy without cardiopulmonary bypass using temporary inflow (caval) occlusion. This method is used when bypass is not available. It is associated with a 50% mortality risk.

c. Transvenous pulmonary embolectomy using a vacuum cup catheter. This newer method holds promise and can be done at the time of partial cardiopulmonary bypass using the femoral vein. It is difficult to remove all of the clot by this method. However, if major occlusive clots are removed, the patient's condition will improve.

IV. PROPHYLAXIS OF PULMONARY EMBOLUS Prophylaxis involves reducing those elements that promote venous thrombosis.

A. Reduce intimal injury

1. No infusions into lower extremity veins.

2. Only buffered, isosmolar infusions into peripheral veins; hypertonic or nonneutral solutions should be administered slowly via a catheter inserted into a central vein.

B. Reduce stasis

1. Encourage early postoperative walking. Getting the patient up to sit in a chair is of no value and actually promotes stasis; the patient must ambulate.

2. Maintain activity in bed with calf and patellar setting exercises and changes in position.

3. Elevate legs 15 degrees when supine. Wrapping the legs with elastic bandages is not effective in increasing venous flow at rest.

C. Reduce hypercoagulability Prophylactic anticoagulation of patients with lower extremity fractures and similar high-risk patients (see above) reduces the risk of pulmonary embolus. Warfarin is the drug of choice for prophylactic anticoagulation and should be continued for a minimum of 3 mo or until the patient is fully active.

V. MANAGEMENT OF PULMONARY EMBOLUS

A. Initial treatment in any suspected pulmonary embolus includes:

1. Immediate **anticoagulation with heparin** to reduce distal propagation of thrombus beyond the embolus.

2. Administration of **oxygen** to increase blood Po_2 and reduce pulmonary artery pressure.

B. Classify patients for further management into three groups on the basis of clinical findings.

1. Group I: no shock or heart failure.

2. Group II: no shock but heart failure exists.

3. Group III: in shock without use of vasoactive drugs.

C. Treatment of group I patients: no shock or heart failure

1. Confirm diagnosis with lung scan or angiogram.

2. High-risk patients need inferior vena cava interruption. Ligation or umbrella placement is performed because these patients have a high risk of recurrent pulmonary emboli and a high mortality rate with recurrent embolization. Follow with anticoagulation, beginning 24 hr postoperatively.

D. Treatment of group II patients: heart failure, no shock

1. Catheterize; confirm diagnosis with angiogram; measure pulmonary artery or right ventricular end diastolic pressure.

2. Pressure <35 mm Hg; anticoagulation with heparin; treat heart failure. When failure clears, inferior vena cava interruption.

3. Pressure >35 mm Hg; embolectomy may be needed; anticoagulate and observe carefully for 2-3 hr; if not improving, proceed with embolectomy.

E. Treatment of group III patients: in shock

1. If shock does not persist or if it responds readily to minimal doses of vasopressors, treat as for group II: anticoagulate, treat shock and heart failure; when shock and failure clear, perform inferior vena cava ligation.

2. If shock persists with or without vasopressors:

    a. Put on partial cardiopulmonary bypass.

    b. Catheterize, confirm diagnosis with angiogram. Measure pulmonary artery or right ventricular end diastolic pressure.

    c. If diagnosis is confirmed, perform transvenous embolectomy or convert to total bypass and perform pulmonary embolectomy.

VI. SEPTIC PULMONARY EMBOLI

A. Embolus originates from septic thrombophlebitis.

B. Emboli tend to be small and multiple and to produce multiple foci of infection in the lungs.

C. Anticoagulants are contraindicated since they tend to promote hemorrhage into infected pulmonary foci and rupture of mycotic aneurysms.

D. Treatment involves three essential steps:

1. Proximal venous ligation. There is no indication for plication or other partial venous interruption procedures. A pelvic focus of infection is frequent; in this situation gonadal veins also must be ligated.

2. Antibiotics in high doses.

3. Drainage of any closed infection. If the embolus originated in a septic superficial thrombophlebitis, the involved vein segment should be stripped. Hysterectomy and bilateral salpingo-oophorectomy may be indicated for septic abortion or tubo-ovarian abscesses.

VII. BONE MARROW AND FAT EMBOLI

A. Ninety-five percent of fat emboli are associated with fractures, which disrupt venous channels in the bone marrow and allow fat particles to enter the venous circulation. Embolization of bone marrow occasionally occurs following fracture of a major long bone, the pelvis, or the sternum, following median sternotomy, or following multiple soft tissue injuries.

B. Seventy-five percent of the fat emboli are trapped in the pulmonary circulation; depending on their number, they may produce no symptoms or only respiratory symptoms. If the emboli pass on into the systemic circulation, a variety of symptoms may appear, primarily due to cerebral embolization.

C. The fat embolus lodged in the pulmonary capillaries is acted upon by lipase to produce free fatty acids. These fatty acids are toxic and produce disruption of the alveolar capillary membrane and destruction of surfactant, leading to pulmonary edema, pulmonary hemorrhage, and alveolar collapse.

D. Clinical manifestations usually begin 12-96 hr after injury and consist of:

1. Dyspnea and tachypnea, occasionally associated with cyanosis, rales, or a pleural friction rub.

2. Cerebral symptoms, such as confusion, delirium, or coma.

3. Petechial hemorrhages are found primarily on the chest wall, axillae, flanks, and subconjunctivas. Retinal petechiae also may be seen on fundoscopic examination.

4. Fever, usually up to 38.8°C (102°F).

E. Laboratory findings include:

1. Lipuria. Fat in the urine is seen in 60% of cases of fat embolism, usually within the first 3 days.

2. Elevated serum lipase is found in 50% of cases of fat embolism, usually after 3 days.

3. Chest x-ray is either normal or reveals bilateral stippled or fluffy pulmonary infiltrates.

4. ECG occasionally may show evidence of right heart strain.

5. Hematocrit fall is common and thought to be related to pulmonary hemorrhage.

6. Low Pa_{O_2} with compensatory respiratory alkalosis is a consistent finding in fat embolism.

F. Treatment consists of:

1. Correction of hypovolemia.

2. Gentle splinting and immobilization of fractures.

3. Respiratory support with oxygen.

4. Parenteral steroids. Methylprednisolone, 125 mg IV, followed by 80 mg every 6 hr for 3 days. Antacids are given concomitantly to help avert GI bleeding.

5. Alcohol and heparin also may be given IV but their use is controversial. Heparin promotes lipase activity, whereas alcohol inhibits lipase.

SUGGESTED READING
Hume, M., Sevitt, S., and Thomas, D. P.   *Venous Thrombosis and Pulmonary Embolism.* Cambridge, Mass.: Harvard University Press, 1970.
McIntyre, K. M., Sasahara, A. A., and Sharma, G. V. R. K.   Pulmonary thromboembolism: Current concepts. *Adv. Intern Med.* 18:199, 1972.

18. MANAGEMENT OF BURNS

The probability of survival of thermally injured patients with burns between 20% and 60% of the total body surface has improved over the past decade. The introduction of adequate topical chemotherapy, the use of biological dressings, and the recognition and prevention of complications are responsible for this improvement.

I. INITIAL CARE

A. History A thorough history is obtained at the initial contact with the patient. This can be accomplished while performing a physical evaluation or initiating treatment.

1. History related to the burn: the date and time of burn; method of injury, e.g., flame, electrical, or chemical; how caused, e.g., house fire, scald, explosion, or airplane crash; whether in an open or closed space. Previous treatment also should be ascertained.

2. Additional historical factors of importance include known allergies, medications the patient may be taking, preexisting diseases such as diabetes, and prior operations. A review of systems may yield information concerning associated injuries or underlying diseases which the patient may not initially remember.

B. Physical examination

1. **Estimate the severity and depth of injury** Appropriate fluid replacement is dependent on the accuracy of this estimate.

   a. **The Rule of Nines** is an easily remembered guide to the extent of injury in adults, allotting 9% for each upper extremity, 18% for each lower extremity, 18% for the anterior trunk, 18% for the posterior trunk, and 1% for the genitalia. A major source of error in the Rule of Nines is the relative difference of surface areas in children when compared with adults. A more precise estimate of the extent of injury may be obtained by using the Lund and Browder burn diagram (Fig. 18-1) which corrects body surface area for age.

   b. **Classify the depth of injury** as either partial thickness or full thickness. Partial-thickness injuries have remaining epithelial elements which, if protected from infection, will spontaneously re-epithelialize the area of burn. Partial-thickness injuries are characterized by erythema, ves-

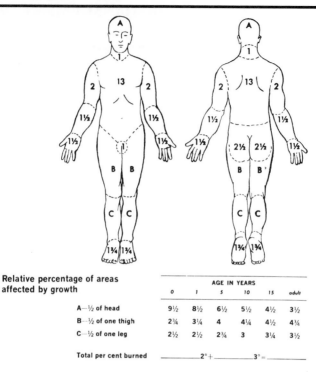

Relative percentage of areas affected by growth	AGE IN YEARS					
	0	1	5	10	15	adult
A—½ of head	9½	8½	6½	5½	4½	3½
B—½ of one thigh	2¾	3¼	4	4¼	4½	4¾
C—½ of one leg	2½	2½	2¾	3	3¼	3½
Total per cent burned		2°+		3°=		

Figure 18-1. Plotting and estimating extent of burn. The accompanying tabulation allows adjustments for the relatively larger head surface area in children. (From "Guide to Initial Therapy of Burns," Subcommittee on Burns of the Committee on Trauma of the American College of Surgeons, Bulletin of the A.C.S., May–June, 1964.)

icle or bulla formation, and pain. Full-thickness injury indicates destruction of all epithelial remnants and will require autograft wound closure. Full-thickness injuries may be charred or pearly white in color, anesthetic, and dry with parchmentlike eschar and underlying thrombosed blood vessels. Scald burns in young children commonly are full-thickness rather than partial-thickness injuries.

2. General examination   A thorough physical examination to identify associated injuries and coexisting illnesses is essential.

C. Criteria for admission to hospital

1. Patients with burns of the face, hands, feet, or perineum.

2. Children with burns of greater than 10% of the total body surface or any component of full-thickness injury.

3. Adults with partial-thickness injury greater than 15% or full-thickness injury greater than 2% of the total body surface.

4. Patients with suspected inhalation injury.

5. Patients with electrical burns, however small.

D. Initial management

1. **General**   Assess the adequacy of **ventilation.** Establish secure IV lines, preferably in an unburned area. Insert a Foley catheter and **measure urine output** hourly; urine output in an adult should be 30–50 ml/hr; in children, urine output should range from 0.5–1.5 ml/kg/hr. Insert a **nasogastric tube** for gastric decompression to help prevent vomiting and aspiration.

2. **Tetanus immunization**   If there has been no prior immunization against tetanus, or the prior immunization history is unknown, administer 250–500 units of human tetanus immune globulin IM for immediate passive protection in adults and, in addition, 0.5 ml of tetanus toxoid to begin primary immunization. Primary immunization must be completed according to schedule (see Sect. VI, Chap. 14). In patients with adequate prior tetanus immunization, an 0.5-ml tetanus toxoid booster is sufficient.

II. IV REQUIREMENTS   A variety of resuscitation formulas have been described to estimate fluids required to replace intravascular volume and restore cardiac output. The assessment of adequacy of volume restoration is based on frequent examination of the patient, the level of consciousness and orientation, vital signs, evidence of peripheral perfusion, urinary output, and body weight. The laboratory determinations of value are serum and urine osmolality, serum and urine electrolytes, and the hematocrit. After adequate urine output, peripheral perfusion, and blood pressure are established, fluids are replaced according to need as determined by the physical examination and laboratory determinations.

A. First 24 hr

1. **Adults**   Colloid solutions are no more effective for intravascular repletion than crystalloid solutions in the first 24 hr post burn; thus, colloids are no longer recommended in the first 24 hr. Resuscitation fluids are calculated as:

2 ml/kg/% burn of crystalloid
plus
2,000 ml of 5% dextrose in water

administered one half in the first 8 hr, one quarter in the next 8 hr, and one quarter in the last 8 hr.

a. A 70-kg man with a 50% burn would require 7,000 ml of crystalloid plus 2,000 ml of 5% dextrose in water, a total of 9,000 ml of fluid estimated for the first 24 hr; one half, or 4,500 ml, administered in the first 8 hr, and one quarter, or 2,250 ml, administered in each succeeding 8-hr period.

2. **Children**   Surface area is greater in relation to body weight in children so that evaporative losses are proportionately greater. The basic calculation, however, is the same:

$$\textbf{2 ml/kg body weight/\% burn of crystalloid}$$
$$\textit{plus}$$
$$\textbf{1,200-1,500 ml of 5\% dextrose in water/m}^2$$

Rapid administration of dextrose in water in children, who have a relatively small intravascular volume, may cause rapid hemodilution, cerebral edema, and convulsions. Total salt and water requirements should be administered so that rapid infusion of hypotonic solutions is avoided.

B. **Second 24 hr**   **One half to two thirds of the fluid volume requirements of the first 24 hr will be needed in this period.** Acute tubular necrosis seldom occurs in the early postburn period in either adults or children; if oliguria or anuria occurs, it is most likely due to inadequate volume replacement. Digitalis should not be used prophylactically, but should be reserved for patients with demonstrated congestive heart failure. Potassium supplementation also is contraindicated in the first 48 hr post burn; if administered, it may cause hyperkalemia.

C. **After 48 hr**   After acute losses have been replaced, the major need is accurate replacement of continuing evaporative losses plus fluids for maintenance. An **estimate of evaporative losses** can be made using the formula:

$$\textbf{(25 + \% burn)} \times \textbf{m}^2 \textbf{ total body surface}$$
$$\textbf{= estimate of evaporative losses/day in liters}$$

An extensively burned individual may require 4,000 ml or more per day of 5% dextrose in water to replace evaporative losses. Potassium replacement now becomes critical as such a patient may excrete up to 300 mEq of potassium per liter of urine. Urine and serum potassium determinations provide the guide to replacement. Whole blood or packed red cells are given to maintain a minimum hematocrit of 35%.

III. **SEDATION AND ANALGESIA**   The most common cause of respiratory arrest in burned patients in the period of resuscitation is narcotic overdose. Full-thickness injury is not painful, although surrounding partial-thickness injury is. **Agitation or distress in a burned patient should be considered as due to hypoxemia or hypovolemia until proven otherwise.** The effect of narcotics administered IM to a hypovolemic patient is unpredictable. Narcotics, if required, must be administered IV, in frequent small doses.

After the acute phase of injury, mild sedation may be required. Sedation should be judiciously employed and the patient examined frequently for evidence of overdose. A somnolent patient is not able to ingest an adequate volume of fluids or calories. In addition, sedatives and hypnotics may accumulate and cause respiratory arrest.

IV. ESCHAROTOMY

A. Extremity   Full-thickness burn produces a nonelastic eschar of heat-denatured skin. When this eschar encircles an extremity, development of subeschar edema may cause vascular compromise resulting in distal ischemia or gangrene.

Escharotomy is the incision of eschar along the medial and lateral aspects of an extremity to relieve vascular compromise and prevent ischemia and gangrene. The incision is made in areas of full-thickness encircling injury and is carried down only through the eschar. Fasciotomy also may be indicated in electrical injury and in patients with prolonged vascular compromise if, after escharotomy, distal pulses fail to return promptly. The Doppler ultrasonic flow meter is a valuable adjunct in determining the presence of distal pulses, especially in children with edematous extremities. In the upper extremity, adequate flow should be checked by ultrasound in the distal palmar arch or digital vessels; in the lower extremity, check the tibialis posterior or dorsalis pedis arteries.

B. Thoracic escharotomy is indicated in patients with encircling full-thickness burn of the trunk with limitation of chest wall excursion. Incisions are made in the anterior axillary line bilaterally, over the midsternum, and transversely at the costal margin.

V. INHALATION INJURY

A. Assessment   Inhalation injury is a **chemical tracheobronchitis** resulting from inhalation of toxic products of incomplete combustion. It may occur in patients burned in a **closed space,** or by the rapid **combustion of petroleum.** Seldom does direct thermal injury of endotracheal or endobronchial mucosa occur. **Live steam** inhalation in a closed space, however, may produce such a true thermal injury. A clinical diagnosis of inhalation injury is made in patients with a compatible history who have bronchorrhea or bronchospasm, who produce carbonaceous sputum, or who become hypoxemic and hypercapnic. There may or may not be thermal injury about the nose or mouth. The roentgenographic changes of inhalation injury may be delayed. A normal chest roentgenogram in the early postburn period does not exclude the possibility of significant inhalation injury. Symptoms of respiratory insufficiency may not occur for 24-72 hr post burn.

B. Treatment of inhalation injury is graded according to the severity and progression of symptoms and signs. Vigorous pulmonary toilet with postural drainage, nasotracheal suction or bronchoscopy, IV bronchial dilators, therapeutic antibiotics, arterial blood gas monitoring, intensive specialized nursing care, and steroids may play roles in the therapy of full-blown inhalation injury syndrome. Hypercapnia is the indication for ventilatory support.

C. Tracheostomy   The indications for tracheostomy in thermally injured patients are no different than in other patients. Upper airway obstruction, inability to handle secretions, management of associated injury such as flail chest, or severe inhalation injury causing inadequate ventilation as evidenced by hypercapnia are indications for tracheostomy. The mere existence of facial edema or burn, unless there is definite upper airway obstruction, is not an indication for a tracheostomy. Tracheostomy should be an elective procedure performed over an endotracheal tube in the operating room with adequate suction, light, and help.

VI. THE BURN WOUND

A. General   Attention is turned to the burn wound after adequate ventilation is insured and hypovolemic shock is being corrected. Gentle cleansing of the entire burn wound is performed, including debridement of superficial bullae, vesicles, and loose remnants of skin.

B. Parenteral antibiotics   Parenteral antibiotics do not affect the major area of burn wound infection, the subeschar interface between viable and nonviable tissue. The burn wound is relatively avascular because of thromboses and, similar to an abscess, is excluded from the circulation. The emergence of superinfection with *Candida*, fungi, and resistant bacteria contraindicate the use of prophylactic antibiotics. The burn wound should be examined frequently for the occurrence of infection. **Systemic antibiotics should be reserved for specific indications** such as the occurrence of pneumonia, septicemia, or other infection, and, if the infection is life-threatening, may be started while awaiting results of culture and sensitivity studies. Antibiotic therapy should be guided by the results of cultures and tissue biopsy. **If areas of hemorrhage are noted, biopsy should be performed to rule out invasive burn wound sepsis.** Other causes of hemorrhage in the burn wound are local trauma, fungal invasion, and disseminated intravascular coagulation.

C. Topical chemotherapy   The era of adequate topical chemotherapy was heralded in 1964 with the introduction of 10% mafenide (Sulfamylon) and 0.5% silver nitrate soaks. Subsequently, 1% silver sulfadiazine was approved as a topical agent for thermal injury. Each topical agent has its own inherent bacteriological and metabolic advantages and disadvantages.

 1. **10% Sulfamylon acetate cream** penetrates intact eschar. It is applied without dressings, leaving the wound visible, since Sulfamylon cream is bacteriologically less effective when dressings are applied. Sulfamylon is applied twice daily over the entirety of the burn wound with a sterile, gloved hand. In the first 2 wk after injury, the entirety of the burn wound should be cleansed and examined every day. After the eschar begins to separate, debridement should be performed on a daily basis. In children, apply Sulfamylon more than twice daily in order to cover the burn wound adequately. *Pseudomonas aeruginosa* has not developed resistance to this agent. Side effects of Sulfamylon are:

   a. Discomfort, primarily in areas of partial-thickness injury and easily controlled by mild analgesia.

   b. Hypersensitivity (atopy) in 6-7% of patients; symptoms respond to antihistaminic (diphenhydramine) and the Sulfamylon applications are continued.

    c. Delayed eschar separation, a consequence of suppression of subeschar bacterial growth.

    d. Acid-base disturbances consisting of early bicarbonate diuresis, decreased hydrogen ion excretion, increased urinary pH, decreased ammonia excretion, increased urinary flow caused by the solute diuresis, and increased urinary sodium and potassium excretion. If the arterial pH in patients treated with Sulfamylon is measured, respiratory alkalosis will be noted as long as pulmonary function is adequate. However, if atelectasis or pneumonia supervene, the pH may rapidly shift, reflecting an uncompensated metabolic acidosis. Sulfamylon should be discontinued and an alternative agent, such as 0.5% silver nitrate or 1% silver sulfadiazine, should then be chosen.

2. 0.5% silver nitrate is an effective topical chemotherapeutic agent if applied early after the burn. This agent is not absorbed through the eschar. If applied after subeschar colonization has occurred, it is not as effective as an absorbable agent. No hypersensitivity has been demonstrated to silver nitrate. It is painless and no resistance of bacteria has developed. Six to eight layers of four-ply 9-in. dressing gauze thoroughly soaked with the silver nitrate solution are applied to the wound and held in place with a circumferential dressing. The dressing must be kept wet by reapplication of silver nitrate solution as needed. The dressings are changed daily. The disadvantages of the silver nitrate method are:

    a. Silver nitrate stains everything with which it comes in contact.

    b. Leaching of sodium, chloride, and calcium into the hypotonic silver nitrate dressings leads to electrolyte loss.

    c. Absorption of hypotonic fluid by the patient, leading to water excess.

    d. Immobilization by the occlusive dressings which may restrict adequate joint motion.

3. 1% silver sulfadiazine recently has been approved for topical use in burn therapy. It has the advantage that it is not painful on application. The wound is visible as with Sulfamylon treatment as it is used in open fashion. The motion of joints can be maintained. Additional bacteriological experience will determine its adequacy.

D. Biological dressings include cadaver allograft, human amnion, and various forms of xenograft (porcine or canine). The functions of biological dressings are:

1. Permit debridement of full-thickness wounds immediately after eschar separation.

2. Promotion of healing of deep partial-thickness burns.

3. Protection and coverage of granulation tissue while awaiting donor site healing in extensive burns.

4. Preparation of recipient site for autograft.

5. Temporary coverage of open wounds prior to delayed primary or secondary closure.

Biological dressings are not used on full-thickness wounds prior to eschar separation because they promote invasion of viable subeschar tissue by bacteria and fungi, with resultant septicemia.

Cadaver allograft is the best temporary biological dressing, although availability is limited. Substitutes, such as porcine xenograft, may be acquired as needed or, in lyophilized form, may be stored. Biological dressings should be removed and reapplied when subgraft suppuration occurs. In addition, cadaver allografts should not be left on a wound for longer than 4-5 days to prevent vascularization ("take") of the graft.

E. **Invasive burn wound sepsis** is invasion of viable subeschar tissue by bacteria or fungi. The syndrome classically was described involving *P. aeruginosa.* The symptoms and signs of invasive burn wound sepsis include development of hemorrhage within the burn wound, hypothermia, ileus and subsequent gastric dilation, disorientation or obtundation, and, finally, cardiovascular collapse. The mortality of invasive burn wound sepsis exceeds 95%.

Prevention is the keynote of therapy and involves adequate topical chemotherapy, prevention of maceration of the burn wound, maintenance of adequate intravascular volume and blood pressure, and timely closure of the burn wound by autografting. After cardiovascular stability is achieved with IV resuscitation, extensively and circumferentially burned patients must be turned regularly or otherwise mobilized to prevent maceration of the burn wound. Frequent inspection of the burn would will identify areas of hemorrhagic change. Biopsy of suspect hemorrhagic areas to include subjacent and adjacent viable tissue should be performed to establish a diagnosis of burn wound invasion.

If a diagnosis of bacterial burn wound invasion is made, therapy is excision of the areas of invaded burn wound, appropriate systemic antibiotics (most commonly carbenicillin and gentamicin in maximum therapeutic dosage), blood and tissue cultures to identify the offending organism and its antibiotic sensitivities. The role of *Pseudomonas* immune human globulin remains to be established in the prevention and treatment of invasive burn wound sepsis.

F. **Skin grafting**   The goal of therapy of a burned patient is to sustain the patient until wound closure can be achieved. Burn wound closure is accomplished either by healing of the partial-thickness wound or by autograft coverage of the full-thickness wound. After the separation of eschar in the full-thickness wound, the use of cadaver allografts to prepare granulation tissue for autografting will help insure a take of autografted tissue. If the burn wound is properly prepared, it will not be necessary to utilize sutures to hold autografts in place. If possible, freshly autografted wounds should not be wrapped in dressings but be left exposed so that subgraft vesicles may be drained promptly and not allowed to lift the entire autograft from the wound.

Systemic antibiotics are begun preoperatively to prevent beta-hemolytic streptococcal infection of donor or recipient sites and are discontinued 3–4 days postoperatively. This prophylactic regimen is aimed only at control of beta-hemolytic streptococci; thus, low-dose penicillin therapy is usually prescribed.

G. Curling's ulcer

1. About 12% of burn patients will develop massive upper GI hemorrhage from stress ulceration of the stomach and duodenum. Approximately 45% of the multiple ulcers are located in the stomach, 45% are in the duodenum, and 10% are combined gastroduodenal ulcerations. Ninety percent of patients who develop Curling's ulcers are septic.

2. **Diagnosis**   Hemorrhage from upper GI bleeding initially may be insidious or brisk and be manifest by hematemesis or melena. An upper GI series frequently fails to demonstrate the shallow ulcer. Gastroscopy, after the stomach has been cleared of blood and clots, is the most reliable diagnostic procedure.

3. **Nonoperative treatment** includes iced saline lavage to clear the stomach of blood and clots, volume repletion, and correction of underlying factors such as septicemia.

4. **Indications for operation** are:

   a. Acute loss of 1,500–2,000 ml of blood.

   b. Fall of the hematocrit to 25% or below.

   c. Acute blood loss causing syncope.

   d. More than 1,000 ml of blood/24-hr period required after initial correction of hypovolemia.

   e. In children, acute replacement of approximately 50% of estimated total blood volume.

   The operation of choice in burn patients with stress ulceration of the GI tract is vagotomy plus removal of the ulcer, which most often dictates partial gastrectomy. If the ulcer is not removed in patients with continuing stress, such as infection, the incidence of rebleeding and perforation is significant.

H. Electrical injury

1. Electrical injury may cause considerable subcutaneous and subfascial injury without initial evidence of skin damage, except at entrance and exit points. In addition, if clothing becomes ignited, there may be associated thermal injury.

2. The resuscitation formulas described above based on the extent of thermal injury cannot be applied to patients who have incurred electrical injuries.

    a. Lactated Ringer's solution is given at a rate to maintain urine output at 70 ml/hr to help prevent deposition of the hemochromogens liberated by extensive electrical injury and thus obviate acute tubular necrosis.

    b. Fasciotomy is indicated in patients who have vascular compromise of electrically injured extremities.

    c. Antibiotics should be begun early after injury. The drugs selected should be effective against microaerophilic streptococci and gram-negative rods.

    d. Debridement of devitalized tissues should be performed after cardiovascular integrity is reestablished. All nonviable tissue must be excised. The cutaneous thermal component of the wound should be treated like any other thermal injury.

    e. Associated injuries, such as vertebral and long bone fractures or other injuries that may be incurred as a result of a fall, are common with electrical injury.

SUGGESTED READING

Curreri, P. W., Asch, M. J., and Pruitt, B. A., Jr.   The treatment of chemical burns: Specialized diagnostic, therapeutic, and prognostic considerations. *J. Trauma* 10:634, 1970.

McManus, W. F., Eurenius, K., and Pruitt, B. A., Jr.   Disseminated intravascular coagulation in burned patients. *J. Trauma* 13:416, 1973.

Moncrief, J. A.   Burns. *N. Engl. J. Med.* 288:444, 1973.

Pruitt, B. A., Jr., and Silverstein, P.   Methods of resurfacing denuded skin areas. *Transplant Proc.* 3:1537, 1971.

19. PEDIATRIC SURGERY

Improvement in surgical techniques and anesthesia and better understanding of physiology and the pathological processes that occur in infants have lowered the mortality and complication rates of anomalies, malignant tumors, surgical infections, and traumatic lesions peculiar to the pediatric patient.

I. **GENERAL CONSIDERATIONS** During the first 4-6 days of life, the full-term infant is particularly hardy and will withstand a major operation well, provided his unique physiology is taken into account.

A. **Fluids and electrolytes**

1. Because of high total body water content (700 ml/kg body weight; blood volume 88 ml/kg), the newborn infant needs minimal maintenance fluids during the first days of life.

2. Beyond the immediate postnatal period, infants normally exchange water and metabolites rapidly. Abnormal losses through the GI tract may result in dehydration and electrolyte depletion within a few hours.

3. Fluid administration during an operation should be no more than 5 ml/kg/hr up to a maximum of 15 ml/kg.

4. Maintenance fluid requirements suggested in Table 19-1 cover insensible water losses and urine output during health. Replacement of abnormal losses of fluids and electrolytes is calculated by reference to Table 19-2.

5. IV fluid orders for children are written to cover 8-hr periods only, and if the infant is in a critical condition, are rewritten every 4 hr.

6. Fluid deficit is estimated by observation of (a) body weight, (b) tissue turgor, (c) sunken eyes, (d) mucous membrane moisture, (e) quality of pulse, and (f) urine output. An infant in shock from dehydration, blood loss or sepsis will be pale, listless, and hypothermic.

7. Blood volume must be expanded rapidly in severely dehydrated infants using plasma, electrolyte solution, or blood; 20 ml/kg can be safely "pushed" rapidly IV. Further therapy is calculated by estimation of the degree of dehydration and observation of improvement of the infant measured by pulse, respiration, skin color, urine output, electrolytes, and weight.

TABLE 19-1. Maintenance IV Fluid Therapy (Premature, Newborn, and Older Children)

Condition and Weight	Water (ml/kg/24 hr)	Calories (Cal/kg/24 hr)	Sodium (mEq/kg/24 hr)	Potassium (mEq/kg/24 hr)	Chloride (mEq/kg/24 hr)	Expected Urine Output (ml/kg/24 hr)
Premature	40	50	0.5	0.5	0.5	30 ml total in first 24 hr
Newborn						
First week	50-60	60	0.5	0.5	0.5	30-110
After first week	100-110	100-110	1.5-2.0	1-1.5	1.5	30-110
Older Infants						
1-10 kg	100	100	1.5-2.0	1-1.5	1.5	30-110
11-20 kg	1,000 ml + 50 ml/kg for wt over 10 kg	1000 Cal + 50 Cal/kg for wt over 10 kg	...	...	...	...
21 kg and over	1,500 ml + 20 ml/kg for wt over 20 kg	1500 Cal + 20 Cal/kg for wt over 20 kg	...	...	...	...

TABLE 19-2. Composition of Abnormal External Fluid Losses in Infants

Fluid	Sodium (mEq/liter)	Potassium (mEq/liter)	Chloride (mEq/liter)	Protein (gm/100 ml)
Gastric	50	10	100-150	. . .
Pancreatic	130	10-15	90-120	. . .
Small intestinal	120	5-15	90-120	. . .
Bile	130	5-15	90-120	. . .
Ileostomy	100-130	5-15	50-100	. . .
Diarrhea	10-90	10-80	20-100	. . .
Sweat				
Normal	10-30	3-10	10-35	. . .
Cystic fibrosis	50-130	5-25	50-110	. . .
Burns	140	5	110	3-5

8. Losses from suction, fistulas, or diarrhea are measured every 8 hr and replaced promptly.

9. **Parenteral alimentation**   An infant or child who needs IV fluids for more than 1 wk (e.g., chronic ileus, obstruction, sepsis), one in whom protein losses will continue for an indefinite period (e.g., fistulas, peritonitis, burns, ileitis), or a recently operated infant in whom these conditions are apt to occur (e.g., gastroschisis, massive intestinal resection) is started on parenteral hyperalimentation to reduce protein depletion and susceptibility to infection. A Silastic IV catheter is inserted into the superior vena cava via the jugular or subclavian vein. Enough protein, nonprotein calories, electrolytes, vitamins, and minerals are given to maintain positive nitrogen balance and to replace previous and continuing losses. Maintenance of asepsis in the infusion system is of critical importance.

10. Plasma or albumin is used more frequently in infants and smaller children than in adults for conditions such as shock, sepsis, and burns. Plasma loss is tolerated poorly by infants owing to their rapid metabolic rate and relatively large body surface area. Albumin maintains colloidal osmotic pressure. There is suggestive evidence that plasma proteins are utilized for nutrition to a greater extent than in adults. Albumin usually is replaced in amounts of 10-20 mg/kg/day, but amounts of 50-75 mg/kg/day have been given in severe situations.

11. Blood replacement is necessary when there is acute or chronic blood loss.

    a. **Normal blood volumes** are: infant, 85 ml/kg, and child, 75 ml/kg.

    b. **Acute blood loss** is replaced in appropriate amounts to maintain normal vital signs, good skin color, normal temperature, and alertness and to restore a normal blood count.

    c. **Chronic blood loss in newborns** is replaced when hemoglobin drops below 8 gm/100 ml. Replacing blood at higher levels suppresses the normal bone marrow response of newborns who have a physiological hemolysis in the first week of life.

d. Chronic blood loss in older infants and children is replaced when the hemoglobin drops below 9 gm/100 ml. Anemic patients are susceptible to infection, heal wounds poorly, do not feel well, and eat poorly. Packed red cells, 10-15 ml/kg, are given slowly, followed by a blood count. As infants often are severely vasoconstricted, they may need more blood than originally estimated.

12. Hypoglycemia is a frequent problem in newborn infants following trauma, operation, or sepsis. Blood sugar is measured whenever irritability, twitching, or convulsions occur. Postoperatively, neonates are maintained on 10% glucose solution for several days to prevent hypoglycemia. A serum calcium concentration below 7 mg/100 ml requires treatment with an IV drip of 200 mg calcium gluconate/kg/day, with one fourth of the total given in the first 30-60 min.

B. Temperature control

1. Hypothermia may develop rapidly, particularly in premature infants. Infants respond to cooling with increased heat production, but their relatively large surface area and minimal subcutaneous fat permit excessive heat loss. Shock, sepsis, anesthesia, and application of surgical preparation solutions accentuate heat loss. Hypothermia produces increased oxygen need; if not corrected, it results in acidosis, hypoglycemia, and hyperkalemia. If severe hypothermia is present postoperatively, respiratory depression or arrest may occur. An incubator set at 32°C (90°F) is used during diagnostic and therapeutic procedures in premature infants. During operation, a warming pad is used and the temperature is monitored; skin preparation is limited and is followed by prompt draping.

2. Sudden hyperthermia under anesthesia leading to convulsions is potentially fatal. Heroic efforts (e.g., iced alcohol bath) to reduce the temperature are indicated. Most commonly, hyperthermia occurs in a febrile infant whose dehydration was inadequately corrected preoperatively; in rare instances, hyperthermia occurs without clues to its etiology. Adequate attention to preoperative rehydration and to reduction of fever and tachycardia decreases the incidence and severity of this problem.

C. Respiratory problems

1. The airway of an infant is small, the tidal volume may be only 15 ml, and the upper airway dead space is proportionately large (2 ml/kg). Thus, the infant has a narrow margin of respiratory reserve.

2. Small amounts of laryngeal edema or mucus may cause serious obstruction. Attempts to compensate through tachypnea soon result in fatigue and combined respiratory and metabolic acidosis.

3. Never restrain an infant flat on his back; the hazard of aspirating saliva or vomitus is great.

4. Every ½ hr postoperatively, change the infant's position and stimulate a cry and cough with pharyngeal suctioning. Direct tracheal suctioning with use of a laryngoscope sometimes may be necessary.

5. High humidity generated by an ultrasonic nebulizer is effective in thinning tracheobronchial secretions and reduces insensible water loss. Ultrasonic nebulization requires special monitoring in premature infants. Infants may "soak up" water in a humid atmosphere and develop water intoxication. Weigh the infant periodically and use ultrasonic nebulization intermittently.

6. Laryngeal edema following prolonged endotracheal intubation may result in hoarseness or stridor. This is treated with humidification and parenteral steroid therapy. Skillful use of a Silastic endotracheal tube may obviate the need for tracheostomy.

7. Tracheostomy is performed for retraction, restlessness, or air hunger that cannot be managed by intubation. Tracheostomy in a small infant is a difficult procedure and must be done with adequate exposure, assistance, and equipment in the operating room. Passage of an endotracheal tube allows control of the airway and facilitates location of the small soft trachea. Ordinary silver tracheostomy tubes are not suitable for small infants because they often are too long, occlude the carina, and have a high-resistance narrow bore. Plastic or Silastic tubes can be cut to the appropriate length and are well tolerated. If respiratory distress occurs after a tracheostomy, immediately take a chest x-ray to rule out pneumothorax or pneumomediastinum.

D. GI Tract

1. A newborn infant normally passes a large meconium stool within the first few hours of life. Swallowed air reaches the rectum within 12-18 hr; a prolongation of this time is expected in premature infants and in any infant who has an anoxic episode during delivery. X-rays also may demonstrate a "double bubble" in premature infants, a sign seen in congenital duodenal obstruction; further x-rays and evaluation are needed before such a diagnosis is established.

2. Infants under 1 yr of age swallow a considerable amount of air during feedings and sucking; it is normal to see air in the small intestine on abdominal x-rays.

3. Gastric emptying is rapid in infants. Clear liquids may be given by mouth to infants under 1 yr up to 4 hr before a scheduled operation. A routine order for "NPO after midnight" deprives a baby of water long enough to produce dehydration and fever.

E. Indications for antibiotics (Table 19-3)

1. Sepsis, suspected sepsis, peritonitis, pneumonitis, meningitis, and wound infections.

2. Thoracic and cardiac operations, intestinal resection or anastomosis, gastroschisis and ruptured omphalocele, genitourinary procedures when infection is present.

3. Patient on respirator.

4. Prophylaxis preoperatively in rheumatic heart disease, cystic fibrosis, and immunological disorders (e.g., Wiskott-Aldrich syndrome, agammaglobulinemia).

5. Antibiotics are not used routinely in full-term healthy infants undergoing clean upper abdominal operations (e.g., duodenal obstruction), repair of unruptured omphalocele with primary closure, gastrostomy, nephrectomy, or resection of intra-abdominal cysts and tumors.

II. SURGICAL CONDITIONS IN THE NEWBORN

A. Airway or pulmonary emergencies (see Table 19-4)

1. Cyanosis with tachypnea, dyspnea, stridor, intercostal retraction, or nasal flaring is cause for alarm and indicates need for prompt diagnosis and treatment.

2. **Diagnosis of an airway problem** involves the following routine:

   a. Place the infant in an Isolette with oxygen and high humidity. Start IV 10% glucose in water. Oral and tracheal suctioning is used as necessary. With respiratory arrest or pending arrest, the infant requires assisted ventilation.

   b. Observe the infant's breathing pattern. Measure vital signs. Auscultate the chest. Examine the head, neck, abdomen, and neurological system.

   c. Pass a catheter into each nostril and down the esophagus into the stomach.

   d. Take a portable upright chest x-ray including abdomen.

   e. Measure blood gases and CBC. Correct severe acidosis with sodium bicarbonate.

   f. Electrolytes, BUN, blood sugar, calcium, bilirubin, and ECG are performed if indicated.

   g. Blood, cord, and tracheal cultures are obtained.

h. A careful review of the family history and the course of the mother's pregnancy, labor, and delivery is obtained.

i. The diagnosis is usually obvious by this time unless an unusual cardiac or vascular lesion exists. Cardiac catheterization and urgent surgical therapy may be necessary.

TABLE 19-3. Antimicrobial Drugs Frequently Used in Pediatric Surgery

Drug	Dosage	Comments
Aqueous penicillin	Newborn: 60,000 units/kg/day IV q12h Older infant: 25,000–50,000 units/kg/day IV or IM q4-6h	Single most useful agent for gram-positive cocci and enterococci
Ampicillin	50-200 mg/kg/day IV or IM q4-6h (oral use causes diarrhea in very young)	Gram-positive cocci, *H. influenzae,* some strains of *E coli,* salmonella, shigella; use with kanamycin or gentamicin in sepsis and peritonitis
Cephalothin	50-100 mg/kg/day IV or IM (painful) q4-6h	Gram-positive cocci, including coagulase-positive staphylococci, *E. coli, Klebsiella, P. mirabilis;* use with kanamycin or gentamicin in sepsis and peritonitis
Methicillin	100-200 mg/kg/day IV or IM q4-6h	Coagulase-positive staphylococci
Oxacillin	50-100 mg/kg/day PO q6h	Coagulase-positive staphylococci
Kanamycin	15 mg/kg/day IM q12h	Many gram-negative organisms except *Pseudomonas;* use with penicillin or ampicillin
Gentamicin	Premature and first 5 days of life: 3-5 mg/kg/day IV or IM q12h After 5 days of life: 3-7.5 mg/kg/day IV or IM q8h	*Pseudomonas,* gram-negative rods, gram-positive cocci; use with penicillin or ampicillin in sepsis and peritonitis
Erythromycin	25-40 mg/kg/day orally	Use in patients allergic to penicillin; *Bacteroides* infections
Lincomycin	Premature and first 5 days of life: 3-5 mg/kg/day IV or IM q8-12h; 30 mg/kg/day PO q6h	Use in patients allergic to penicillin; *Bacteroides* infections
Clindamycin	10-40 mg/kg/day IV or IM q6h	Primary drug for *Bacteroides* infections
Chloramphenicol	50-100 mg/kg/day IV q6h	Use in life-threatening infections when other effective drug not available
Polymixin B	1.5-2.5 mg/kg/day IV or IM q8-12h	*Pseudomonas* infections
Colistin (polymixin E)	3-5 mg/kg/day IM q6-12h	*Pseudomonas* infections
Neomycin	50-100 mg/kg/day PO in 6 divided doses	Bowel prep; necrotizing enterocolitis in newborn
Sulfisoxazole	150-180 mg/kg/day PO q4-6h; 100 mg/kg/day IV or IM q8-12h	Do not use under 2 mo of age; urinary tract infections
Nitrofurantoin	6 mg/kg/day PO q6h	Urinary tract infections
Nystatin	2 cc (200,000 units) qid	Oral *Candida* infections (thrush)

TABLE 19-4. Respiratory Distress in the Newborn

Condition	Symptoms	Physical Findings	X-ray Findings	Comments
Airway obstruction				
Choanal atresia	Apnea and cyanosis at rest, relieved with crying	Catheter will not pass nose		Early operative correction
Pierre Robin syndrome	Retraction, choking with feedings	Small jaw, midline cleft palate, retrodisplaced tongue		Prone position, tube feeding
Lingual thyroid or cyst	Tachypnea, retraction	Palpable mass at base of tongue, head retracted		May need temporary tracheostomy; excise mass
Macroglossia	Noisy obstructive breathing	Large tongue (actual) or small mouth		Suspect Down's syndrome, cretinism, Beckwith's syndrome. Treat primary condition; partial glossectomy occasionally required
Vocal cord paralysis	Tachypnea, retraction, stridor, poor cry	Laryngoscopy is diagnostic		Tracheostomy if bilateral
Subglottic stenosis	Wheeze, poor cry, retraction	May be visible on laryngoscopy	Stenosis seen on lateral views of neck and chest	Tracheostomy, dilation
Vascular ring	Wheezing, choking on feeding	Head may be retracted	Indented esophagus on barium swallow, aortography	Divide anomalous artery
Neck mass (cystic hygroma, hemangioma)	Tachypnea, retraction, stridor, poor cry	Laryngoscopy is diagnostic		Excision
Esophageal atresia, with or without tracheoesophageal fistula	Choking on feeding, excessive salivation	Unable to pass nasogastric tube into stomach	Blind pouch (contrast medium); gas in stomach with fistula	Repair
"Tension" lesions (pulmonary displacement)				
Pneumothorax	Progressively severe tachypnea, cyanosis, tachycardia, retraction	Absent breath sounds, mediastinal shift	No lung markings on affected side	Needle aspiration; may need chest tube if condition persists after aspiration

342

	Symptoms	Physical findings	Radiographic findings	Treatment
Diaphragmatic hernia	Same as above	Scaphoid abdomen, no breath sounds on side of hernia	Intestine in chest on affected side	Nasogastric tube; endotracheal tube with positive pressure; O_2; IV $NaHCO_3$; immediate operation
Congenital lung cyst; lobar emphysema	Same as above	Mediastinal shift	Radiolucency, possibly with air-fluid level on affected side	Thoracotomy and excision (lobectomy)
Empyema or pyopneumothorax	Same as above	Fever, absent breath sounds, dullness	Opacity or air-fluid level	Diagnostic thoracocentesis, then chest tube; specific antibiotics (organism usually *Staphylococcus*)
Eventration of diaphragm	Same as above	Dullness, absent breath sounds on affected side	Elevated diaphragm	Thoracotomy and repair if condition severe
Pulmonary insufficiency				
Atelectasis or pneumonia	Progressively severe tachypnea, cyanosis, tachycardia, retraction	Dullness, absent breath sounds on affected side	Opacification of involved lung	Tracheal suction, antibiotics, humidity, nebulization
Hyaline membrane disease	Same as above	Rales, rhonchi, diminished breath sounds	Ground glass appearance, air bronchograms	Same as above; may need assisted ventilation; measure blood gases as needed
Wilson-Mikity syndrome	Same as above	Same as above	Same as above	Same as above; appears after prolonged course of respiratory distress and oxygen therapy
Cardiac failure	Same as above	Same as above	Rales, enlarging liver, diminished urinary output, edema	Digitalis, diuretics; cardiac surgery may be necessary if severe cyanotic lesion present
Abdominal distention (e.g., intestinal obstruction, peritonitis, sepsis, paralytic ileus)	Respiratory distress with grunting respirations; vomiting bile	Abdominal distention, scanty diarrheal stools or obstipation	Elevated diaphragm, dilated loops of intestine with air-fluid levels	Antibiotics; nasogastric tube; fluid replacement; operation, if indicated

3. **Esophageal atresia** with or without a tracheoesophageal fistula is suspected when excessive salivation is present at birth and persists. Feedings produce coughing, choking, or cyanosis. A catheter passed into the nares meets an obstruction 8-10 cm from the lips and will not pass into the stomach. A chest x-ray demonstrates the catheter in the neck and upper chest. A small amount (½ ml) of barium inserted through the catheter into the upper esophagus demonstrates esophageal atresia. Aspirate the barium immediately. Air in the GI tract confirms the presence of an associated tracheoesophageal fistula. The absence of air suggests atresia without a fistula.

   Put the infant in a semisitting position. A small constant suction catheter is placed in the proximal esophageal pouch to remove saliva. Humidity, oxygen, and antibiotics are used to treat pulmonary infection. An operation is performed as soon as pulmonary sepsis has cleared.

4. **Diaphragmatic hernia** is particularly serious in an infant because the mediastinum is mobile and readily displaced, causing severe respiratory embarrassment. Suspect a diaphragmatic hernia in a newborn with respiratory distress, a scaphoid abdomen, and a shifted apical cardiac impulse. A chest x-ray will demonstrate air-filled loops of intestine in the pleural cavity with mediastinal displacement. This lesion rarely may be confused with a congenital lung cyst; if the infant's condition is not severe and the diagnosis really is not clear, an upper GI series may be done. Immediate surgical repair is required. An abdominal approach is preferred. The viscera are reduced into the abdomen, the diaphragm repaired, and any rotational anomaly of the intestine corrected.

B. Intestinal obstruction in the newborn

1. Any infant who **vomits bile-stained material** in the first days of life has intestinal obstruction unless it can be absolutely ruled out.

2. Failure to pass normal meconium stool, passage of bloody stool, and abdominal distention are other features strongly suggestive of intestinal obstruction in a newborn.

3. If intestinal obstruction is suspected, a systematic plan of diagnosis should be followed.

   a. Pass a nasogastric tube and note the amount and character of the aspirate.

   b. Do a complete physical examination, including a rectal examination. The history and physical findings may suggest a cause other than obstruction, e.g., sepsis, birth anoxia, hypothyroidism, or intracranial hemorrhage, for which an appropriate workup is done.

c. Begin IV fluids calculated to include fluid sequestered in the intestine. Determination of electrolyte and acid-base balance is made.

d. Obtain a flat plate of the abdomen and upright films of the abdomen and chest. If air is seen only in the stomach or duodenum but not more distally, duodenal atresia, tight duodenal stenosis, or a rotational abnormality with midgut volvulus is present. Prompt operation is indicated without further studies.

e. If distention is present and films show multiple intestinal loops with air-fluid levels, a gentle barium study of the colon is indicated. A tiny, unused colon seen on contrast enema indicates small-bowel obstruction due to atresia, stenosis, meconium ileus, or, rarely, an internal hernia. Urgent exploration is indicated except in meconium ileus, which may be treated by Gastrografin enemas.

A normal or slightly distended colon may indicate congenital aganglionosis, meconium plug syndrome, or, rarely, a rectal or low colonic stenosis, or a condition not requiring operation. The surgical conditions in which a normal or dilated colon is present do not require urgent operative correction. Meconium plugs commonly pass when the barium is expelled. Hirschprung's disease and its accompanying obstructive symptoms can be controlled by saline irrigation of the colon; a colostomy and biopsy confirmation of the diagnosis is performed electively. Low colonic or rectal stenosis may be amenable to dilation; if not, an operation can be done semielectively.

C. Anorectal malformation

1. Careful inspection of the perineum and genitalia provides correct diagnosis of most anomalies.

2. The critical decision in the newborn is to determine if the anomaly is a "low" or a "high" lesion.

3. Low lesions in boys invariably have a fistula opening in the midline of the perineum either at the usual site of the anus or anterior to it. A limited anoplasty in the newborn period followed by persistent dilations for a month or more provides good results.

4. Low lesions in girls usually present with a fistula to the perineum or to the vaginal fourchette. Dilation usually is adequate initial treatment, although a limited "cutback" procedure may be necessary to give a functionally adequate although ectopic opening. The decision about a later procedure to place the anus in a normal position need not be made until 4-6 yr of age.

5. When no perineal fistula is present in boys the likelihood is great that the lesion is a high one. With high lesions, a fistula into the urethra or, rarely, the bladder, is always present.

6. After 24 hr of age, longer if required for the abdomen to begin to show mild distention, inverted lateral x-rays help to define the level of the anomaly. High lesions are indicated by gas only above a line drawn from the pubis to the sacrococcygeal junction.

7. In high lesions a colostomy (preferably right transverse) is indicated. Definitive reconstruction is technically difficult and is best done between 18–24 mo of age.

D. Abdominal wall defects

1. Omphalocele is the result of embryonic arrest during the period when the GI tract is herniated into the umbilical cord. The clinical presentation is a mass of viscera herniated through the umbilical ring and covered by a membranous sac.

2. Small omphaloceles will close spontaneously if kept protected and painted several times with 0.5% silver nitrate solution. Early operation is also satisfactory if no concurrent problems exist, e.g., prematurity, severe congenital anomaly (especially cardiac), pulmonary problems, or sepsis.

3. Large omphaloceles are more difficult problems. The abdominal cavity is underdeveloped; forceful return of the viscera and complete closure of the abdomen may elevate abdominal pressure, resulting in respiratory insufficiency, impaired venous return, and even compromised circulation to the intestine. Alternatives to immediate closure are, first, apply silver nitrate and wait until sufficient shrinkage of the sac has occurred to permit safe closure (usually 4–6 wk), or, second, cover the viscera with Silon sheet sutured to the full thickness of the abdominal wall. Reduce the sac in size every 2–3 days and after 10–14 days completely remove the sac and close the abdominal wall.

4. Omphalocele may rupture prior to or during delivery. In this event, immediate closure must be carried out. Primary closure is done only if possible without tension; a staged closure using a Silon sheet is very satisfactory.

5. Gastroschisis differs etiologically but presents much the same problem as a ruptured omphalocele. In some instances, primary closure may be done after gentle manual stretching of the abdominal wall; in most instances, staged closure with Silon sheet is preferred management.

E. Abdominal masses in infants and children (Tables 19-5 and 19-6)

1. Abdominal masses in the newborn or very young infant are often asymptomatic and usually benign, but all masses must be considered to be malignant until proven otherwise. Early diagnosis and treatment are essential.

2. The leading cause of death in infants and children is trauma; malignancy is second in frequency. The most common malignancies are Wilms' tumor and neuroblastoma.

3. Abdominal masses occur in all organs and areas of the abdomen. The diagnosis often can be inferred by the location of the mass.

4. Diagnosis is facilitated by the CBC, urinalysis, chest x-ray, and an IVP. A renal scan and cystogram also may be helpful if a kidney is not visualized on IVP. A liver scan may localize extrarenal upper abdominal lesions and liver masses. Careful urinary bladder catheterization in bladder neck obstruction is both diagnostic and therapeutic. Rarely, aortography, inferior venacavography, cystoscopy, retrograde pyelography, and barium studies are necessary.

5. If the infant is healthy and full-term, prompt laparotomy can be undertaken. If urinary or intestinal obstruction exists, rapid intervention is required. If the infant is very premature or ill from another cause, operation should be delayed until improvement has been obtained. Infants suspected of harboring a malignant mass are not operated on if pulmonary metastases are present; preoperative chemotherapy may be required.

F. Masses in the neck (Table 19-7)

1. Neck masses present at delivery only rarely require emergency treatment.

   a. **Cystic hygroma** (lymphangioma) is a soft mass in the anterior cervical triangle which may involve any portion of the neck, parotid region, and cheek, and extend under the tongue and around the pharynx and larynx. Despite their alarming appearance, these masses usually do not cause respiratory or feeding problems. A period of observation, allowing the baby to grow, is worthwhile, as surgical excision is tedious and accompanied by many complications when done in a newborn.

   b. Masses in the **thyroid** are rare. Congenital goiter is the most frequent and usually is due to maternal medications during gestation; these goiters usually subside spontaneously. Occasionally, congenital goiters cause severe respiratory obstruction; subtotal excision is required. Virtually all tumors in the neonatal thyroid are teratomas; they are very rare and require early excision.

2. Neck masses in older children are more common. Their diagnostic features are summarized in Table 19-7.

TABLE 19-5. Abdominal Masses in Infancy

Organ or Area	Lesion	Diagnostic Studies	Treatment
Kidney	Unilateral multicystic kidney	IVP; renal scan (nonfunctioning kidney or obstruction with some function)	Resection
	Hydronephrosis (unilateral or bilateral)	IVP; renal scan; voiding cystourethrogram	Resection or pyeloplasty
	Polycystic kidney (bilateral)	IVP; renal function tests (large cysts)	Supportive
	Tumors (fibromas, mesoblastic nephromas, Wilms' tumor)	IVP	Resection
	Renal vein thrombosis	History of diabetic or toxemic mother and large baby; flank mass on examination; IVP: no visualization; hematuria, thrombocytopenia, anemia	IV therapy; no immediate operation; 5–10% may require later nephrectomy for renal hypertension
Extrarenal (retroperitoneal)	Neuroblastoma	IVP: displaced kidney	Resection; good prognosis if < 1 yr
	Teratoma (rare location)	IVP: displaced kidney	Resection
	Sarcoma	IVP: upper GI series: displaced kidney, stomach, duodenum	Resection; poor prognosis

		Diagnosis	Treatment
Liver	Cysts	Hepatomegaly; liver scan for space-occupying lesions	Resection
	Hemangioma	Liver scan; arteriogram	Biopsy; may develop high output heart failure and thrombocytopenia
	Hamartoma	Liver scan	Resection
	Hepatoma	Liver scan	Hepatic lobectomy if localized
	Glycogen storage disease	Hepatomegaly; abnormal glucose tolerance test	Biopsy
	Hepatitis (neonatal)	Hepatomegaly; liver chemistries	Prefer to make diagnosis without biopsy
Intestinal and mesenteric	Choledochal cyst	Cholangiogram; upper GI series	Resection and anastomosis
	Duplication (large and small intestine)	Barium enema: obstruction or displacement; GI bleeding	
	Mesenteric cyst	Examination (very mobile); barium studies (displacement)	Resection of cyst; may need bowel resection as well
Ovary	Cyst	IVP; barium enema (displacement); mass in lower abdomen	Resection
	Teratoma and other solid tumors	IVP; barium enema (displacement); mass in lower abdomen	Resection
Bladder	Bladder neck obstruction	Pass catheter; voiding cystogram; IVP	Vesicostomy; later definitive operation
	Neurogenic bladder	Infant with meningomyelocele	Usually do not require operation
Vagina and uterus	Hydrometrocolpos	Abdominal midline mass with bladder displacement on cystogram	Vaginal drainage

TABLE 19-6. Malignant Tumors in Infancy

Tumor	Age	Symptoms	Diagnostic Studies	Metastases	Catecholamines	Treatment	Prognosis of Cure
Wilms' tumor	1–4 yr	Abdominal mass, often found by mother; microscopic hematuria in 40%	IVP: calyces distorted	Lung	Normal	Excision Irradiation (begin on day of operation) if lesion beyond capsule Actinomycin D and vincristine	70% 2-yr survival if metastases present; 90% if no metastases present
Neuroblastoma	Less than 1 yr (may appear up to teens)	Abdominal mass; bone pain or proptosis secondary to metastases may be first symptom. Usually crosses midline of abdomen. Also occurs in posterior mediastinum	IVP: kidney or ureter displaced by tumor; bone films and chest x-rays show metastases	Bones, liver, skin	Elevated (diagnostic after operation)	Excision when possible; biopsy when nonresectable	75% cure under 1 yr; overall survival over 1 yr less than 20%
Teratoma	Newborn to 5 yr	Sacrococcygeal, ovarian, or mediastinal mass	Chest x-ray	Generalized	…	Total excision	Good if excised in newborn period; prognosis poor in older child
Hepatoma	Newborn to teens (usually before 2 yr of age)	Upper abdominal mass	Liver scan: space-occupying lesion	Generalized	…	Hepatic lobectomy if localized to one lobe	Less than 10%
Genitourinary rhabdomyosarcoma (prostate, bladder, vagina, uterus)	Newborn to teens (early infancy)	Abdominal mass or external lesions	IVP and cystogram (obstruction may be present)	Generalized	…	Pelvic exenteration if localized; chemotherapy and irradiation preop and postop	20–50%, if localized (depends on site)

350

TABLE 19-7. Neck Masses in Children

Type	Location	Character	Workup	Treatment
Lymphadenitis	Primarily upper lateral neck	Firm, movable, and tender	ENT examination, PPD, chest film, throat culture	Treat primary lesion if present; 7–10 days of antistaphylococcal drugs; incision and drainage if fluctuance develops; biopsy if no response to antibiotics
Lymphoma	Lateral neck, supraclavicular region	Multiple rubbery, nontender nodes	Hemotological investigation, chest film	Biopsy followed by chemotherapy or irradiation, depending on histology
Carcinoma of thyroid	In thyroid or lateral cervical nodes	Hard nodule	History of head or neck irradiation in infancy, chest film, thyroid scan	Total thyroidectomy; node dissection if indicated; thyroxine or ^{131}I
Thyroglossal duct cyst	Midline	Moves with swallowing; "tug" when tongue is protruded	None	If cystic, excise with midportion of hyoid bone; if solid, biopsy to identify midline ectopic thyroid
Branchial cleft cyst	Lateral along anterior border of sternomastoid muscle	Cystic; sinus tract may be palpable	None	Excise with sinus tract

G. Hypertrophic pyloric stenosis

1. Pyloric stenosis usually manifests itself in infants 2-6 wk of age. The diagnosis should be considered in any infant who vomits, although faulty feeding practices account for most instances of vomiting.

2. An infant with pyloric stenosis is hungry and will take a feeding immediately after vomiting. Vomiting varies from mild to forceful and rarely is bile-stained.

3. Give the infant a bottle and observe his abdomen. Peristaltic waves across the upper abdomen from left to right are frequently seen. This sign is highly suggestive but not pathognomonic of hypertrophic pyloric stenosis.

4. The sine qua non of diagnosis is palpation of the enlarged pylorus. It is most commonly felt just to the right of the midline halfway between the xiphoid and umbilicus. Palpation is best done from the baby's left side using the left hand. If the mass is not palpated on the initial examination, the examination should be repeated after an interval. If the mass is not palpated after several attempts by experienced examiners, an upper GI series is obtained. If several examiners have failed to find the pyloric mass, the radiologist usually finds a hiatus hernia, chalasia of the esophagus, or pylorospasm rather than pyloric stenosis. Operation ordinarily should not be done unless a mass is palpated.

5. If vomiting has been prolonged, hypochloremic, hypokalemic alkalosis is common. A solution of 0.45% saline with 5% glucose is begun IV. After the baby voids, potassium chloride is added at a concentration of 40 mEq/liter. Hydration should be restored and acid-base balance brought within normal limits prior to operation.

H. GI bleeding in infants and children

1. Although GI bleeding is frightening in any age group, in children it rarely is life-threatening. The child's cardiovascular system will tolerate acute bleeding better than an adult's. Fifty percent of cases of GI bleeding in childhood will not be diagnosed and will not recur.

2. A child with acute GI bleeding should have blood drawn for a CBC, typing and cross matching, coagulation profile, and liver function studies. An IV infusion is started with lactated Ringer's or normal saline solution. A nasogastric tube is inserted into the stomach to see if blood is present in the upper GI tract. A bone marrow biopsy is performed if leukemia is suspected. Vitamin K, 1 mg, is given to newborns who have not already received it.

3. Barium studies in the acute phase rarely are helpful and will only jeopardize a patient who may become hypovolemic if prolonged studies are carried out in the x-ray department.

4. Blood should be started if there is evidence of shock and a falling hematocrit.

5. A rule of thumb in acute GI bleeding in children is that surgical intervention is carried out when the patient has had one complete exchange of blood volume without cessation of bleeding and there is no evidence of blood dyscrasia or coagulopathy.

6. Acute GI bleeding in children is divided into three groups (Table 19-8):

 a. Newborn (95% of causes are nonsurgical).

 b. One month–2 yr (33% are surgical or serious medical).

 c. Over 2 yr (high percentage of surgical or serious medical diseases).

7. When the patient is stable definitive barium studies (upper and lower GI series with small-bowel follow-through) are performed along with proctoscopy. Obtain stools for specific pathogen culture and examination for parasites. Angiography is just beginning to be used in pediatrics with any frequency.

8. Gastroenteritis should not be considered a cause for GI bleeding until all other causes have been ruled out. Bleeding due to gastroenteritis is rare.

I. Umbilical hernia

1. The great majority close spontaneously.

2. Operation is not advised until age 3 if the defect is greater than 2 cm. If the defect is less than 2 cm, observation is continued until age 5. All defects in females should be repaired at age 5 since later pregnancy may precipitate incarceration. In males, any defect less than 2 cm need not be repaired, as it will close further as abdominal muscles develop in adolescence.

J. Appendicitis   Children react with abdominal pain to a large variety of nonsurgical illnesses. However, the symptom complex of abdominal pain, vomiting, and fever requires that the diagnosis of appendicitis be a prominent consideration. Remember that appendicitis progresses more rapidly in children than in adults. If abdominal pain persists and there is localized lower abdominal tenderness, predominantly right-sided but occasionally midline or slightly to the left, that cannot be explained on the basis of another condition, operation for appendicitis must be undertaken.

K. Constipation

1. Constipation in childhood, although usually not a serious organic problem, can become a serious social and psychological problem for both the child and parents.

TABLE 19-8. Gastrointestinal Bleeding in Infants and Children

Age	Peak Age	More Frequent and Common Causes	Other Causes	Clinical Manifestation and Character of Bleeding	Workup	Treatment
Newborn	1–2 days	Swallowed maternal blood		Vomiting bright red blood	Apt test positive	None
		Hemorrhagic disease of newborn		Patient may be pale, listless	Apt test negative	Vitamin K
		Gastroduodenal ulcer		Patient may be pale, listless	Apt test negative	Blood transfusion; nasogastric irrigation
			Midgut volvulus	Vomiting bile; bloody stool; abdominal distention	X-ray (intestinal obstruction)	Immediate operation
			Duplication	Vomiting bile if obstructed, bloody stool	Barium studies	Operation
			Reflux esophagitis	Vomiting blood	Barium studies	Keep child upright in infant seat; thicken feedings
			Necrotizing enterocolitis	Vomiting bile, bloody stool, abdominal distention. Premature with anoxia or infant on respiratory assistance	Air in wall of intestine, ileus; air in portal vein and biliary tree	IV fluids; antibiotics; albumin; nasogastric suction; operate for perforation

1 mo–2 yr	1–6 mo	Anal fissure		Bright bleeding with hard stool	None	Stool softener
	6–12 mo	Intussusception		Colic; blood in stool (currant jelly); abdominal mass	Barium enema	Hydrostatic pressure with barium enema; operation if barium unable to reduce completely or symptoms longer than 12 hr
	Over 4 mo	Meckel's diverticulum		Hematochezia; anemia	Barium studies normal; sodium pertechnetate scan may be helpful	Operate with second recurrence of massive bleeding and hemoglobin less than 8 gm/100 ml
Over 2 yr	Over 2 yr	Polyp		Bright to dark rectal bleeding	Barium enema; proctoscopy	Remove via proctoscope; if massive bleeding, operate
	2–4 yr	Polyp, Meckel's diverticulum, T&A, epistaxis	Peptic esophagitis	Poor feeder; vomiting; recurrent pneumonia	Upper GI series	Antispasmodics; keep child in infant seat, especially after feeding
	Over 3 yr		Esophageal varices	Vomiting blood (usually with aspirin ingestion or viral infection)		Supportive therapy; occasionally, Sengstaken-Blakemore tube; shunt after 8 yr of age; generally improve with age (good liver function)
	Over 5 yr		Peptic ulceration	Vomiting blood (usually with aspirin ingestion or viral infection)		Supportive therapy; usually operate if blood loss exceeds one blood volume

2. The common type of constipation is functional, without any known causes; motor dysfunction of the colon is suspected but not proved.

3. Onset of constipation occurs with toilet training around 2-3 yr. The child has 1-2 massive stools a week and constant soiling due to fecal impaction and overdistention of the colon. Growth and development are normal. The rectal examination demonstrates stool impacted in the rectum.

4. Hirschsprung's disease, in contradistinction, begins in the newborn period, the rectum usually is empty of stool, and there is a failure of normal growth and development.

5. The diagnosis of functional constipation is made by history, physical examination, and a barium enema which demonstrates a uniformly distended colon without areas of narrowing.

6. Treatment consists of reassurance, keeping the colon relatively empty through daily bowel movements encouraged by stool softeners and suppositories (no laxatives), and prevention of fecal impaction. Suppositories are inserted when the child awakens in the morning in order that he can defecate before leaving for school. With constant treatment, most children develop proper bowel control in 6-18 mo.

SUGGESTED READING
Firor, H. V.   Omphalocele—An appraisal of therapeutic approaches. *Surgery* 69:208, 1971.
Gans, S. L.   *Surgical Pediatrics.* New York: Grune & Stratton, 1973.
Kirtley, J. A., and Holcomb, G. W.   Surgical management of diseases of the gallbladder and common duct in children and adolescents. *Am. J. Surg.* 111:39, 1966.
Potts, W. J.   *The Surgeon and the Child.* Philadelphia: Saunders, 1959.
Stephens, F. D., and Smith, E. D.   *Ano-Rectal Malformations in Children.* Chicago: Year Book, 1971.

20. TRANSPLANTATION

I. KIDNEY TRANSPLANTATION Kidney transplantation is a well-established treatment of patients with end-stage kidney disease unless serious contraindications exist, e.g., ischemic heart disease, advanced arteriosclerosis, malignancy, active autoimmune disease, sepsis, or advanced age. The greatest likelihood of success occurs with living related donors, but cadaver kidney transplantation is desirable in many instances, necessitating active search for potential cadaver donors.

A. Identification and evaluation of potential cadaver donors

1. Persons who have irretrievably lost brain function and whose death appears imminent may be suitable kidney donors. Brain death is customarily diagnosed by a neurologist or neurosurgeon. The criteria include:

   a. Areflexia, including pupillary and eye globe responses (cephalo-ocular reflexes); occasionally deep tendon reflexes may be elicited after brain death.

   b. Total unresponsiveness to painful stimuli.

   c. Absence of respiratory effort.

   d. Where deemed appropriate, a cerebrally silent electroencephalogram.

2. These strict **contraindications** to kidney donation must not be present in a prospective donor:

   a. Malignancy.

   b. Sepsis.

   c. Preexisting renal disease.

3. Renal function must be adequate. Prolonged hypotension and shock are extremely damaging to the kidneys. Diuresis with colloid and crystalloid IV infusions and furosemide (40–500 mg IV push) should be established before accepting the donor.

4. Permission to remove kidneys must be obtained from the next of kin. If the person carried a signed donor card indicating a desire to donate

organs at time of death, such a card is a legal instrument under the Uniform Anatomical Gift Act and organ procurement may proceed without additional permission.

B. Procurement and maintenance of cadaver kidney

1. The donor is taken to the operating room after brain death has been declared. Circulation and respiration must be maintained until organ procurement is under way.

2. Donor is anticoagulated with 2 mg/kg of heparin IV.

3. Ganglionic blockade with phenoxybenzamine is helpful to avert vasospasm in the renal circulation.

4. The kidneys must be removed with care to preserve adequate length of artery, vein, and ureter. Excessive manipulation must be avoided. Removal must be accomplished within 30 min of cessation of circulation.

5. The kidneys are cooled immediately by submerging them in an iced saline bath and flushing with an iced crystalloid solution. An "intracellular" crystalloid solution (Collins' solution or equivalent) may be used if the kidney is to be reimplanted within 8-12 hr. If longer preservation is required, pulsatile perfusion with solutions containing plasma protein is necessary.

C. Evaluation of recipient The uremic patient is evaluated for dialysis or transplantation as follows:

1. Renal function is measured by clearance studies; irreversible renal impairment must be confirmed by these studies.

2. Renal biopsy often is desirable for diagnosis.

3. Lower urinary tract obstruction must be ruled out by history, cystoscopy, retrograde pyelography, voiding cystourethrography, and residual urine determinations, as indicated. If lower tract disease exists, appropriate surgical preparation, such as construction of an intestinal conduit or bladder neck revision, must precede transplantation.

4. A chest x-ray must not show evidence of active tuberculosis or other serious parenchymal or cardiovascular disease.

5. An ECG is taken to evaluate organic and ischemic heart disease.

6. Liver function tests must show no evidence of serious primary abnormality. Viral hepatitis may exclude the patient from transplantation, and dictates extreme caution on the part of all dialysis-transplantation personnel.

7. PPD (second-strength) skin test must be recorded. Uremia may impair reaction to the antigen, so these tests should be performed following dialysis.

8. Evaluation of autoimmune disease must be made by measuring C3 complement, anti-glomerular basement membrane antibody, and antinuclear antibody and by LE cell preparations. Active, progressive autoimmune disease usually precludes transplantation.

9. Social and pertinent psychological profiles must be performed and confirm that the patient will be able to cooperate in the complex treatment regimen.

10. Measures of histocompatibility between donor and recipient must be made, whether the donor source be a family member or a cadaver. Matching is vital when a family member is chosen as donor; both good and bad matches will be present in any family group. A preoperative cross match must be performed in every case, since presensitization of the recipient resulting in development of antibodies to donor antigens will cause hyperacute kidney rejection.

D. Evaluation of living donor

1. The donor must be a blood relative of the recipient.

2. The donor's history and physical examination must be entirely normal.

3. The chest x-ray and ECG must be normal.

4. BUN, creatinine, creatinine clearance, uric acid, cholesterol, alkaline phosphatase, calcium, phosphorus, acid phosphatase, prothrombin time, and liver function tests must be normal.

5. The urinalysis must be within normal limits and urine cultures found negative on three occasions.

6. Hemoglobin, hematocrit, leukocyte count, erythrocyte count, bleeding, and clotting time must be within normal limits.

7. The excretory urogram must be normal.

8. Abdominal aortography must be performed prior to donation to determine the anatomy of the renal arteries. Kidneys with solitary renal arteries are preferred, although successful anastomoses of multiple renal arteries usually can be attained.

E. Preparation of a living donor   In addition to usual measures of preoperative preparation, the following must be accomplished:

1. Special operative permits must be signed indicating the donor's knowledge of the possible consequences of his donation.

2. One unit of blood is withdrawn from the donor several days preoperatively to be held in reserve as an autologous blood transfusion if needed during the operation. Transfusion of banked blood is avoided.

3. The prospective donor is brought to the operating room 1 hr before induction of anesthesia, and IV hydration with 15 ml/kg of Ringer's lactate solution is begun.

4. An indwelling catheter is placed during the operation to permit free urine flow and to record urine output rate.

5. During anesthesia, strict attention is paid to maintenance of normal blood pressure and continuous good hydration.

6. Vasopressors cannot be used.

7. Intermittent IV furosemide is given to maintain a urine output of at least 1.5 ml/min.

8. Immediately prior to removal of the kidney, the donor is anticoagulated with 2 mg/kg of heparin. The left kidney is taken preferentially, all other factors being equal.

9. Following removal, the kidney is flushed by gravity flow (100 cm) with a solution of refrigerated crystalloid solution containing heparin until the renal venous effluent is cold and clear.

F. **Preoperative and operative management of the recipient**

1. The potential recipient is placed on hemodialysis to be prepared for transplantation. Access to the arterial circulation for repeated hemodialysis is achieved with external Silastic AV shunts or internal AV fistulas or shunts which cause "arterialization" of an accessible vein.

2. Baseline hematological data are obtained, including bone marrow aspiration and clotting studies. If leukopenia is detected, a spleen scan should be performed. Splenectomy should be done prior to transplantation if splenomegaly and hypersplenism can be documented.

3. Chest x-ray and cultures of skin lesions, nose and throat, sputum, and urine are obtained.

4. For 1–2 wk preoperatively, the recipient of an elective transplant is given daily baths with a germicidal soap.

5. Preoperative and intraoperative transfusions are administered as needed, using packed washed red cells or frozen blood. Transfusion with whole blood is avoided.

6. The operative permit signed by the recipient must include special indication that he has been made aware of the possible consequences of transplantation.

7. Immunosuppression is begun with azathioprine (Imuran), 5 mg/kg, several hours prior to operation. Azathioprine, 3 mg/kg, is given 12-24 hr after operation. If liver dysfunction occurs, cyclophosphamide is substituted for azathioprine.

8. Prednisone (or IV equivalent, such as methylprednisolone), 5 mg/kg, is given before operation. IV methylprednisolone, 30 mg/kg, is given as one dose during the operation.

9. The renal artery is anastomosed end-to-end to the internal iliac artery, and the renal vein is sutured end-to-side to the common iliac vein. The donor ureter is implanted into the recipient's bladder, or the recipient's ureter may be anastomosed to the pelvis of the transplanted kidney.

10. Postoperative immunosuppression is maintained with azathioprine, 2-3 mg/kg/day, depending on the leukocyte count. Methylprednisolone, 30/mg/kg, is given IV on the first postoperative day, and rapidly reduced by halving on the second and third days. Thereafter, the dose of prednisone is decreased stepwise to 30 mg/day by the twentieth postoperative day. Steroids are given as a single dose once daily. While on steroids the patient is given oral antacid medications.

11. Postoperative laboratory studies

    a. Daily: serum electrolytes, BUN, creatinine, urinalysis, CBC.

    b. Every other day: calcium and phosphorus, blood sugar, urine culture.

    c. Twice a week: bilirubin and liver enzymes, uric acid.

    d. Once a week: serum proteins.

    e. Isotope scanning using the gamma camera is useful to monitor perfusion and function of the transplant.

12. Rejection episodes are characterized by swelling and tenderness of the transplanted kidney, fever, tachycardia, decreased urine output, proteinuria, hypertension, and a rise in BUN and creatinine. Rejection episodes are treated by increasing the dose of steroid to 30 mg/kg given IV for 1-3 days, and by local irradiation to the transplant, 150 roentgens for four doses, not to exceed a total of 600 R. Anticoagulation may be considered if a localized angiopathy in the transplant is suspected.

II. **TRANSPLANTATION OF OTHER ORGANS** Allografting of heart, lung, liver, pancreas, bone marrow, and skin has been successfully accomplished. At the present time, the efforts in transplantation of those organs and tissues are concentrated in a few specialized centers. In these centers, acceptable clinical results are now being achieved with heart, liver, and bone marrow grafts, although wider application of these methods is not yet advisable.

Skin allografts are being used with considerable temporizing success in several burn units, allowing good wound coverage for many weeks until autografts are available. Efforts to transplant the lung and pancreas have been disappointing, with few survivors for even a few months. Newer techniques of pancreas transplantation, with anastomosis of the pancreatic duct to the ureter, are promising, with several patients surviving for more than 1 yr.

Transplantation of cornea in selected patients with blindness due to certain varieties of corneal opacities is a well-established procedure. Corneal cadaver transplants have a high success rate, in part due to the restricted access of antigen from and antibody into the anterior ocular chamber.

SUGGESTED READING

Hamburger, J., Crosnier, J., Dormont, J., and Bach, J. F. *Renal Transplantation: Theory and Practice.* Baltimore: Williams & Wilkins, 1972.

Najarian, J., and Simmons, R. L. *Transplantation.* Philadelphia: Lea & Febiger, 1972.

21. CANCER CHEMOTHERAPY

I. GENERAL COMMENTS

A. Chemotherapeutic agents have been used in the treatment of cancer for more than 1,600 years. Agents such as antimony, mercury salts, and zinc chloride were used locally as caustics or escharotics. Only a little more than a hundred years ago, Sir Astley Cooper was still using arsenic in the local treatment of certain cases of chimney-sweeps' cancer.

B. The **modern approach** to chemotherapy was sparked by the report of Gilman and Philips in 1946 of the use of nitrogen mustard in the treatment of neoplasia. Since then, the number of chemotherapeutic agents and their indications in clinical practice have been rapidly increasing. The major application of currently available drugs is palliative, and cure in patients with solid tumors is rare. The curative role of chemotherapy in patients with lymphomas and other forms of nonsolid tumors is more promising. Furthermore, the role of adjuvant chemotherapy, along with operations or radiotherapy in solid tumors, is becoming increasingly clear.

C. Rationale of chemotherapy   The ideal anticancer drug should selectively destroy cancer cells with minimal or no damage to normal cells. So far, the available agents act on mechanisms common to both normal and neoplastic cells; for that reason, all commonly used drugs produce significant toxicity. Consequently, today's chemotherapy is predominantly used for nonresectable, recurrent, or disseminated cancer.

D. Mode of action   The chemotherapeutic drugs produce their effect at different cellular and subcellular sites. Briefly, the majority of agents act by interfering with the biosynthesis of nucleic acids. This end is achieved either by inactivating cellular enzymes, by substituting some essential amino acids, or by creating an unfavorable environment for cellular growth and division. Some drugs are called *cyclic active* because they are dependent on a phase of cell cycle DNA metabolism.

E. Mechanism of action of anticancer drugs at the cellular level   The available anticancer drugs have distinct mechanisms of action which may vary at different drug concentrations and in their effects on different types of normal and cancer cells. In general, DNA acts as the selective template for the production of specific forms of transfer, ribosomal, and messenger RNA. DNA, in directing the formation of specific sequences of messenger RNA, determines which enzymes will be synthesized on the RNA template. The enzymes in turn are responsible for the structure, metabolic activity, proliferative rate, and function of the cell.

1. **Drugs that modify nucleic acid biosynthesis** Certain antimetabolites inhibit the biosynthesis of the nucleic acids. Antimetabolites with this mechanism of action are useful in some forms of cancer; 6-mercaptopurine and 6-thioguanine prevent purine ring biosynthesis and interconversion of the purine bases. Methotrexate inhibits folic acid reductase to block the reduction of folic acid to tetrahydrofolic acid. 5-Fluorouracil is metabolized to its deoxynucleotide form to inhibit the enzyme thymidylate synthetase, which also is involved in the methylation of deoxyuridylic acid to thymidylic acid.

2. **Drugs that modify DNA function** Interference with the structure of DNA (alkylating agents, procarbazine) or its function (actinomycin D, daunomycin, and adriamycin) disorganizes and disrupts the cell.

3. **Drugs that inhibit protein synthesis** L-Asparaginase acts in a unique manner to hydrolyze asparagine to aspartic acid; certain neoplastic cells, unable to make asparagine and, therefore, dependent on a supply in the circulating blood, cannot grow if that supply is destroyed by the enzyme. Normal cells synthesize L-asparagine and thus appear to be unaffected by the L-asparagine deficiency.

4. **Drugs that arrest mitosis** These agents, all plant alkaloids, have the ability to arrest mitosis in metaphase. The *Vinca* alkaloids disorganize the mitotic spindle to arrest cell division. While this is the most characteristic effect of the *Vinca* alkaloids, they probably act also by other mechanisms, since vincristine differs from vinblastine pharmacologically and therapeutically. Vincristine is more effective in acute leukemia and vinblastine in Hodgkin's disease than are other plant alkaloids.

5. **Steroid hormones** Unphysiological doses of exogenously administered steroid hormones alter hormonal balance in the patient and modify the growth of some cancers arising from tissues particularly susceptible to hormonal influences. The mechanism whereby the steroid hormones stimulate or inhibit cellular growth and function is not clear; an important mechanism may be interference with cell membrane receptors for growth stimulation.

F. **Cell cycle-specificity of anticancer drugs** In addition to differences in biochemical mechanisms of action, anticancer agents differ in the point in the cell cycle at which they influence cell growth and replication. In this respect, drugs fall into **three general classes:**

1. **S-phase-specific** These are agents whose sole or principal mechanism of action is inhibiting DNA synthesis, which occurs in the S-phase for all cells. They cause marked inhibition of growth of cells in culture and in animal tumors. Recent evidence suggests that this may also be true for some human tumors.

2. S-phase-specific, self-limited Some agents (e.g., 6-mercaptopurine, methotrexate) are capable of inhibiting DNA synthesis. However, their breadth of action produces inhibition of RNA and protein synthesis also. These latter effects slow the cell cycle and prevent cells from entering the highly sensitive S-phase. Thus, they are only relatively S-phase specific.

3. Cycle-nonspecific Certain agents (e.g., alkylating agents, antibiotics) exert a direct effect on DNA and thus their activities are not enhanced by administration during the S-phase. The steroid hormones, L-asparaginase, and certain agents with specific effects (e.g., o.p'-DDD) appear also to be cycle-nonspecific.

G. Application of cell kinetics in planning of chemotherapy Studies of the kinetics of the cell cycle have suggested optimum dose schedules for the use of cycle specific agents. Combination of cycle-specific and cycle-nonspecific agents, appropriately timed, appears to provide therapeutic effects superior to those achieved with other schedules. Consideration of cell cycle specificities and the biochemical mechanisms of action of antitumor drugs seems important in designing therapeutic programs.

II. ADMINISTRATION OF CHEMOTHERAPEUTIC DRUGS (Table 21-1)

A. Dosage and toxicity. As a general rule, the dose for each drug is given either in milligrams or micrograms per kilogram of body weight; however, in children and obese patients, a dose based on square meter of body surface area is preferable. In patients in whom the possibility of spurious weight gain due to edema exists, the dose should be calculated on the basis of ideal weight of the individual.

With many cytotoxic drugs, the therapeutic margin between an effective dosage and a severely toxic one may be quite narrow or even nonexistent; careful inquiry and frequent laboratory evaluation are necessary to detect the earliest signs of toxicity. It is important to realize that the **production of toxicity is not mandatory to induce objective regression.** Yet, in patients who fail to respond, at least mild toxicity must be demonstrated before it can be stated that enough of the drug has been given.

In general, anticancer drugs produce a common pattern of toxic reactions, including bone marrow depression, oral ulcerations, damage to intestinal mucosa, alopecia, and hypogonadism. These deleterious effects vary in intensity and extent with different agents. The frequency of drug administration and the dosage should be altered or stopped according to the severity of toxic manifestations.

B. Assessment of response

1. Objective response

a. Reduction in measurable tumor mass, determined either by actual measurements of the dimensions of the tumor or by measurement of the diameters of the lesion in radiographs. A decrease of at least 50% of the tumor mass can be considered a reliable index of response.

TABLE 21-1. Dosage and Toxicity of Commonly Used Anticancer Chemotherapeutic Agents

Agent	Dosage	Tumor	Toxicity
Alkylating agents			
Nitrogen mustard	0.4 mg/kg total IV	Lymphomas, lung cancer, Kaposi's sarcoma, malignant pleural effusion and ascites	Nausea, vomiting, anemia, leukopenia, thrombocytopenia
Thiotepa	0.8 mg/kg total IV	Lymphomas, lung cancer, Kaposi's sarcoma, malignant pleural effusion and ascites	Nausea, vomiting, anemia, leukopenia, thrombocytopenia
Chlorambucil	0.2 mg/kg/day PO	Cancer of ovary, testes, and breast	Toxicity unusual; leukopenia, thrombocytopenia, anorexia, bone marrow depression (late)
Cyclophosphamide	50–200 mg/day PO or 3–5 mg/kg IV for 10 days	Burkitt's lymphoma, squamous and epidermoid carcinoma	Toxicity unusual; oral lesions, leukopenia, thrombocytopenia
Phenylalanine mustard	4–6 mg/kg/day PO	Melanoma, thymoma, Ewing's tumor	Systemic leukopenia, thrombocytopenia, nausea, vomiting; perfusions: local and vascular injury
Triethylenemelamine	10–15 mg total IV	Retinoblastoma	Leukopenia, thrombocytopenia
Antimetabolites			
Methotrexate	2–5 mg/day PO or 50 mg IV infusion	Choriocarcinoma, testicular ovarian tumors, and mesenchymal tumors	Mucositis, nausea, vomiting, leukopenia, thrombocytopenia
5-Fluorouracil	5–15 mg/kg/day IV	GI and pancreatic carcinoma, ovarian and breast carcinoma	Alopecia, mucositis, nausea, vomiting, leukopenia, thrombocytopenia
6-Mercaptopurine	2–5 mg/kg/day PO	Acute and chronic leukemia	Therapeutic doses usually well tolerated, excessive doses cause bone marrow depression
Cytosine arabinoside	3 mg/kg/day IV for 6–21 days	Acute and chronic leukemia	Bone marrow depression, megaloblastosis, leukopenia, thrombocytopenia
Antibiotics			
Actinomycin D	12 μg/kg/day IV for 5 days	Wilms' tumor, choriocarcinoma, testicular and carcinoid tumors	Alopecia, nausea, vomiting, leukopenia, thrombocytopenia
Mithramycin	25 μg/kg/day IV for 5 days	Intracerebral tumors	Bleeding diathesis, thrombocytopenia, leukopenia
Bleomycin	0.25 mg/kg/day IV or IM for up to 5 days or IV twice weekly for up to 5 wk	Epidermoid and squamous cancer of head and neck, lung and esophagus	Mucocutaneous ulcerations, alopecia; pulmonary fibrosis in approximately 5% of patients
Adriamycin	50–75 mg/m² single or divided doses, or 0.65 mg/kg/day for 3 days	Breast, colon, lung, and bladder carcinoma	At cumulative doses over 600 mg/m², stomatitis, GI disturbances, alopecia, bone marrow depression, cardiac toxicity

Drug	Dosage	Indication	Toxicity
Plant alkaloids			
Vincristine	0.015–0.05 mg/kg IV once weekly	Lymphatic leukemia, neuroblastoma, rhabdomyosarcoma, and lymphomas	Nausea, vomiting, leukopenia, thrombocytopenia
Vinblastine	0.1–0.2 mg/kg IV once weekly	Hodgkin's lymphomas, mycosis fungoides	Alopecia, neurotoxicity, leukopenia, nausea, vomiting
Steroid compounds			
Stilbestrol	15–30 mg/day PO		Feminization, nausea, vomiting, vaginal bleeding, fluid retention
Testosterone propionate	100 mg IM 3 times weekly		Masculinization, polycythemia
Hydroxyprogesterone caproate	500 mg IM 3 times weekly		Nausea, vomiting, diarrhea
Prednisone	15–60 mg/day PO		Cushingoid appearance, upper GI bleeding, emotional disturbance
Medroxyprogesterone acetate (Provera)	1,000 mg/wk PO		Nausea, vomiting, leg edema
Miscellaneous			
Procarbazine	50–300 mg/day PO	Hodgkin's disease	Bone marrow depression, leukopenia and thrombocytopenia, mental depression
Imidazole carboximide	4–6 mg/kg/day IV for 10 days	Melanoma and lung cancer	Nausea, vomiting, bone marrow depression
Hydroxyurea	1–2 gm/day PO	Chronic myelogenous leukemia and melanoma	Bone marrow depression
BCNU	100–200 mg/m^2 total PO over 2–5 days	Melanoma, adenocarcinoma of lung, lymphoma, glioblastoma multiforme	Bone marrow depression, leukopenia, thrombocytopenia
CCNU	100–130 mg/m^2 total PO; repeat in 6–8 weeks	Melanoma, adenocarcinoma of lung, lymphoma, glioblastoma multiforme	Bone marrow depression, leukopenia, thrombocytopenia
L-Asparaginase	200–1,000 mg/kg IV 3–7 times weekly		Anorexia, weight loss, somnolence, lethargy, confusion, hypoproteinemia (including albumin and fibrinogen), hypolipidemia and hyperlipidemia, abnormal liver function tests, fatty metamorphosis of the liver, pancreatitis (rare), azotemia, lymphopenia, and thrombocytopenia (usually mild and transient)

b. Prolongation of survival: This must be computed and compared with the natural history of a given tumor.

2. Subjective response of the patient as a whole, that is, relief of symptoms and improvement of performance.

C. Systemic chemotherapy   Continuous or interrupted IV and oral administration are the most frequently used modes of cancer chemotherapy. The choice of the route of administration depends primarily on the rate of absorption and the structure of the agent. Certain drugs are effective only when given IV, e.g., nitrogen mustard and actinomycin D. These agents are particularly irritating when they inadvertently infiltrate the subcutaneous tissue. The absorption of 5-fluorouracil from the GI tract is irregular, and therefore toxic manifestations are difficult to anticipate or control.

D. Solid tumor response to chemotherapy   After prolonged trial and error, it is now generally agreed that some guidelines can be devised regarding the effectiveness of chemotherapy for solid tumors. Table 21-2 lists the types of cancer presently considered responsive to chemotherapy.

E. Local chemotherapy

1. Topical application   Preparations of certain anticancer agents (5-fluorouracil and methotrexate) are used in the treatment of superficial or multiple skin cancers. These drugs produce a temporary severe local reaction at the site of application. Usually, preparations containing 5% 5-fluorouracil in hydrophilic ointment or 1-5% in propylene glycol are used.

TABLE 21-2. Solid Tumors Responding to Chemotherapy

Type of Cancer	Drug(s)	Expected Cure Rate
Prolonged survival or cure		
Choriocarcinoma	Methotrexate	70%
	Actinomycin D	
	Vinblastine	
Neuroblastoma	Actinomycin D	5%
	Cyclophosphamide with surgery and radiotherapy	
Wilms' tumor	Actinomycin D with surgery and radiotherapy	40%
Testicular tumors	Actinomycin D	40%
	Methotrexate plus chlorambucil	2-3%
Burkitt's tumor	Cyclophosphamide	50% apparent cure
Palliation and prolongation of life		
Breast cancer	Hormones, alkylating agents, 5-fluorouracil, vincristine, prednisone, methotrexate	20-40% response
Prostate	Estrogen, castration	70%
Head and neck tumors	Bleomycin	5-10% response

Note: Tumors of the ovary, endometrium, and GI tract, sarcomas, and melanomas occasionally respond, but the probability of response is uncertain.

2. **Perfusion chemotherapy** involves the administration of the drug through an artery after isolating the blood supply to a tumor-bearing area. The technique is used chiefly in the extremities. Circulation to the area is maintained by an extracorporeal circuit which includes an oxygenator and a heat exchanger. The purpose of this method is to increase the drug concentration reaching the tumor, while protecting the host from the toxic effects of high dosage.

In recent years, attention has been directed to the part played by temperature and hyperoxygenation in improving results. Normothermic and, occasionally, hyperthermic perfusion prevents vasospasm and possibly permits better circulation in the tumor. Hyperoxygenation seems to be effective in the treatment of tumors recurrent after radiotherapy. Complications of perfusion therapy include damage to the vessel wall, hemorrhage, and gangrene.

3. **Intracavitary chemotherapy**   Chemotherapeutic agents are introduced into a body cavity to achieve direct contact with cancer cells. Agents such as nitrogen mustard or thiotepa are used in treating malignant pleural effusion or ascites. These agents also may be injected intrathecally or into a viscus to produce a cytotoxic effect on existing cancer deposits or to prevent implants at an anastomosis.

There is usually some systemic absorption, but side effects are fewer than after systemic administration. Another advantage is that failure of intracavitary therapy to control effusion does not preclude subsequent trials with systemic chemotherapy, radiotherapy, or radioactive isotopes.

4. **Infusion chemotherapy**   Anticancer drugs are injected intra-arterially without attempting to recover the drug from the venous end. By this route, a high concentration is delivered to the tumor, but the agent will be dispersed in the general circulation, producing systemic effects. Infusion is at a slow rate by means of an electric pump or, if the patient is ambulatory, a portable pump.

Infusion can be carried out through the external carotid artery or one of its branches for tumors of the head and neck; through the hepatic artery for liver neoplasms; and through the hypogastric artery for pelvic tumors. To counteract the systemic toxicity of the drug, an antidote, e.g., citrovorum factor, in the case of methotrexate therapy, or thiol, in the case of mustard therapy, is given. Catheter misplacement, bleeding, and leakage are technical problems encountered with this method of administration.

F. **Combination chemotherapy**   Combination of two or more compounds, usually with different mechanisms of action, is being widely used. These agents are given sequentially or together at individual lower dosage. The advantages of this regimen are believed to be less cumulative toxicity and aversion of tumor resistance to a single agent. In the treatment of testicular neoplasms, a combination of antinomycin D and chlorambucil has been used. Triple therapy with the addition of methotrexate to the above two drugs has also been tried. Currently, four- and five-drug therapy is being evaluated for treating soft-part sarcomas and other solid tumors. Although final results are not yet available, such combinations appear to produce less toxicity and better therapeutic effects than does single drug therapy.

22. VENOUS DISORDERS OF THE LOWER EXTREMITIES

I. FACTS AND DEFINITIONS

A. Anatomy There are three venous systems in the legs: superficial, deep, and perforator.

1. The **superficial** system includes all the subcutaneous venous vessels. The major superficial channels are the greater and lesser saphenous veins. The greater (long) saphenous system drains the superficial tissues of the medial and posterior aspects of the lower leg and thigh and empties into the common femoral vein at the groin. The short saphenous system drains the superficial lateral aspect of the leg and empties into the popliteal vein in the upper portion of the popliteal space. The superficial system can be sacrificed without resulting in signs of venous insufficiency.

2. The **deep** venous system includes the multiple channels draining the muscular tissues of the calf and thigh, and the popliteal, deep femoral, and common femoral veins. The deep venous system is essential to the viability of the leg.

3. Connecting the superficial and deep systems are the communicating **perforator** veins. The majority of these channels join the greater saphenous system and are found in a regular series on the medial aspect of the lower extremity. There are usually one or two perforators above the knee, three or four between the knee and the ankle, and one perforator (the arch vein) just below the medial malleolus.

4. All three venous systems possess biscuspid valves which, when competent, permit flow only toward the heart. When in an upright position, the hydrostatic pressure in the veins of the lower extremity is limited to the height of the blood column between two adjacent venous valves.

B. Pathology

1. Pathological changes in venous disease involve:

   a. Dilation and elongation.

   b. Intrinsic occlusion by thrombosis with or without inflammation.

   c. Extrinsic venous occlusion.

2. Elements (Virchow's triad) promoting venous thrombosis:

   a. Increased coagulability of the blood, which may follow trauma, be secondary to anemia or polycythemia, or be present for undetermined reasons.

   b. Stasis of blood in the lower limb, which may occur secondary to heart disease, dehydration, immobilization, and incompetent valves.

   c. Intimal damage, which results from trauma, venipuncture, IV infusion, or infection. Intimal injury causes a reduction in fibrinolytic activator activity within the vessel wall and reduces the intrinsic capacity of the vessel to inhibit thrombus formation.

3. **Primary varicose veins** are manifested by bilateral dilation and elongation of the superficial system. The deep and perforator venous systems are normal, i.e., their valves are competent and functioning.

4. **Secondary varicose veins** also involve dilation and elongation of the superficial venous system. Involvement is often unilateral. The perforator or the deep venous systems are incompetent.

5. **Superficial phlebitis** refers to inflammation of a subcutaneous vein, either previously normal or varicose. The perforator and deep venous systems are not involved.

6. **Thrombophlebitis** refers to inflammation and thrombosis of the deep venous system. The perforator veins sometimes are also involved. The superficial system usually is not involved. Inflammation causes the clot to adhere to the vein wall and, therefore, pulmonary embolization is not frequent.

7. **Phlebothrombosis** refers to thrombosis of the deep venous system not accompanied by immediate signs or systems of inflammation. The superficial veins are not involved. The most frequent sign is edema of the involved limb. Since the inflammatory reaction in phlebothrombosis is not severe, adherence of clot to vein wall is more tenuous and the danger of pulmonary embolization is increased.

II. PRIMARY VARICOSE VEINS

A. Etiology and incidence

1. This is the most common venous disorder of the lower extremity, and it affects 10% of the population, three fourths of the patients being young women.

2. Varicosities result from incompetence of proximal valves in the affected veins. Dilation of the vein prevents the valve cusps from meeting, allowing increased hydrostatic pressure to be transmitted to the next lower

segment of vein. Progressive distal dilation and valve incompetence result in the varicosity.

3. Factors predisposing to varicose veins are:

   a. Hereditary defects in the venous structure.

   b. Occupations requiring standing in place for long periods.

   c. Pregnancy and other conditions causing increased intra-abdominal pressure.

   d. Old age, resulting in loss of tissue elasticity.

   e. Obesity.

B. Clinical features

   1. **Symptoms are usually minimal**   "Ugly-appearing legs" is the usual presenting complaint. A thorough history and physical examination are imperative so that one will not blame a few varicose veins for all leg symptoms. Symptoms, when present, are usually of aching, tiredness, a sense of fullness in the leg when upright for long periods of time, and nocturnal muscle cramps. All cramps and leg pains must be differentiated from claudication due to arterial insufficiency.

   2. The major sign of primary varicose veins is the presence on inspection of tortuous, dilated venous channels. These most commonly involve the posterior communicating arch joining the greater and lesser saphenous systems. Peripheral pulses should be evaluated. Edema may prevent adequate palpation, but the portable Doppler ultrasound device can be used to detect arterial flow.

   3. **Complications** of longstanding varicosities are:

      a. Pain from superficial thrombosis.

      b. Edema of the leg.

      c. Dermatitis (brawny induration and pigmentation).

      d. Ulceration, usually in the area of the medial malleolus.

      e. Hemorrhage.

C. Pertinent tests

   1. Evaluation begins with a thorough history and physical examination. Special attention should be given to the peripheral arterial system.

   2. **Trendelenburg's test**   Valvular incompetence is determined by allowing the varicose veins to fill from above.

a. With the patient supine, elevate the limb to 65 degrees and allow the veins to empty by gravity aided by gentle manual milking. Apply a rubber tourniquet high on the thigh to occlude superficial vein flow.

b. Have the patient stand; record the time and direction in which the veins fill.

c. If the varices remain empty for more than 20 sec, valves in the communicating veins are competent. If the veins fill rapidly with the tourniquet in place, there is incompetence of valves in the communicating veins, probably including the small saphenous vein. If, when the patient is standing, the tourniquet is removed and rapid filling of veins from above is noted, incompetence of valves of the great saphenous vein is conformed.

d. Engorgement and pain in the leg with the tourniquet in place mean that the deep venous system is severely compromised.

3. **Test for adequacy of deep vein flow**   If the history suggests previous episodes of venous thrombosis, i.e., previous pain and swelling, the capacity of the deep venous system to carry the necessary volume of blood flow should be tested. The leg is firmly wrapped from the ankle to the thigh with an elastic bandage to occlude the superficial system; the patient walks for 5 min to exercise the leg. If the deep veins are unable to carry the blood flow, severe pain may result. Such deep vein insufficiency is rare but, when present, is a contraindication to ligation or excision of varices. Pain more usually indicates a recent active process of deep vein thrombosis.

4. **Venograms** are of aid in evaluating the perforator vein system. Whenever Trendelenburg's test indicates perforator incompetence and the position of the incompetent perforators cannot be determined by palpation, venograms should be obtained. Dye must enter superficial veins only through the incompetent perforators if they are to be identified with accuracy. Therefore, dye must be injected only into the deep venous system. The usual technique of injection through a dorsal vein of the foot with a tourniquet about the ankle is often successful in visualizing incompetent perforator veins; sometimes sufficient dye leaks under the ankle tourniquet to fill the superficial varicosities, and the presence of incompetent perforator veins cannot be determined with accuracy. In such cases, specific visualization of only the deep and perforator venous systems can be obtained by injecting 5–10 ml of 50% meglumine diatrizoate (Hypaque) or 60% meglumine iothalamate (Conray) directly into the marrow cavity through the medial malleolus. Such injections cause severe pain, so that regional or general anesthesia is required, a drawback to widespread use of malleolar venography.

5. A **Doppler ultrasound** device, especially a portable model, can be used to detect flow in the femoral and popliteal veins; one listens to the variation in the flow sounds in these vessels with respiration or Valsalva's maneuver. Accuracy of this test below the popliteal vein is not very good.

6. Impedance plethysmography is becoming increasingly available as a non-invasive detector of competence of the deep venous system. There is, however, a high incidence of false-positive results with this method.

D. Nonoperative treatment

1. Primary varicosities should not be treated with sclerosing agents. Small noncommunicating veins that remain after ligation and stripping can be injected with sclerosing agents such as sodium morrhuate.

2. Pregnancy Varicosities during pregnancy should be treated nonoperatively. Early prenatal instruction in prevention and reduction of aggravating causes should be given. If a woman has had symptoms progressing with each pregnancy, ligation and stripping can be performed on the third postpartum day and the patient discharged on the sixth postpartum day. No difference or difficulties with regard to safety, complications, or results are encountered with such treatment, as compared with operations in nonpregnant women.

3. The principles of nonoperative treatment are:

a. Wear firm elastic support from toe to thigh whenever upright. Elastic stockings should be put on before getting out of bed in the morning.

b. Avoid prolonged periods of standing or sitting.

c. Sleep with the foot of the bed elevated 6-8 in.

d. Avoid trauma to the affected limb.

e. Avoid circular constricting garments such as tight girdles and circular garters.

f. Elevate legs above the level of the heart for 20 min three times each day.

E. Operative treatment

1. Indications

a. Cosmetic—improvement of appearance.

b. Symptomatic varicosities.

c. Anatomical or symptomatic progression of varices while on nonoperative therapy.

d. Stasis ulceration.

e. Superficial thrombophlebitis present less than 48 hr.

f. Recurrent varicosities.

2. Varicosities should be marked the evening before operation. A **marking solution** that will not come off during skin preparation can be made by the pharmacist: pyrogallol, 500 mg; 40% ferric chloride solution, 4 ml; acetone, 5 ml; alcohol, qs ad 10 ml. The solution is applied with an applicator stick; it darkens as it dries.

3. Standard operative treatment of varicose veins is high ligation at the saphenofemoral junction and stripping of the greater saphenous system from the saphenofemoral junction to the ankle. If the short saphenous system is involved, it is ligated at the saphenopopliteal junction and stripped from the external malleolus to the point of ligation. Ligation alone is not sufficient therapy; the varicose veins must be stripped. Dilated tributaries of the long or short saphenous trunks should also be stripped. Any remaining dilated vessels may be dealt with postoperatively by injection of sodium morrhuate or a similar sclerosing agent.

4. Postoperatively, pressure bandages are applied from the toes to the groin and are maintained for 7-10 days. An elastic stocking should then be worn until 3-4 wk after the operation.

5. Ambulation with assistance is begun the day of operation. While ambulating, leg movement is to be constant. Sitting or standing promotes venous stasis and should not be permitted.

6. Discharge from the hospital is usually on the third or fourth postoperative day.

7. Complications of stripping and ligation

   a. Hematomas can be prevented by placing the patient in the Trendelenburg position, by expressing blood from the wound before closure, and by using an elastic bandage. Drainage usually is not needed. Postoperatively, the foot of the bed should be elevated to reduce venous pressure when the patient is in bed.

   b. Infection and wound breakdown. Careful operative technique is imperative. Stasis ulcers should be clear of signs of acute inflammation before operation. If infection is present, broad-spectrum antibiotics are used, but antibiotics are not used routinely.

   c. Patchy numbness. Superficial nerves are sometimes interrupted with stripping. If the saphenous and sural nerves are spared, minimal numbness will result. Restoration of sensation usually occurs in 6-12 mo.

   d. Early recurrence may be caused by:

      (1) Failure to recognize and strip an accessory saphenous vein joining the common femoral vein.

      (2) Failure to recognize and strip an incompetent small saphenous vein.

(3) Failure to deal adequately with incompetent perforator veins.

e. Ligation of the femoral artery occurs in inexperienced hands but can be obviated by adequate knowledge of groin anatomy.

f. Deep venous thrombosis and pulmonary embolism occur rarely.

III. SECONDARY VARICOSE VEINS

A. These varicosities are caused by high venous pressures applied to the superficial venous system as a result of:

1. Deep venous insufficiency with incompetence of the perforator veins.

2. Congenital or acquired AV fistula.

B. Secondary varicosities **usually are unilateral.** There is often a **history of thrombophlebitis or trauma.** Usually there will be clinical signs of deep venous insufficiency (edema, dermatitis, stasis ulcer) as well as the presence of superficial varicosities.

C. **Nonoperative therapy** is instituted with the use of elastic supports. Since the patient requires elastic stocking support because of deep venous insufficiency, stripping of superficial varicosities is not necessary in most cases. In certain cases, if the deep system has recanalized, superficial veins can be removed, but the patient should be warned of probable recurrence, continued postphlebitic symptoms, and the continuing need for elastic stocking support.

D. Post-traumatic AV fistulas are treated by resection of the fistulous communication. Congenital fistulas usually are multiple and respond poorly to operative intervention; varicosities should be treated nonoperatively in most cases. Only where localized fistulas can be demonstrated do excision of the fistula and stripping of the associated varicose veins yield a good result.

E. Late sequelae in the postphlebitic leg are discussed in Section **VII,** p. 382.

IV. SUPERFICIAL VENOUS THROMBOSIS

A. **Phlebitis migrans** is a disorder characterized by recurrent attacks of thrombophlebitis involving segments of previously normal superficial veins. The cause is unknown. The typical patient is usually a man under 45 years of age. He complains of pain, redness, tenderness, and swelling of a segment of superficial vein, usually in the leg but sometimes on the trunk or arm. After an acute episode, remission may last several years. Many cases of Buerger's disease (thromboangiitis obliterans) begin with this disorder. Treatment is symptomatic; elastic support of inflamed leg veins is helpful. Smoking should be banned. Persistently active cases may need long-term anticoagulation therapy. Steroids are of no benefit.

B. **Thrombophlebitis in varicose veins** usually presents as firm, tender, reddened nodules or as red streaks overlying varicosities which were previously soft and painless. If the patient is seen shortly after onset, high ligation and stripping will remove the inflamed vein segments and abort the episode of thrombophlebitis. After 48 hr of symptoms, the inflammatory reaction makes stripping impossible. Treatment then consists of reassurance, medication for pain, anti-inflammatory drugs (aspirin; phenylbutazone in more severe cases), elastic bandage support to control edema, and active use of the leg as soon as pain will permit. Antibiotics and anticoagulants are not needed. When the acute process has subsided, ligation and stripping can be done. When there is involvement of the greater saphenous system at the saphenofemoral junction, division of the saphenous vein is indicated to prevent extension as a femoral thrombophlebitis.

C. Thrombophlebitis may also be secondary to an IV infusion, or be a response to such conditions as thromboangiitis, bacterial or viral infection, lupus erythematosus, and forms of vascular allergy. Heparin can be used to reduce the inflammatory reaction rapidly. Aspirin, where not contraindicated (duodenal ulcer, allergy, or concomitant heparin therapy), in large doses of 3–5 gm/day is effective. Edema is controlled with elastic bandages.

V. PHLEBOTHROMBOSIS

A. Often there are no apparent reasons for the onset of phlebothrombosis. It is sometimes found in association with abdominal cancers, especially those involving the body and tail of the pancreas. Polycythemia and Buerger's disease can be initiating causes. Phlebothrombosis may follow dissection of the popliteal space for arterial reconstruction or graft. Much of the leg swelling labeled "edema of arterial reconstruction" is, in fact, phlebothrombosis. Prolonged bed rest, trauma, and major operation are other situations with a high risk of development of phlebothrombosis.

B. Phlebothrombosis may be difficult to recognize clinically because of its **minimal local and constitutional signs. Pulmonary embolus may be the first indication of its presence.**

C. Bland thrombosis may progress to a more inflammatory state of symptomatic thrombophlebitis. Otherwise, local symptoms are only mild discomfort and stiffness in the calf of the leg on active motion together with unilateral swelling. *Note: this condition rarely causes postoperative fever.*

D. Early recognition by daily examination of the legs of every patient confined to bed for whatever reason is the main factor in successful prevention of pulmonary emboli.

E. **Diagnosis**   Newer methods make documentation easier, but a high index of suspicion still is needed. Invasive diagnostic methods include **venography.** The noninvasive diagnostic methods are Doppler **ultrasound** and impedance **plethysmography.** Of great help in high-risk patients is the ^{125}I-**fibrinogen test** which relies on incorporation of radioactive fibrinogen into a newly forming clot. This results in increased detected radioactivity over the area of clot formation. The thyroid must be blocked preoperatively by Lugol's solution. 100 microcuries of ^{125}I-labeled human fibrinogen is injected IV several hours after operation. Baseline counts are obtained over the thyroid, heart, and leg 1 hr after injection. Daily leg counts or scans then can be made up 10 days after injection.

F. Anticoagulation therapy is designed to limit the local condition and prevent emboli. Heparin is the drug of choice. A baseline coagulation profile should be obtained of clotting time, prothrombin time, and partial thromboplastin time. Heparin then can be given IV in dose of 10,000–12,000 units. Two hours later the clotting time should be longer than 20 min; if it is less, increase the dose of heparin. Continue to administer 5,000 units of heparin IV every 4–6 hr to maintain the clotting time at one and a half to two times normal. Alternatively, the partial thromboplastin time can be used to guide heparin therapy, keeping the PTT above 60 sec. Heparin therapy is continued until symptoms have disappeared and the patient is fully ambulatory.

Warfarin then can be started orally, at least 48 hr before stopping heparin. Warfarin is started with doses of 30, 20, and 10 mg on successive days if the baseline prothrombin time is normal. Lower loading doses are used if initial prothrombin values are low. The dose of warfarin is then adjusted to keep the prothrombin time in the range of two to two and a half times normal. Anticoagulation should be continued for at least 6 wk, and possibly up to 6 mo in high-risk patients.

G. Other important treatment measures:

1. Maintenance of adequate hydration.

2. Bed rest without massage or active exercise of the legs.

3. Elevation of the foot of the bed on 8-in. blocks.

4. Wrapping the legs while the patient is in bed is not necessary.

5. Local heat: may be used for symptomatic relief, but does not influence resolution of the thrombus.

6. Ambulation: may begin 1–2 days after all local signs have disappeared. Elastic stockings or wraps should be applied when the patient is upright.

H. Complications of phlebothrombosis:

1. Pulmonary emboli, often resulting in sudden death.

2. Pulmonary hypertension from repeated emboli, with resulting cor pulmonale.

3. Progression of the phlebothrombosis to more severe deep thrombophlebitis or to iliofemoral phlebothrombosis.

4. Indications for vena caval ligation are discussed in Section **III.B,** Chapter 17.

I. Prevention   Preoperative, intraoperative, and postoperative measures to prevent phlebothrombosis should be considered, especially in high-risk patients. Ambulation, support hose properly worn, intraoperative flexion of limbs by electrical stimulation or pneumatic compression have proved to be beneficial. The prophylactic value of heparin ("minidose") is unproved; it can neither be recommended nor condemned.

VI. THROMBOPHLEBITIS

A. Etiology and incidence

1. Deep vein thrombophlebitis has the same etiological factors as phlebothrombosis. The local picture and late results are modified by the presence of inflammation in the vein wall and surrounding tissue.

2. The onset is usually rapid. Initial pain of thrombotic occlusion is probably a result of reflex arterial spasm which causes a transient pallor similar to that of arterial insufficiency, followed by the plethora and edema of venous occlusion.

3. Incidence is about 2% following major operations, with a higher incidence in genitourinary and gynecological procedures. Onset is usually between 3 and 10 days after operation.

4. The more intense the inflammatory reaction, the more fixed the thrombus becomes; however, it is not true that an inflammatory thrombophlebitis can never produce a pulmonary embolus.

5. In the usual case of deep venous thrombophlebitis, the veins of the calf and deep posterior tibial system are involved. The thrombus may extend or involve the popliteal vein in patients with more severe symptoms.

B. Signs and symptoms

1. The **earliest signs,** which should raise a suspicion that thrombophlebitis is present are:

   a. Assumption of the **"frog-leg" position** of the involved extremity. The position is similar to that of a patient with a fractured hip: leg externally rotated, knee flexed.

   b. **Tenderness** usually can be elicited by careful palpation of the posterior calf, popliteal fossa, or inguinal region.

   c. Tenderness to pressure over the instep of the foot.

2. Other early symptoms are calf heaviness and aching pain on movement of the calf muscles or thigh.

3. Obstructive signs resulting from the occluding thrombus include:

    a. Swelling, especially in the loose connective tissue around the ankle, popliteal fossa, or suprapubic area.

    b. Mild to deep cyanosis after initial vasospasm has subsided.

    c. Increased warmth of the affected limb or segment.

    d. Distention of superficial veins, more noticeable when the limb is dependent.

4. Tenderness is evaluated by compression of the calf against the tibia resulting in pain (Pratt's sign) or calf pain resulting from dorsiflexion of the foot (Homan's sign). The calf muscles are tender and doughy, with a tightness not unlike abdominal guarding in acute appendicitis.

5. Extensive deep vein thrombosis involving the major veins draining the leg is called **iliofemoral thrombophlebitis.** In order to produce classic milk leg, or **phlegmasia alba dolens,** the common femoral vein above the deep femoral vein must be thrombosed. Involvement of the external iliac vein up to and including the junction of the internal iliac vein is sometimes present. The leg is swollen, pale or mottled, and cool. Although the main deep venous channels are occluded, small veins in the lower extremity remain patent, so that some routes of venous drainage from the limb via collateral channels are available. Phlegmasia alba dolens usually does not carry a risk of extensive gangrene.

    In **phlegmasia cerulea dolens,** the entire venous collateral bed of the leg is thrombosed in addition to thrombosis of the iliofemoral system up to and involving the first portion of the inferior vena cava. Drainage of blood from the leg is seriously impeded. The leg is massively swollen, exquisitely tender because of ischemic pain, cold, and deeply cyanotic. Gangrene is an imminent threat.

C. Differential diagnosis

1. Acute lymphangitis can occur in lymphedema. In addition to swelling, chills, fever, and red streaks are noted.

2. Rupture of the gastrocnemius, adductor, or quadriceps muscle can give excruciating pain. A subcutaneous hematoma distal to the rupture site appears a few days later. A gap usually can be felt between the ruptured, retracted muscle and its tendon.

3. Cardiac or renal edema causes swelling of the legs. Usually there are no other signs of venous disease.

4. Saphenous neuritis may give pain, but the leg is not swollen.

5. Radiculitis and sciatica may cause pain in the thigh or calf. Painful trigger zones in the back, reproduced by various movements of the back and leg, differentiate these conditions from phlebitis.

6. Arthritis and bursitis can produce reflex muscle spasm and diffuse pain in the leg.

7. If serious doubt exists, the diagnosis can be confirmed and the lesion localized by phlebography, ^{125}I-fibrinogen uptake, or ultrasound scanning.

D. Treatment

1. Prophylaxis involves preventing stasis by early ambulation, elevating the foot of the bed or operating table, avoiding long periods of sitting with the legs bent, and maintaining adequate hydration.

2. Treatment   The aim of treatment is limitation and early resolution of the acute phase and prevention of late sequelae. All cases with involvement limited to the channels distal to the popliteal vein should be managed nonoperatively as outlined for cases of phlebothrombosis. Early residual symptoms of edema, heaviness, and fatigue will decrease over a 6–12-mo period. At this point the patient must be impressed again with the need for continual care of the damaged leg:

a. Continual wearing of elastic stockings from morning to night.

b. No standing for more than 30 min. Elevation of the leg for 15 min after standing.

c. Active leg exercises as an hourly habit.

d. Elevation of the leg when sitting and elevation of the foot of the bed when sleeping.

e. Avoidance of irritation, bruises, etc., of the affected leg.

3. Thrombectomy, especially in cases of iliofemoral thrombosis, gives good symptomatic results if done within 48–72 hr after onset of symptoms, but does not influence the incidence of late postphlebitic sequelae. Thrombectomy is no longer widely used; reliance is placed on adequate anticoagulation therapy until symptoms subside. Anticoagulation therapy should continue for at least 6 wk; if the ileofemoral system is involved, therapy should continue up to 6 mo.

VII. THE POSTPHLEBITIC SYNDROME

A. The degree of resolution of a thrombus in the deep venous system is unpredictable. The clot may lyse, organize, recanalize, grow by apposition, or break loose.

B. A postphlebitic leg is the result of resolution of a thrombus in a large vein, such as the iliofemoral or popliteal vein, by means of recanalization of the thrombus. The lumen becomes patent, but deep venous insufficiency develops as a result of destruction of the venous valves.

C. The uninterrupted hydrostatic pressure head from the right atrium to the toes is transmitted to the tissues of the leg every time the patient stands.

D. Pressure in the veins at the ankle is 10 times normal and may reach twice the mean arterial pressure in the subcutaneous tissues about the ankle. This causes transudation of fluid under pressure from the intravascular to the interstitial space. The result is stasis, intractable induration, chronic edema, pigmentation, eczema, and ulceration. Incompetent perforators develop, are probably the cause of chronic ulcers in the ankle region, and also lead to secondary varicosities. Cellulitis is commonly superimposed.

E. The diagnosis is established by a previous history of deep vein thrombosis. The patient may become aware of symptoms 2 mo-25 yr after the initial episode of phlebitis.

F. Slight trauma to the leg resulting in a nonhealing ulcer is common. Ulcers, however, must be distinguished from other ulcer-producing entities such as arterial insufficiency and syphilis. Clinical examination and laboratory tests should be made to rule out diabetes, syphilis, hypoprothrombinemia, splenic disease, hemolytic anemia, and erythema induratum.

G. The ulcers and skin changes always are in the lower two thirds of the inner side of the leg or the lower third of the outer side of the leg. When dependent, the involved leg is more cyanotic than its mate.

H. **Treatment**   The best treatment is prevention. After the postphlebitic syndrome has developed, only palliative and symptomatic therapy is available, since the damage is irreparable. Treatment must compensate for persistent venous hypertension by leg elevation and constant elastic support.

I. Chronic leg ulcers are first treated by bed rest and elevation. Infection in the ulcer is controlled by giving antibiotic therapy based on culture and sensitivity studies together with local wound care. Other important treatment measures are physiotherapy and exercise in bed, control of excessive weight, and general treatment of the patient's health. After 10-14 days, ambulate the patient. Apply compression bandages to the leg (Unna boot or zinc oxide paste bandage); change them every 7-14 days. After these bandages have been applied, most patients can return to work unless their job entails prolonged standing. The ulcers usually will heal slowly over a 3-12-wk period. If edema is prevented and soft tissue protected, the leg should remain well but is never really cured.

J. Operative therapy may be required at some time during treatment. Operative treatment implies prior control of excessive edema and infection, and may include:

1. Stripping superficial varices and ligating incompetent perforators under and near the leg ulcer.

2. Grafting the ulcer if it is large and fails to heal. Grafting is useless if the basic cause of the ulcer is not treated at the same time, i.e., ligation of incompetent perforators. Permanent firm external support after grafting is imperative.

SUGGESTED READING

Bergan, J. J., and Yao, J. S. T.   Vascular surgery. *Surg. Clin. North Am.* 54:1, 1974.

23. COMMON ANORECTAL DISORDERS

I. CLINICAL EXAMINATION

A. The history

1. The patient comes in fear or pain, or both. Be reassuring and gentle.

2. Pay particular attention to the following:

   a. **Pain**   Type? During, before, or after bowel movement? Itching?

   b. **Change in bowel habits**   Diarrhea? Constipation? Combination of both?

   c. **Protrusion**   When? Is underclothing soiled? Is protrusion constant? After straining or defecation? Does prolapsed tissue reduce spontaneously? With manipulation? Not at all?

   d. **Bleeding**   Bright? Dark? Pink on the paper? Mixed with stool? Dripping after defecation?

B. Preparation

1. The outpatient should be prepared for examination with a Fleet enema administered in the knee-chest position the night before; repeat the enema the following day, 1-2 hr prior to examination.

2. Preparation for immediate examination requires two Fleet enemas administered to the patient in the knee-chest position. This enema may cause increased secretion of mucus. If the patient is apprehensive or in extreme pain, diazepam (Valium), 5-10 mg, or meperidine (Demerol), 50 mg, or both, can be given parenterally 1 hr prior to examination.

3. **Position** of patient

   a. **Knee-chest position**   Patient's left arm folded across the chest; left shoulder touching the table; head turned to the right; knees slightly apart, allowing the sigmoid colon to hang free. Tilt the proctoscopic table into a head-down position.

   b. **Sims's position**   Patient lying on the left side; buttocks over the edge of the bed or table; right leg drawn up.

C. Examination of the patient involves the following steps:

1. **External examination**   Try to localize any point of tenderness that might indicate a deep-seated infection; look for fissures, fistula tracts, excoriations, skin tags, hemorrhoids, or other abnormalities.

2. **Digital examination**   Using a lubricated finger cot, note size of prostate or position of cervix; the amount of redundant internal hemorrhoidal tissue, as well as the presence of polypoid or hard masses; and areas of pain or tenderness. The posterior quadrant of the rectum just internal to the anal canal is often overlooked; be sure to examine this area. Never use an instrument before performing a digital examination of the anal canal and rectum.

3. **Anoscopic examination**   Insert the instrument and check all four quadrants of the anal canal, particularly posteriorly and anteriorly.

4. **Proctoscopic examination**   Insert the sigmoidoscope to 24 cm, watching carefully for abnormalities. Never force the scope, particularly in patients with previous pelvic operations. During withdrawal, rotate the eyepiece end of scope in a wide circle to visualize all the bowel mucosa. Be prepared to do a biopsy of mucosa or excise a polyp and to fulgurate with cautery. Never take a biopsy specimen of a "polyp" without first applying pressure to its base; it might be an inverted diverticulum.

II. ANORECTAL DISORDERS

A. Anal fissure

1. **Acute severe pain begins during defecation,** usually with passage of a bulky or hard stool. The pain will last from a few minutes to several hours. The episode may be accompanied by slight bleeding, but the predominant symptom is pain.

2. An acute anal fissure will appear as a **narrow V-shaped raw split** in the mucosa of the anal canal. The apex of the mucosal split is in the rectum. Eighty percent of acute fissures are located posteriorly and can be seen readily on external examination if lateral traction is placed on the buttocks.

3. There is marked **spasm** of the anal canal and exquisite pain when a digital examination is performed.

4. A trial of stool softeners, sitz baths, and Proctofoam-HC enemas is the initial therapy. Early acute cases respond well.

5. **Chronic anal fissure** presents as a diagnostic triad of an enlarged anal papilla, generally a midline linear anal ulcer, and a sentinel pile. Surgical correction consists of a superficial transection of the external sphincter, and excision of the hypertrophied papilla and skin tag.

6. Pruritus ani is a very common anal problem frequently associated with poor hygiene, excessive alkalinity of the stool, fistulas, fissures, anal warts, and hemorrhoids. Other etiological factors may be parasites, fungal infections, allergies to nylon and Dacron, and metabolic disorders, such as diabetes. Treatment consists of elimination of the etiological factor and the use of topical hydrocortisone (Cort-Dome ½%).

B. Hemorrhoids

1. Acute thrombotic hemorrhoids

a. There is an acute onset of pain, unrelated to the patient's activity. A mass outside the anus can be felt by the patient.

b. A small vessel at the mucocutaneous junction has ruptured, causing hemorrhage into the subcutaneous tissues of the anal canal.

c. Inspection shows an extremely tender dark purplish nodule at some point on the anal verge. If present for more than a few hours, the overlying skin may be necrotic.

d. The mass should have an ellipse of skin excised to evacuate the clot. Local anesthesia may be used, but in many cases pain is so intense that incision without an anesthetic causes no increase in pain. Relief of most of the pain occurs rapidly following evacuation of the clot. Hemostasis is achieved by pressure. If necessary, cautery or catgut sutures may be used. Apply ice bags for 24 hr; then begin sitz baths, compresses, and stool softeners.

2. Acute prolapsing edematous hemorrhoids

a. There usually is a history of symptomatic hemorrhoids in the past. Following defecation or straining, a prolapsed mass of hemorrhoids can be felt outside the anus. Digital reduction of the hemorrhoids, if attempted, is unsuccessful.

b. The prolapsed hemorrhoids become progressively more engorged, edematous, and extremely painful.

c. Inspection shows an edematous purplish mass surrounding the anus.

d. Treatment consists of rest in bed in the prone position. If possible, the bed should be tilted 15 degrees head-down, so that the buttocks and legs are elevated. Compresses are applied to the prolapsed hemorrhoids and adequate doses of analgesic drugs administered. When the acute episode has subsided, hemorrhoidectomy usually is indicated.

3. Internal hemorrhoids

a. These are the common chronic variety of hemorrhoids. They are varicose veins of the submucosal internal hemorrhoidal plexus. As the varices enlarge, the overlying mucosa becomes redundant. Enlargement may progress to involve the submucosal venous channels of the anal canal and perianal skin (external hemorrhoids).

b. The etiology of hemorrhoids is unknown but may be related to chronic constipation, pregnancy, man's bipedal upright position, or the great American habit of reading in the bathroom.

c. Complaints are of protrusion during defecation producing discomfort; of protrusion with straining, coughing, lifting, or other daily activity, producing soiling of undergarments and pruritus ani; or of bleeding during defecation. Symptoms in a given patient are not constant, but tend to come and go intermittently. The protruding hemorrhoids cause irritation and discomfort, but usually not pain.

d. Frequently the patient will describe manually reducing the hemorrhoidal tissue following defecation, coughing, or lifting heavy objects. Examination will reveal markedly redundant external hemorrhoidal tissue and the examining finger will feel redundant internal tissue. Anoscopic examination reveals marked dilation of the internal hemorrhoidal vessels.

e. Hemorrhoids are common. Therapy is directed at regulation of bowel habit and perianal hygiene. Operation is reserved for persistently and chronically symptomatic patients. Constipation is to be avoided. The patient should drink plenty of fluids. Prescribe a stool softener, such as dioctyl sodium sulfosuccinate (Colace) or dioctyl calcium sulfosuccinate (Surfak), and, if necessary, a bulk laxative. A sitz bath or use of Tucks pads for thorough cleansing of the perianal skin should follow every defecation.

f. Outpatient or office treatment by the application of elastic bands (Barron ligator) and the use of cryosurgery are useful methods in skilled surgical hands.

g. Hemorrhoidectomy is reserved for those patients who have constant rather than episodic complaints, whose symptoms cannot be managed on the nonoperative regimen outlined above, and who demonstrate a nearly complete rosette of hemorrhoidal prolapse on straining.

C. Prolapse

1. Mucosal prolapse   This condition is often an extension of hemorrhoidal disease. It also occurs, without large hemorroids, in debilitated elderly patients. Only the mucosa prolapses, so that the walls of the prolapsed mass are thin. The prolapse is circumferential, the anal opening is located centrally, and the prolapse is rarely larger than 4 in. even with straining. Excision of the redundant mass with end-to-end approximation of the mucosa is indicated.

2. Intussusceptive rectal prolapse   This type of prolapse involves all layers of the rectal wall, not just the mucosa. It starts as an intussusception of rectum into itself; on straining, the mass protrudes out of the anal canal. This type of prolapse is also circumferential, but there is a palpable groove between the prolapsed mass and the wall of the anal canal. The rectal opening is located centrally. The walls of the prolapsed mass are thicker than in simple mucosal prolapse. In patients who are acceptable operative risks, excision of the prolapsed tissue and end-to-end approximation of each layer of the rectum should be done. In older and debilitated patients, use of a Thiersch wire is advised. A #20 silver wire is placed subcutaneously, approximately 3 cm around the rectum, the prolapse is reduced, and the wire is tightened sufficiently to prevent recurrence of the prolapse but still permit passage of stool. The wire seldom becomes infected, but if it does it can be removed in the surgeon's office without any great difficulty.

3. **Sliding rectal prolapse (complete rectal procidentia)**   This is really a sliding hernia of the pouch of Douglas into the rectum and then out of the anal canal. As the hernia protrudes, it turns the anterior wall of the rectum and anal canal inside out. The anterior wall of the prolapse is much thicker than the posterior wall since it contains the sliding peritoneal sac. Because of its asymmetrical development, the rectal opening points posteriorly. Operative repair of this type of rectal prolapse is a major undertaking whether done through the abdomen, through the perineum, or by a combined approach. The underlying cause is a defect in the pelvic diaphragm (levator ani) which must be repaired. The redundant bowel sometimes needs to be excised; if not, it should be anchored intraabdominally.

D. Cryptitis

1. The patient complains of discomfort in the anal area following defecation.

2. Digital examination usually yields negative results. Anoscopic examination shows a markedly dilated V-shaped anal crypt without ulceration. Eliminate constipation and use Proctofoam-HC. This condition does not need operative treatment; but if symptoms persist, biopsy of the crypt should be done to rule out a malignancy.

E. Perirectal abscess

1. These abscesses originate as infections in anal glands or crypts. A break in the mucosa, caused by necrosis resulting from the infection or trauma, permits the infection to extend into the perirectal tissues.

2. The abscess may be located in one of the following areas:

   a. Beneath the anorectal mucosa or the perianal skin, but superficial to the anal sphincter muscles—submucosal, subcutaneous, and mucocutaneous abscesses.

   b. Between the internal and external sphincters—intermuscular abscesses.

   c. Lateral to both sphincters and below the levator ani muscle (pelvic diaphragm)—ischiorectal abscess.

   d. Above the levator ani muscle—pelvirectal abscess.

3. The main symptom is pain. Examination reveals a tender mass, usually fluctuant, with edema and inflammation of the overlying tissues.

4. Treatment involves incision and drainage. If the patient has signs of systemic toxicity (chills, fever, leukocytosis), administer a broad-spectrum antibiotic. Except for small submucosal and subcutaneous abscesses, incision and drainage should be performed in the operating room under general or regional anesthesia. Local anesthesia is never sufficient to permit adequate exploration of a significant perirectal abscess. A linear or cruciate incision is made over the area of maximum tenderness and fluctuance. A sample of the pus should be obtained for culture and antibiotic sensitivity tests. An instrument or a finger is inserted into the abscess cavity; all internal loculations are broken up and the initial incision is extended so that the cavity is wide open. The cavity is then lightly packed with gauze. The patient is placed on ice packs and pain-relieving drugs for 24 hr and then given routine sitz baths. In the great majority of cases (95%) the abscess resolves, leaving an anal fistula.

F. Anal fistula

1. *Fistula* means "pipe" or "reed"; in this case, it refers to the narrow sinus tract left behind by a resolving perirectal abscess.

2. There is an internal opening in the base of an anal crypt. The external opening is in the perianal skin.

3. Fistulas with posterior external openings have their internal orifice in the posterior midline; fistulas with anterior external openings have radially located internal openings or may run as a horseshoe fistula to open internally in the posterior midline.

4. Anal fistulas must be either unroofed or excised in toto. Otherwise, the perirectal abscess will recur.

G. Condylomata acuminata (venereal warts)

1. These are moist, warty, whitish lesions located at the anal verge. Additional lesions may be located within the anal canal or rectum. They grow very rapidly and cause a great deal of local irritation.

2. These lesions occasionally are mistaken for carcinoma; a specimen taken for biopsy will settle this issue.

3. Small lesions may be treated with podophyllum resin. Cover the surrounding normal skin with petroleum jelly, then paint the condyloma with 20% podophyllum resin in tincture of benzoin. Repeat this treatment weekly until the lesion is obliterated.

4. Cryosurgery in skilled hands has shown promising results.

5. Larger lesions should be excised. There will be a surprisingly large artery supplying the condyloma. Be prepared. Following excision, the base of the lesion should be fulgurated or ligated.

H. Hidradenitis suppurativa

1. Perianal glands become chronically infected with staphylococci, leading to persistent drainage, maceration, and scarring. The process is similar to that seen in the axillae.

2. Wide excision of the involved skin and subcutaneous tissues is required.

I. Pilonidal cyst and sinus

1. This is an **acquired, not an embryological, condition** in nearly every case. The process is a foreign body reaction to an ingrown hair in the intergluteal cleft complicated by secondary infection.

2. The patient complains of pain and drainage. Affected patients are usually men who are hairy, overweight, and have a job that necessitates sitting.

3. This lesion is commonly overtreated. Proper treatment can be carried out in the surgeon's office or outpatient clinic. A generous area around the sinus should be shaved. Local anesthesia is used, with 1% or 2% Xylocaine with epinephrine infiltrated over the sinus tract. The tract is probed and incised to unroof the entire sinus. There invariably is a collection of hair and debris which should be removed. The wound is packed open and kept packed until healed.

4. In recurrent cases, excision of the sinus tract is required. Following excision, the wound is packed open and allowed to granulate and close secondarily. Only in an exceptional case, with multiple burrowing sinus tracts, will radical excision of all the tissues of the intergluteal cleft be required. Such operations are associated with considerable morbidity and are not needed for most cases of pilonidal sinus.

J. Carcinoma of the anus

1. Squamous carcinoma usually presents as an ulcer. The patient notices a little blood on the paper or feels a lump. There is little pain. Tuberculous and syphilitic ulcers should be differentiated; biopsy gives the answer.

2. The skin surrounding the ulcer usually is indurated because of intracutaneous lymphatic spread of the cancer or because of inflammation from infection.

3. Metastases occur via the lymphatics both laterally to the iliofemoral nodes and upward to the perirectal and mesocolic nodes with equal frequency.

4. Basal cell carcinoma and melanoma also may originate in the perianal epidermis or in the anal canal. Primary adenocarcinoma arising in rectal mucosa below the anorectal ring frequently spreads downward and may appear clinically as carcinoma of the anus.

K. Radiation proctitis

1. Bright red bleeding and tenesmus may occur early following radiation treatment involving the pelvis. Low colonic obstruction caused by fibrous rectal stricture appears later.

2. Proctoscopic examination in the early stages will show irritable, friable mucosa at 6–18 cm from the anal verge. In later stages there may be marked stenosis, usually about 12–14 cm from the anus.

3. Early treatment consists of steroid retention enemas at bedtime each evening for 1 wk; then repeat the proctoscopic examination. In case of late proctitis with stricture, colostomy may be necessary if the stricture cannot be resected.

L. Fecal impaction

1. Impaction is the most common cause of obstructive bowel symptoms in elderly patients. Impaction also occurs in patients following rectal surgery, in orthopedic patients in traction or body casts, and in neurotic children and adults.

2. Paradoxical diarrhea may occur around an obstructing impaction.

3. A digital examination quickly makes the diagnosis.

4. Treat by manual digital breakdown of the bolus. Pass a rubber catheter beyond the mass and administer an oil-retention enema. Follow with Fleet enemas until the rectum is clear.

5. Acute impactions in elderly patients can be treated with caudal anesthesia—but stand clear!

M. Benign polyps

1. Any lesion that projects into the lumen of the bowel is a polyp. Polyps with a stalk are pedunculated; those without a stalk are sessile.

2. About 75% of all polypoid lesions of the entire large bowel can be seen through a 20-cm sigmoidoscope.

3. About 10% of patients over 45 yr of age harbor one or more polyps.

4. Less than 1% of adenomatous polyps contain a focus of true (i.e., invasive) carcinoma. Up to 40% of villous adenomas, on the other hand, will contain foci of invasive carcinoma.

5. Polyps seen through the sigmoidoscope should be biopsied.

a. First, be sure the lesion is a polyp and not an inverted diverticulum. Push on the base; an inverted diverticulum can be returned to an everted position.

b. Polyps that lie above the peritoneal reflection (12 cm from the anal verge) should be biopsied only by a skilled operator.

c. Excise the polyp in toto, including all the stalk, together with a small rim of surrounding normal mucosa. Bleeding can usually be controlled by maintaining pressure on the biopsy site with a cotton pledget for 3 or 4 min. If bleeding continues, cauterize the bleeding point.

d. A barium enema examination of the colon, using air contrast technique, should be carried out in every patient. Polyps will be found proximally in up to one of every four otherwise normal patients and in every case of Gardner's syndrome and familial polyposis. The barium enema should be done either before or 10 days after excision biopsy of a polyp. Spasm, edema, or blood clots may confuse interpretation of the films if x-rays are done in conjunction with the biopsy.

III. GENERAL PRINCIPLES OF TREATMENT

A. Always check the results of current therapy. If the patient were improving, he might not be there to see you.

B. Sitz bath   Not more than 6 in. of comfortably warm water in a tub, three or four times a day for not more than 15 or 20 min.

C. Compresses   Wet cloth over the anal area with hot water bottle or covered heating pad. If neither a bottle nor a pad is available, taping a piece of plastic across the buttocks will contain body heat.

D. If warm compresses do not give improvement, use an **ice bag** or homemade ice pack (three cubes of ice wrapped in a wet facecloth).

E. For **pain,** use one of the compounds combining aspirin and codeine.

F. Suppositories are seldom of any value in rectal conditions, except psychologically. An anesthetic suppository with hydrocortisone will, in rare cases, be of benefit in a patient with extremely large, edematous internal hemorrhoids.

G. Diet is an important element of management. The foods listed in Table 23-1 should be avoided until the wound is healed and the patient is symptom-free.

IV. PREOPERATIVE AND POSTOPERATIVE CARE

A. Preoperative orders are generally left by the anesthesiologist. If not, meperidine, 100 mg, and atropine, 0.4 mg, usually are given 1 hr prior to operation.

TABLE 23-1. Foods to Avoid in Anorectal Disease

Nuts	Citrus fruits and juices
Fatty foods	Corn
Coffee	Any foods with seeds
Alcohol, including beer and wine	Popcorn
Spices	Excessive amounts of cheese and milk

The patient should fast from bedtime the evening before. A Fleet enema administered in the knee-chest position is given at bedtime and repeated 2 hr before the operation.

B. Postoperative management

1. **Drains**   Occasionally it may be necessary to place a small, lubricated rubber drain in the anal canal to give warning of hemorrhage.

2. **Diet**   Fluids are restricted until the patient voids and then may be progressed to a liquid diet and usually a general diet the following morning.

3. **For pain**   Dihydromorphinone (Dilaudid), 1-2 mg every 3-4 hr for several days. Acetaminophen (Tylenol) with 30 mg of codeine every 3-4 hr may be used for less severe pain.

4. **For sleep**   Secobarbital (Seconal), 100 mg.

5. **A tranquilizer,** such as chlordiazepoxide HCl (Librium), 10 mg qid, is started immediately.

6. **Metamucil,** 1 tablespoon with water bid, for 2 wk.

7. **Petrogalar,** 30 cc bid, until first bowel movement, then once daily for 2 wk, unless the patient has diarrhea.

8. If **urinary retention** occurs, use a Foley catheter for a minimum of 48 hr. Cranberry juice, 240 ml twice a day, will help keep the urine pH acidic.

9. The day following the operation, the patient is given warm **wet compresses. Sitz baths** are given the next day.

10. **Avoid enemas and rectal examinations;** they produce pain.

11. **Surfak,** 1 or 2 capsules hs, is helpful in producing a soft, formed stool. If by the end of the fourth postoperative day a bowel movement has not occurred, insert a pediatric Fleet enema; repeat if necessary.

12. The patient should be seen weekly until the wound is healed. Keep the patient on sitz baths and Proctofoam-HC tid.

24. CUTANEOUS AND SUBCUTANEOUS TUMORS

I. PRINCIPLES

A. Benign tumors are removed either for cosmetic reasons or because of their premalignant potential. Malignant tumors are removed because they threaten life or limb.

B. The surgical management of these tumors varies as widely as the lesions themselves. Be familiar with all the etiological possibilities in each case. Management of benign lesions is generally obvious and simply handled. Malignant tumors often are complex and are "masqueraders." The complications of initial mismanagement are awesome and frequently tragic.

C. Resection of probably malignant tumors, exploration of undiagnosed masses, skin grafts, and similar procedures must be performed in the operating room. These are not to be done in the office or outpatient clinic.

D. A surgical field large enough to encompass any eventuality must be prepared.

E. Local anesthesia, using ½% Xylocaine, is recommended for minor biopsies or cosmetic corrections. After a negative history of agent sensitivity has been obtained, the anesthetic should be injected circumferentially around the lesion to form a field block. Epinephrine solution may be incorporated in the anesthetic to prolong its effect and to aid hemostasis. Do not use epinephrine in diabetic patients or in treating lesions of the hand or foot.

F. The surgeon must be alert to possible complications of local anesthesia. Supportive facilities for oxygen administration, endotracheal intubation, IV fluids, and defibrillation, as well as ancillary personnel must be available. Drugs such as epinephrine (1:1,000 solution), Benadryl, hydrocortisone, and short-acting barbiturates may be needed to counteract allergic reactions or cardiovascular collapse and should be available in any area where local anesthetics are used.

G. The incision should be made around the lesion and prolonged as an ellipse along skin tension lines in order to effect the most cosmetic closure (see Chap. 25). Wide undermining of the skin will permit closure without tension. If the wound is large, a skin graft may be needed. Procedures probably necessitating a skin graft always must be done in the operating room.

H. The entire specimen must be totally excised, either for diagnostic biopsy purposes or tumor "cure." Very large or bulky lesions may require preliminary incisional biopsy. Resection through tumor-free tissue should be verified by frozen-section examination of the wound margins in all cases of proved or suspected malignancy. Benign specimens should be preserved promptly in a 10% formalin or an alcohol solution, as appropriate.

I. Minimal tissue handling of both specimen and adjacent margins is the rule.

J. After a suspected malignant tumor—even one of low grade—has been removed, new instruments should be utilized in the wound closure. Complete hemostasis, of course, is imperative.

K. A conforming dressing of minimal pressure generally should be affixed over the wound.

II. SPECIAL PROBLEMS   Even though the surgeon exercises good judgment and is familiar with cutaneous and subcutaneous neoplasms, exploration of tumors in certain locations is extremely hazardous and warrants special consideration.

A. Subcutaneous tumors of the wrist and hand   Neoplasms in the subcutaneous tissues of the wrist and hand are generally benign but complex in nature. They include ganglia arising from tendon sheaths, joint capsules, or articular surfaces, giant cell tumors, tuberculosis of joints, etc. Because most of these lesions involve vital hand structures, indicated surgical resection always must be done in the operating room under regional block or general anesthesia and with tourniquet control of the operative field.

B. Tumors of the neck   Subcutaneous masses in the region of the neck rate as the most difficult diagnostic and technical problems in surgery. Actually, the possibilities are far too numerous to list in this chapter. The lesions range from benign embryonal arrest cysts and aberrant glandular tissue to aneurysms to primary or metastatic malignancies. Tumors of this area frequently require an exhaustive workup and maximal surgical judgment and skill in the operating room.

C. Skin and subcutaneous lesions of the midline   Tumors and lesions of the midline deserve special consideration because of the frequency of complications when treated by a novice. Congenital abnormalities, such as a thyroglossal duct cyst or sinus, frequently signal unexpected findings, such as an ectopic thyroid. There is an increased incidence of malignancy in dorsal midline giant nevi. Increased or aberrant vascularity may be anticipated in resection of many midline tumors.

D. Cirsoid aneurysm   This lesion is an abnormal AV communication of extremely high flow rate, of congenital or post-traumatic etiology, and usually progressive. The lesion may occur in any location, but most frequently it involves the subcutaneous tissue over the calvaria. In this location, multiple arterial and venous vessels may be involved, as well as perforating channels through the tables of the skull. Excision is the only therapy for a cirsoid aneurysm. However, such pulsatile masses always must be explored in an operating room, with adequate help, facilities, and anesthesia, because of the danger of massive hemorrhage. The most advantageous surgical approach is to raise a U-flap, individually ligate the feeding vessels as they are encountered, and, finally, resect the central aneurysm, after which the flap is closed.

III. BENIGN TUMORS   In contrast to malignant lesions, the physical appearance of the benign neoplasms of the skin and subcutaneous tissues is usually very characteristic and such tumors are easily identified. Seldom is microscopic evaluation necessary except for confirmation of the clinical diagnosis or to rule out the possibility of malignant degeneration. Cosmetic or functional improvement is the primary reason for removal of these lesions.

A. Keratoses

1. **Senile keratoses** and cutaneous horns are patches of roughened epidermis covered with scales or crusts and found especially in aged individuals. Carcinomatous degeneration occurs rarely. Lesions suspected to be malignant should be excised.

2. **Seborrheic keratoses** are dark brown in color, elevated, rather well delineated, and oily to touch. Generally, seborrheic lesions are observed in protected areas of the body. For cosmetic purposes, electrodesiccation or excision may be considered.

B. Pigmented nevi

1. **Intradermal and compound nevi** are the common nevi of adulthood. Cosmetic improvement is the principal indication for removal.

2. **Giant pigmented nevi** should be resected if location and donor (skin) sites permit because of their cosmetic disfigurement and the possibility of malignant melanoma.

3. **A junctional nevus** is darkly pigmented and sometimes elevated; it arises from the epidermal-dermal junction and is a precursor of melanoma. These nevi should be excised.

4. **Any nevus that exhibits any of the following features should be excised with wide margins** (margins equaling the tumor diameter up to a maximum of 5 cm):

   a. Change in pigmentation.

   b. Appearance of a pigmented ring or spots in surrounding apparently normal skin.

   c. Increase in size.

   d. First appears after puberty.

e. Located on the palm or sole.

f. Subjected to frequent trauma.

C. Warts

1. These troublesome lesions present in all age groups. They occur as a papillary type (verrucous) on any skin surface or on the sole of the foot (plantar). They are due to a viral infection of the dermis.

2. The most rapid and reliable methods of treatment are complete electrocoagulation or limited excision with electrocoagulation of the subcutaneous base. If the lesion is large and over a joint or weight-bearing surface, turn a rotation flap to close the wound in order to give a painless and functional skin surface.

D. Sebaceous cyst

1. These are retention cysts arising in a plugged sebaceous gland. When located on the scalp, such a cyst is called a wen.

2. These cysts are very liable to become infected, usually with staphylococci.

3. Effective treatment involves the complete removal of the cyst wall; otherwise, the cyst will recur.

4. Small sebaceous cysts, particularly if infected, can be treated on an outpatient basis by making a small incision into the cyst, evacuating its contents, and inserting a few crystals of silver nitrate. After a few days the cyst wall shrivels up and can be grasped with a hemostat and removed.

5. Larger sebaceous cysts must be excised in the operating room. Dissect around them to remove all cyst wall, together with a small ellipse of the overlying skin which includes the plugged pore. If infected, these larger cysts should be incised, the contents evacuated, the cyst lightly packed open, and the patient started on antibiotics. A few days later, when infection is controlled, the cyst wall should be excised.

E. Epidermal inclusion cyst

1. Small bits of epithelium are carried to a subcutaneous position as a result of trauma; then further growth produces a small hard knot.

2. These cysts may be excised if they cause symptoms or cosmetic disfigurement.

F. Lipoma

1. Lipomas are common, benign, soft, encapsulated subcutaneous fatty tumors. They may be found anywhere on the body, but are most frequent on the upper back.

2. Lipomas are characteristically movable but are loosely attached to surrounding structures.

3. Lipomas that are growing in size and are cosmetically disfiguring, or that interfere with normal function because of their location, should be excised.

G. Neurofibroma

1. Neurofibroma may occur as an isolated single subcutaneous tumor or, more usually, as multiple tumors of varying size accompanied by pigmented café-au-lait spots of the skin (Recklinghausen's disease).

2. Neurofibromas are soft, freely movable, often pedunculated tumors which are easily deformed by pressure.

   a. Tumors arising from cranial or sensory nerve roots may produce symptoms of cerebellopontile angle tumor or of paresis.

   b. Sarcomatous degeneration of one or more tumors occurs in 5-10% of patients with neurofibromatosis.

   c. Other tumors develop with increased frequency in these patients: meningioma, glioma, and pheochromocytoma.

3. Excision of all single lesions, and excision biopsy of a readily accessible lesion in cases of multiple neurofibromatosis, should be done to confirm the diagnosis. Any lesion suspected of malignant degeneration or any that seriously interferes with function should be excised.

4. Attempts by excision of many tumors to improve the cosmetic appearance of patients with multiple neurofibromatosis are fruitless, since new crops of neurofibromas may appear throughout the patient's lifetime.

H. Ganglia

1. Ganglia are the most common tumors found in the hand. They are cystic in nature and arise from generative synovial tissue of either tendon sheath or articular surfaces. Occasionally, they originate from tendon fibers per se. A past history of trauma or abuse is elicited in more than one third of cases.

2. These lesions occur most frequently on the dorsum of the wrist, the volar aspect of the fingers and distal palm, and the dorsum of the foot.

3. A ganglion should be excised if it causes pain or interferes with function.

I. Keloid

1. The keloid is a benign hypertrophy of scar due to excessive development of collagen in the reparative phase of healing of the primary wound.

2. This tumor has a high incidence rate in blacks. Keloid is an obvious diagnosis from the findings and past history.

3. Optimum cosmetic results are achieved when excision and closure are done after treatment with steroid injections into the lesion has brought about partial involution of the keloid. Additionally, injection of steroids is made into the wound margins at the time of excision and, in some cases, systemic steroids may be continued postoperatively.

J. Hemangioma

1. Capillary hemangiomas produce the familiar port-wine stain in skin and seldom demonstrate progressive tendencies. In fact, modest involution is often noted throughout childhood. The use of paste makeup coverings is usually satisfactory.

2. Cavernous hemangiomas present in various forms ranging from the slightly elevated strawberry nevus to large, purple, multilobular tumors. As a general rule, these neoplasms tend to involute spontaneously in infancy and early childhood, so that expectant nonoperative management is satisfactory in most cases. If very large, they may be associated with thrombocytopenia. Rapid growth rarely may necessitate combined radiotherapy, infusion of sclerosing solutions, and staged surgical resection in selected cases. The arterial and venous tributaries should be controlled before the neoplasm is resected.

K. Glomus tumor (glomangioma)

1. The glomus neoplasm is a singular tumor of uniform glomus cells fed by a discrete afferent artery and containing an efferent vein.

2. It is found over joints, the coccyx, or the scapula, and in the nail beds of the fingers. It should be resected.

L. Lymphangioma

1. Lymphangiomas are found in a variety of forms: a single nodule (simplex), diffuse opalescent, verrucous nodules (circumscriptum), and large, deforming cavernous masses (cavernosum).

2. When a cavernous lymphangioma occurs in the neck, it is called a cystic hygroma.

3. All varieties of lymphangiomas appear in infancy or early childhood and many undergo spontaneous involution as the child grows.

4. If these lesions become infected or interfere with breathing, deglutition, or other function, they should be excised. The larger defects remaining after excision of these tumors are best closed with delayed rotation flaps.

M. Dermoid cyst

1. Dermoid cysts may occur as a subcutaneous mass. The usual location is the periorbital tissues; most patients are children. Dermoid cysts are never attached to skin but often are attached to or extend through bone.

2. While dermoids are benign, an experienced surgeon should explore suspected lesions, since many have intracranial or meningeal attachments in the nasofrontal area. Excision is the only indicated treatment.

N. Xanthomas

1. These yellow lesions of the skin or mucous membranes are universally benign and consist of coalescent foci of lipid histiocytes in slightly raised papules or plaques.

2. Xanthomas may serve as signals of diabetes or hyperlipemia. Otherwise, they appear to be innocuous, and the only indication for excision is cosmetic.

O. Keratoacanthoma

1. This lesion arises from any dermal squamous tissue, usually in areas of sun exposure. It is characterized by cornified squamous hyperplasia, often with central necrosis—grossly and microscopically similar to squamous cell carcinoma. Generally, it is considered benign and self-limiting; however, often keratoacanthoma is rapid-growing and highly invasive. Metastases have been noted.

2. The keratoacanthomas must be recognized early and wide local resection is imperative because of its rapid growth, invasive nature, and possible confusion with squamous carcinoma.

IV. MALIGNANT TUMORS   Cutaneous cancer is the most frequently encountered malignant neoplasm. These lesions, along with those occurring in the subcutaneous tissues, range from very low grade malignancy to the most aggressive and unpredictable kinds of carcinoma.

A. Basal cell carcinoma

1. This skin cancer is most commonly encountered on the face, neck, and other areas of chronic exposure to sunlight, chemicals, or trauma.

2. Grossly, the lesion may be a single, discrete, erythematous nodule or, in a more advanced stage, a rodent ulcer with raised, pearly margins. Basal cell tumors typically are umbilicated or have cystic central ulceration or erosion. An unusual variety of this tumor is multicentric in character, simulating dry, scaly eczema.

3. Histologically, the tumor is identified by nests of basal cells in an alveolar or cylindromatous pattern accompanied by central necrosis.

4. Either excision or irradiation is equally effective treatment of small lesions. Large lesions should be widely excised and closed primarily or with split-thickness skin grafts or rotation flaps. Adequate excision is curative, as basal cell carcinoma rarely metastasizes. Irradiation is preferred for lesions in sites such as the puncta of the eyelid.

B. Squamous cell carcinoma

1. This malignant tumor frequently occurs in the skin. It also may arise in any mucous membrane composed of squamous cells (primary or metaplastic), such as bronchial, buccal, and genitourinary mucosa. Approximately 75% of squamous cell carcinomas occur on the head and neck, with the lower lip being the most frequent site on the face in middle-aged or older patients.

2. This lesion has a special predilection for development in areas of chronic irritation or trauma such as a burn scar (Marjolin's ulcer).

3. Squamous cell carcinoma presents in two typical forms, papillary and ulcerating. The former appears as a small reddish papule with modest scaling and progresses slowly into a large multilobular exophitic neoplasm. The ulcerating form has raised indurated margins and tends to be more aggressive, with marked propensity for invasion of adjacent tissues and relatively early lymphatic metastasis.

4. Microscopically, the tumor is easily identified by irregular nests of epidermal cells demonstrating varying degrees of anaplasia that infiltrate the entire dermis. Occasionally, combined elements of basal cell and squamous cell tumors are observed simultaneously.

5. Treatment involves wide resection. Since this lesion may spread by direct extension, via lymphatics or along nerves, consideration also should be given to regional lymphatic dissection.

C. Malignant melanoma

1. Melanoma is an infrequent but dangerous and unpredictable malignancy. A surgical intern or uninitiated resident should seek consultation when he suspects that a lesion may be a melanoma.

2. The lesion generally occurs in the skin but may arise from either ectodermal or mesodermal tissues; thus, rare sites of origin are occasionally seen, such as the retina of the eye and the GI tract.

3. Junctional cell nevi, especially those located on the sole, palm, and genitals, may degenerate to malignant melanoma. Trauma and hormones appear to be influential in causing malignant degeneration of junctional nevi.

4. Melanoma rarely is observed before puberty except in association with giant pigmented nevi, where the primary malignancy rate ranges from 3–10%.

5. Any increase in the growth of a nevus, sudden increase of pigmentation, spontaneous ulceration, or induration at the base of nevus may be an indication of malignant transformation. Variations of the classic pattern include diffuse satellite formation and nodular, amelanotic lesions.

6. Microscopic diagnosis offers little difficulty; anaplastic melanocytes with large nucleoli and bizarre mitotic figures universally are present invading all dermal layers.

7. Because metastases occur via intradermal and subdermal lymphatic pathways as well as via the vascular system, optimum treatment includes wide resection of the original lesion. Perfusion of an extremity harboring a melanoma with phenylalanine mustard is beneficial. Dissection of the appropriate regional nodes is done either immediately or within 3 wk of the initial operation.

D. Sarcomas

1. These lesions occasionally are found as subcutaneous nodules, especially in the lower extremities. Sarcomas vary greatly in histological composition, even within the same tumor, but they all originate from mesenchymal tissue and most of the subcutaneous malignant tumors prove to be spindle cell fibrosarcomas.

2. Between 50 and 60% of the reported cases of fibrosarcoma occur on the lower extremities; approximately 25% are noted on the arms. They occur in all age groups, but the greatest incidence is in the third and fourth decades of life.

3. Fibrosarcomas develop as small, firm, generally painless nodules that grow slowly for long periods of time and may become very large before the patient seeks care.

4. Fibrosarcoma may masquerade as a hematoma, sebaceous cyst, lipoma, or fibroma. Whenever fibrosarcoma is a definitie possibility, narrow excision must not be contemplated. If the lesion cannot be excised with wide margins, an incisional biopsy with margins confined within the tumor is done.

5. Treatment by en bloc surgical excision with a 5-cm margin of surrounding normal tissue offers slightly better than a 50% 5-yr cure rate. In an extremity, achieving an adequate border may involve amputation.

6. Since the primary mode of metastasis of this tumor is hematogenous, lymph node dissections should be performed only when nodes are involved clinically. Fibrosarcoma responds poorly to chemical agents, irradiation x-ray, and radium implantation.

25. MINOR SURGICAL TECHNIQUES

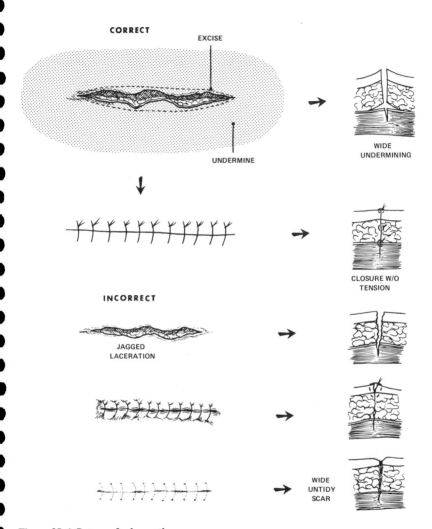

CORRECT

EXCISE

UNDERMINE

WIDE UNDERMINING

CLOSURE W/O TENSION

INCORRECT

JAGGED LACERATION

WIDE UNTIDY SCAR

Figure 25-1 Suture of a laceration.
Never shave eyebrows or the scalp; it is usually not necessary to shave around any laceration. Smear sterile lubricating jelly on hair to hold it away from the wound. Wear cap, mask, and gloves. Gently wash skin surrounding the laceration with iodophor detergent solution or a hexachlorophene soap. Use sterile towels to set up a sterile field. Establish anesthesia by infiltration of wound margins or use a field block. Cleanse the wound, remove foreign matter, excise irregular wound margins, and debride all nonviable tissue. Undermine all but superficial lacerations to reduce tension. Undermine on the trunk and extremities in the plane between subcutaneous fat and superficial fascia; in the scalp, undermine in the plane just external to the galea; in the face, undermine in the midst of the subcutaneous fat. Suture each layer of the wound with fine sutures. Remove skin sutures as soon as possible.

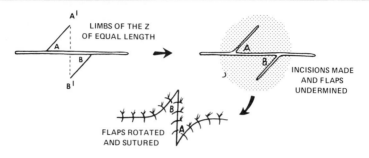

Figure 25-2 Technique of a Z-plasty.
If there is tension along the length of a clean laceration, or if the wound crosses a flexion crease, a Z-plasty may be a helpful maneuver to relieve tension.

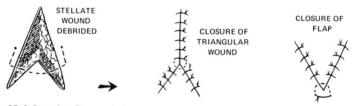

Figure 25-3 Suturing flaps and tips.
Necrosis of the tip of a flap is avoided by use of the "tip stitch," a modified mattress suture which is brought subcutaneously away from the tip so that pressure is not exerted on the tip when the suture is tied.

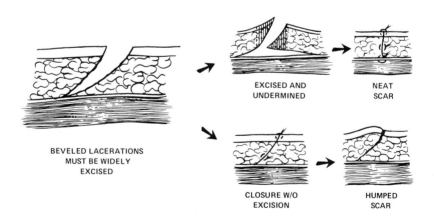

Figure 25-4 Closure of a beveled laceration.
To avert a hump of tissue resulting from contraction of scar, excise a beveled wound to create vertical wound margins and undermine it widely before closure. If the laceration is very deep, excise it in steps at each major layer of the wound.

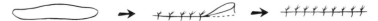

1.   DOG EARS CAN BE EXCISED (THIS WILL LENGTHEN THE SCAR)

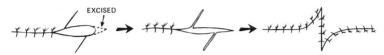

2.   Z-PLASTY AS ALTERNATIVE

Figure 25-5 Closure of round and ovoid wounds.
Direct suture closure of an ovoid wound sometimes results in a "dog ear." Excision of the dog ear will make the wound longer. Alternatively, a Z-plasty can be used to manage the dog ear; this makes the wound area wider.

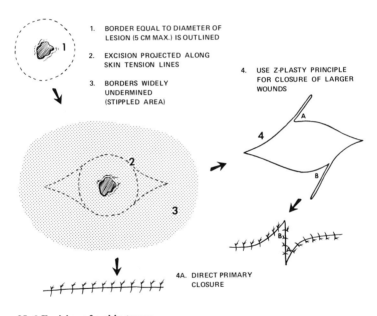

1.   BORDER EQUAL TO DIAMETER OF LESION (5 CM MAX.) IS OUTLINED

2.   EXCISION PROJECTED ALONG SKIN TENSION LINES

3.   BORDERS WIDELY UNDERMINED (STIPPLED AREA)

4.   USE Z-PLASTY PRINCIPLE FOR CLOSURE OF LARGER WOUNDS

4A.   DIRECT PRIMARY CLOSURE

Figure 25-6 Excision of a skin tumor.
Benign skin lesions can be excised with little or no margin. Lesions suspected of malignancy should be excised with a margin equal to the diameter of the tumor, up to a maximum margin of 5 cm. Prolongation of a circular wound by excision of small triangles at either end, together with wide undermining, often permits primary closure. Alternatively, use a Z-plasty.

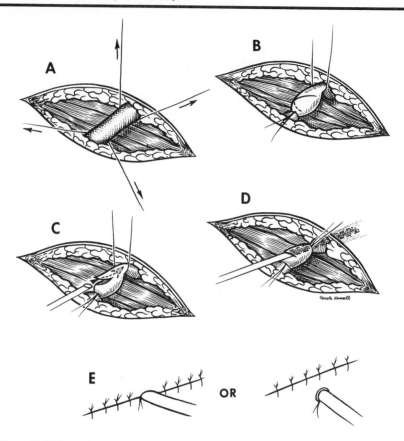

Figure 25-7 Venous cutdown.
In infants, the great saphenous vein just anterior to the medial malleolus or the external jugular vein in the neck are the preferred sites for a cutdown. In adults, the antecubital vein at the elbow or the cephalic vein in the upper arm are preferred, although any accessible vein may be used. Apply a tourniquet proximal to the cutdown site. Prepare a sterile field; incise the skin transversely, dissect out the vein and pass two ligatures around it (A). Tie the distal ligature (B) and place it on gentle traction. Make a beveled transverse incision halfway through the vein (C); release the tourniquet. Insert the venous catheter; tie the proximal ligature around the vein and catheter (D). Suture the wound, tying the catheter in place (E), and apply a dressing.

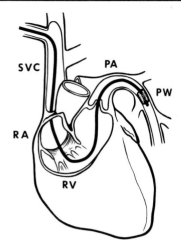

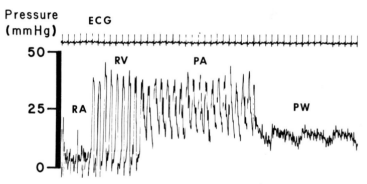

Figure 25-8 Insertion of Swan-Ganz catheter.
Prime the catheter with heparinized saline (1 unit/ml), insert it via an antecubital vein cutdown (see Fig. 25-7) and pass the catheter via the brachial (medial) branch to the subclavian vein. Initial passage is facilitated by facing the curved tip of the catheter toward the humerus. Advance the catheter to the superior vena cava, rotate it 180° so that the curved tip faces the midline, then half inflate the balloon with air. Connect the primed catheter to a pressure transducer and monitor pressure on an oscilloscope or recorder. Gently advance the catheter, observing the pressure tracing to identify the location of the catheter tip.

With the catheter tip in the superior vena cava (SVC), the pressure is low, usually less than 20 mm Hg; deflections are negative and coincide with respiration. When the right atrium (RA) is entered, pressure is unchanged but deflections become positive and correspond with the heartbeat. Complete inflation of the balloon, then continue advancing the catheter through the right ventricle (RV) and into the pulmonary artery (PA). Watch the ECG for premature ventricular contractions which result from impingement of the catheter tip in the myocardium; if PVCs occur, withdraw a little, then gently advance again. After the catheter tip enters the pulmonary artery, advance it to a wedge position (PCW), then deflate the balloon.

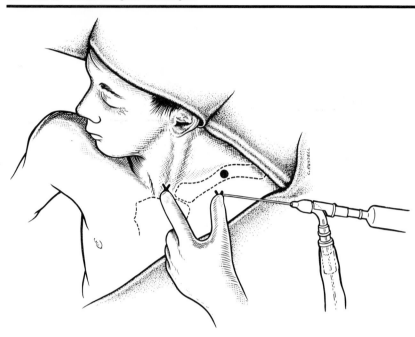

Figure 25-9 Subclavian venous catheterization.
Place the patient in Trendelenburg position, prepare the skin, and set up a field using sterile towels. Observe strict aseptic techniques throughout the catheterization. Insert the needle-catheter assembly (Advanset, Bard) through a point 3 cm below the middle of the clavicle, aiming at the center of the suprasternal notch. Place a small button of local anesthetic at the skin puncture site; deeper tissues are not anesthetized. Keep the needle horizontal and advance it while maintaining slight suction in the syringe. Entry into the subclavian vein is signaled by abrupt appearance of blood in the syringe; advance the needle an additional 2-3 mm. Confirm the presence of the needle tip in the vein by ability to freely aspirate and reinject blood. Hold the outer sheath in position, withdraw the needle, and advance the inner catheter into the superior vena cava. Spray the skin surrounding the puncture site with tincture of benzoin. Dress the catheter with antibacterial ointment and several layers of gauze covered completely with adhesive tape. Anchor the catheter to the external surface of the dressing with additional adhesive tape.

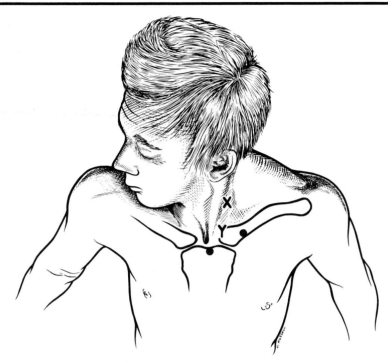

Figure 25-10 Landmarks for internal jugular venous catheterization.
Needle is inserted at the posterior border of the sternocleidomastoid muscle, halfway between the mastoid process and the head of the clavicle (X), and is directed between the clavicular and sternal heads of the muscle (Y).

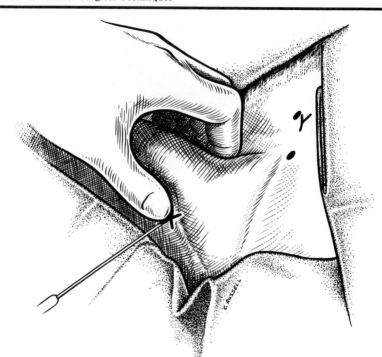

Figure 25-11 Insertion of internal jugular venous catheter.
The drawing is of the right side of the patient; the head would be to the left of the drawing. The sternocleidomastoid muscle is grasped firmly and elevated slightly to fix the internal jugular vein. The needle-catheter assembly is passed deep (posterior) to the sternocleidomastoid muscle to enter the vein. Landmarks are illustrated in Figure 25-10. Other details of technique are identical with subclavian catheterization (see Fig. 25-9).

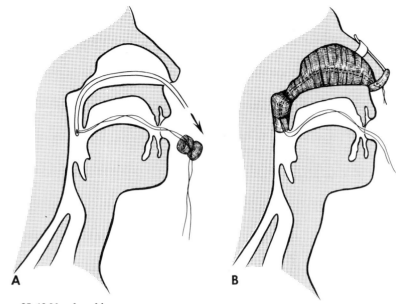

Figure 25-12 Nasal packing.
A gauze roll is drawn into the nasopharynx as a posterior pack (A). Alternatively, a Foley catheter is used, the inflated balloon acting as the posterior pack. Then the anterior pack is placed, filling the nose (B).

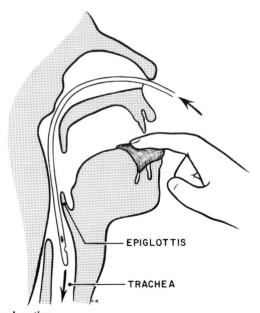

EPIGLOTTIS

TRACHEA

Figure 25-13 Nasotracheal suction.
Insert the rubber catheter through the nose, extend the head, pull the tongue gently forward to open the epiglottis, and advance the catheter while the patient takes a deep breath. Sometimes a coudé tip catheter is needed.

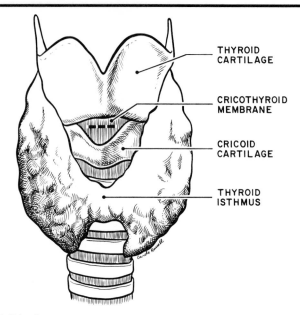

Figure 25-14 Cricothyrotomy.
An airway can be established quickly and safely by puncture of the cricothyroid membrane (broken line). In an emergency, it is faster than a tracheostomy.

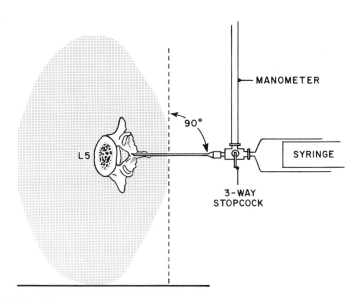

Figure 25-15 Lumbar puncture.
Lumbar puncture in acute head injury requires precautions to prevent loss of fluid or a sudden drop in pressure. The needle is passed through the skin with the bevel facing the patient's side. When the needle engages the interspinal ligament, the obturator is withdrawn and a saline-filled manometer and syringe are connected. When the subarachnoid space is entered, only a small volume of fluid will enter or leave the manometer; there is no change in CSF pressure.

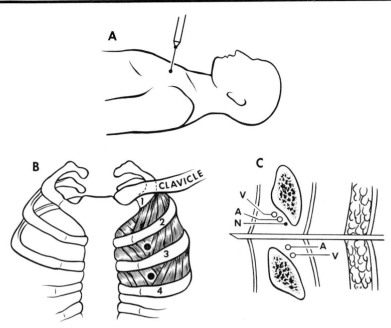

Figure 25-16 Needle thoracentesis.
In suspected **tension pneumothorax,** a needle is inserted anteriorly (A) through the second or third interspace in the midclavicular line (B). The needle should pass through the middle of the interspace to avoid intercostal blood vessels (C). To remove an **effusion,** the patient sits upright; the needle is passed through the seventh or eighth interspace in the mid or posterior axillary line. In this latter technique, since the blood vessels all are in relation to the inferior border of the rib, the needle should pass immediately above the next lower rib.

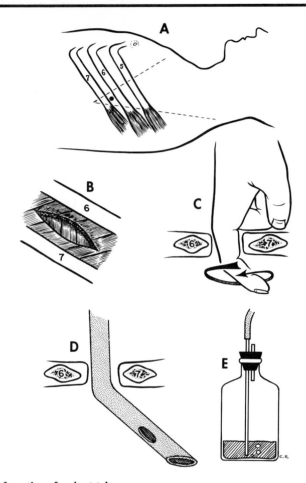

Figure 25-17 Insertion of a chest tube.
A chest tube can be placed quickly and safely in an emergency through the sixth intercostal space in the midaxillary line (A). This location avoids major nerves and overlying muscles. A 2-3 cm incision is made in the midinterspace and carried partially through the intercostal muscles (B). Entry into the pleural space is completed by blunt dissection with a clamp. A sterile gloved finger is inserted into the chest to clear adhesions, clots, etc. (C). The finger is withdrawn and a 32-35 Fr chest tube is inserted (D) and connected to water seal drainge (E). The wound is sutured. The small induced pneumothorax clears immediately. The major advantage of this method is its safety in inexperienced hands.

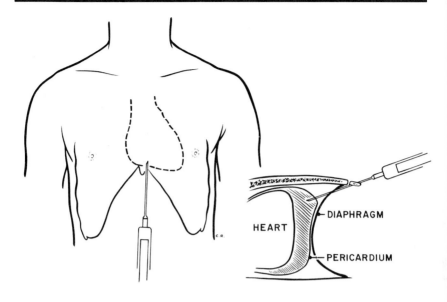

Figure 25-18 Needle pericardiocentesis.
A 14- or 16-gauge Angiocath needle is inserted between the xiphoid and the left costal margin at an angle of about 30 degrees from the body wall and is advanced straight superiorly while suction is maintained on the syringe. ECG lead II can be connected to the steel needle and will accurately identify when the epicardium is touched. If blood returns from the pericardial sac, leave the outer plastic cannula in place.

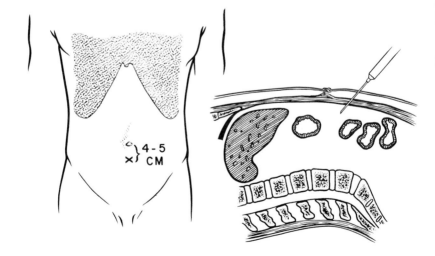

Figure 25-19 Abdominal diagnostic paracentesis.
An 18-gauge IV catheter unit is used. The needle is inserted in the midline, about 4-5 cm below the umbilicus, and the inner catheter is advanced into the peritoneal cavity. If fluid does not return immediately, 100-200 ml of normal saline solution is run into the abdomen over 5 min using an IV drip set. The IV tubing and bottle are then lowered to the floor to siphon fluid from the abdomen.

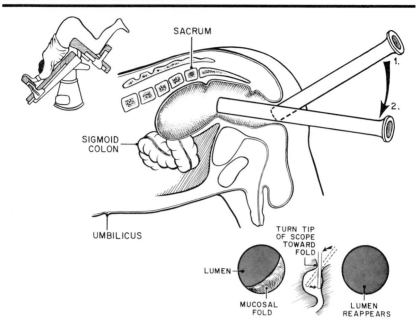

Figure 25-20 Sigmoidoscopy.
Place the patient in head-down position (top insert). Digital rectal examination always is done as the first step.

Insert the sigmoidoscope through the anus, aiming at the patient's umbilicus (1). Advance only 3-4 cm, stop, rotate the scope (2), remove the obturator, and insert the eyepiece. Advance the scope under direct vision, turning the tip slightly *toward* each successive mucosal fold (lower insert). If the lumen is not apparent, withdraw the scope a little. Avoid insufflating air unless absolutely necessary. At about 15 cm the sigmoid colon curves to the left; because of this angulation or fixation of the bowel by disease, it is not possible to pass the scope beyond this point in about 30 percent of patients.

Attention during insertion is directed to safe, smooth passage of the scope. Attention during withdrawal is directed to careful scrutiny of the mucosa; use a rotary or spiral motion as the scope is slowly withdrawn.

INDEX

The user of this book will find very few of the conventional kinds of cross-references in the Index. Because it is a reference manual, the authors wished to provide as direct access as possible to the information contained in it. Therefore, the indexer has attempted to include all alternate terms for any main entry as separate entries (e.g., Trauma; Wounds, rather than Wounds. See Trauma, or vice versa). Where See also references seem to be absolutely necessary, the indexer has attempted to bring together related material by referring from one entry to the subentries under another, similar, entry (e.g., Bicarbonate [HCO₃] See also subentries in this index under Sodium bicarbonate [NaHCO₃]) and, where there are no subentries, by giving page references for the item referred to (e.g., Operative procedures. See also Surgery, minor, techniques of, 405-418).

Wherever possible, names of drugs listed in this index are generic, followed by proprietary names in parentheses.

intravenous, in diabetic management, 246, 248
after head injury, 13
of heparin, 317
and thrombophlebitis, 378
of radiopaque medium, in obstructive uropathy, 228
in tube feeding, 216
Inhalation injury
defined, 329
treatment of, 329
Injury, reactions following, 301, 302. *See also subentries under* Trauma; *and specific types of injuries, e.g.,* Abdominal injuries/trauma, 28–36
Innervation, sensory, of hand, 69
Insulin
and coma, 47
crystalline
in ketoidosis, 249
in preoperative diabetic management, 247
for diabetic patient, 245, 246, 249
in hyperglycemia, of tube feeding, 217
and serum potassium, 191
Intensive care unit, in postoperative care, 153
Intermittent positive pressure breathing (IPPB), 238, 240
postoperative, 156
preoperative, 155
Intestinal obstruction, 125–141
abdominal pain in, 103
age incidence of, 106, 126
causes of, 127, 128–129, 134–135
in cervical injury, of newborn, 20
closed-loop, 129, 132, 135, 138, 139
defined, 126
general considerations, 125–126
long intestinal tubes in, 132–133, 134, 170
nasogastric tubes in, 132
operative treatment of, 134
paralytic, 137–138
clinical features in, 131
defined, 126
pathophysiology of, 127–130, 135
prime findings of, 109
simple mechanical type
clinical features of, 131, 135–136
in colon, 126, 131, 134–138
in small bowel, 126, 127–134, 136–137
strangulation type, 138–140
causes of, 138–139
clinical features of, 131
defined, 126

pathophysiology of, 139–140
signs and symptoms, 140
treatment of, 140
treatment of (general), 132–134, 136–137
types of, 126
vascular ileus, 140–141
clinical features in, 131
Intestines, trauma of, management of, 35–36
Intracaval umbrella device, in venous interruption, 319
Intracellular fluid (ICF), 184
Intracranial pressure, in head injuries, 14
signs of increase in, 15–16
Intraluminal pressure
in colon obstruction, 135
in paralytic ileus, 137
in small-bowel obstruction, 129
Intraocular injuries, 52–53
Intraocular pressure, in ocular trauma, 53
Intubation
Baker tube, 168
Cantor tube, 168
chest tubes, 172–174. *See also subentries under* Chest tube(s)
common bile duct, T-tubes, 171–172
endotracheal
in acute respiratory insufficiency, 238
in aspiration pneumonia prevention, 178
in chest injury, 22
complications of, 239, 240
in facial injury repair, 12
in head injury, 13
in infants, 339
in trauma, 1
Johnston tube, 168
long intestinal tube, 168–170
complications of, 169–170
technique of, 168–169
Miller-Abbott tube, 168
nasogastric, 166–168
in burn management, 327
in coma, 49
for gastric emptying, 178
in gastrointestinal bleeding, of infants, 352
in intestinal obstruction, 132
in massive gastrointestinal hemorrhage, 120
in postoperative vomiting, 147
in shock, 4
in stomach injuries, 35
in tube feeding, 213
Sengstaken-Blakemore tube, 170–171
tracheal, in respiratory arrest, 98
Intussusception
differential diagnosis, 106–107
reverse, in long-tube therapy, 170

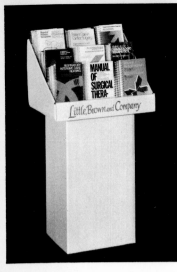

THE LITTLE, BROWN

MANUAL SERIES

Titles in Little, Brown's Manual Series are readily available at all medical bookstores throughout the United States and abroad. You may also order copies directly from Little, Brown and Company, 34 Beacon Street, Boston, Massachusetts 02106, by simply tearing out, filling in, and mailing this postage-free card.

NAME_____
(Please print)

STREET_____

CITY_____ STATE _____

ZIP CODE _____

ORDERS FOR LESS THAN $10.00 MUST BE PREPAID. PUBLISHER PAYS POSTAGE AND HANDLING CHARGES ON ALL ORDERS ACCOMPANIED BY A CHECK. (Please add sales tax if applicable.)

☐ Bill me.
☐ Check enclosed.

The prices listed above are Little, Brown and Company prices as of the printing of this particular book and are subject to change at any time without notice. In no way do they reflect the prices at which books will be sold to you by suppliers other than Little, Brown and Company.